SBAs for the MRCS Part A

SBAs for the MRCS Part A
A Bailey & Love Revision Guide
Second Edition

Vivian A. Elwell
BA (Hons), MA (Cantab), MBBS, MRCS, FRCS (Neuro. Surg.)
Consultant Neurosurgeon and Spinal Surgeon
Brighton and Sussex University Hospitals NHS Trust, Brighton

Jonathan M. Fishman
BA (Hons), MA (Cantab), BM BCh (Oxon), PhD, MRCS (Eng),
DOHNS (RCS Eng), FHEA, FRCS (ORL-HNS)
Consultant ENT Surgeon, University College London Hospitals NHS
Foundation Trust (UCLH) and Honorary Clinical Lecturer, University
College London, London

Rajat Chowdhury
BSc (Hons), MA (Oxon), BM BCh (Oxon), MRCS, FRCS, FBIR, PGCME
Consultant Musculoskeletal Radiologist, Oxford University Hospitals
NHS Foundation Trust, Oxford

All Managing Directors of Insider Medical Ltd.

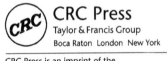

CRC Press
Taylor & Francis Group
Boca Raton London New York

CRC Press is an imprint of the
Taylor & Francis Group, an **Informa** business

CRC Press
Taylor & Francis Group
6000 Broken Sound Parkway NW, Suite 300
Boca Raton, FL 33487-2742

Printed on acid-free paper

International Standard Book Number-13: 978-1-138-50199-7 (Paperback)

Library of Congress Cataloging-in-Publication Data

Names: Elwell, Vivian A., author. | Fishman, Jonathan M., author. | Chowdhury, Rajat, author.
Title: Single best answers (SBAs) for the MRCS Part A / Vivian A. Elwell, Jonathan M. Fishman, Rajat Chowdhury.
Other titles: SBAs and EMQs for the MRCS Part A | SBAs for the MRCS part A
Description: Second edition. | Boca Raton : CRC Press, 2019. | Includes index. | "A Bailey & Love revision guide." | Preceded by SBAs and EMQs for the MRCS Part A. 2011.
Identifiers: LCCN 2018013793| ISBN 9781138501997 (pbk. : alk. paper) | ISBN 9781315144672 (e-book)
Subjects: | MESH: General Surgery | Examination Questions
Classification: LCC RD37.2 | NLM WO 18.2 | DDC 617.0076--dc23
LC record available at https://lccn.loc.gov/2018013793

Visit the Taylor & Francis Web site at
http://www.taylorandfrancis.com

and the CRC Press Web site at
http://www.crcpress.com

Also by Vivian A. Elwell, Jonathan M. Fishman, and Rajat Chowdhury

OSCEs for the MRCS Part B: A Bailey and Love Revision Guide (2nd Edition)

SBAs & EMQs for the MRCS Part A: A Bailey and Love Revision Guide (1st Edition)

OSCEs for the MRCS Part B: A Bailey and Love Revision Guide (1st Edition)

The Insider's Guide to the MRCS Clinical Examination

By three methods we may learn wisdom:
first, by reflection, which is noblest;
second, by imitation, which is easiest;
and third by experience, which is the bitterest.

Confucius, 551 BC–479 BC

For all our past, present, and future patients

Contents

Preface to the Second Edition

This book has been written as an accompaniment to *Bailey and Love's Short Practice of Surgery,* 27th Edition and targeted for the MRCS Part A examination, which is the first part of the Intercollegiate MRCS Examination. The examination syllabus, format, and content are common to The Royal College of Surgeons of Edinburgh, The Royal College of Surgeons of England, and The Royal College of Physicians and Surgeons of Glasgow. This examination is designed and set by the Royal Colleges of Surgeons to test the knowledge, skills, and attributes acquired during core surgical training.

From September 2018, the Intercollegiate MRCS Part A examination will comprise two MCQ papers taken on the same day. The first paper (Applied Basic Sciences) will be 3 hours and the second paper (Principles of Surgery-in-General) will be 2 hours in duration. Both papers will be in a single best answer (SBA) format. A minimum mark must be obtained in both papers, in addition to attaining the total pass mark, to obtain an overall pass in the Intercollegiate Part A Examination. Successful completion of the Intercollegiate Part A Examination qualifies the trainee surgeon to enter the Intercollegiate Part B Objective Structured Clinical Examination.

This book, now in its second edition, is based on our highly successful *Insider Medical MRCS Courses* and the feedback obtained from countless candidates who have sat for the examination. We have carefully selected those high-yield topics that are likely to be faced in the examination and offer methods to tackle the challenges that they may pose. We have drawn from our breadth of experience of teaching at both the undergraduate and postgraduate levels and have identified common pitfalls.

A thorough understanding of applied basic science and the ability to problem-solve underpins surgical science and sets the foundation for future surgical practice. Whilst it is not feasible to cover the complete syllabus within the remit of this book, we have selected the most important and high-yield topics to facilitate examination study and revision. The style of questions is typical of those found in the real examination and will therefore serve well as mock papers. We are confident that this book will assist and help focus any trainee surgeon in their revision for the MRCS Part A examination, and in doing so, refine their analytical approach to all areas of their surgical practice.

Vivian A. Elwell

Jonathan M. Fishman

Rajat Chowdhury

Acknowledgements

This book would not have been possible without the ongoing support of the following individuals:

Mrs. Carole D. Elwell, Dr. Nigel Mendoza, Mr. and Mrs. John Cervieri Jr., Dr. and Mrs. George Leib, Mr. and Mrs. Lawrence Flick, Dr. Sandra Ginsberg, Dr. David Fishman, Mrs. Wendy Fishman, Dr. Galia Fishman, Master James Fishman, Miss Emily Fishman, Mr. and Mrs. Ashit Chowdhury, and Dr. Madhuchanda Bhattacharyya.

About the Authors

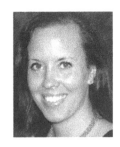

Vivian A. Elwell, BA (Hons), MA (Cantab), MBBS, MRCS, FRCS (Neuro. Surg.) is a consultant neurosurgeon at the Brighton and Sussex University Hospitals NHS Trust. She has a special interest in complex spinal surgery. She obtained her bachelor's degree in biological sciences from Columbia College, Columbia University (New York) and her master's degree from the University of Cambridge. She then earned a Bachelor of Medicine and Bachelor of Surgery from the Imperial College School of Medicine, London.

She held posts in Accident and Emergency, Orthopaedics, Neurosurgery, and General Surgery within her surgical rotation at St Mary's Hospital, Imperial College, London. She completed her neurosurgical training on the North Thames Neurosurgery Training Programme in London. Thereafter, she completed the Central London Senior Spinal Fellowship. She is committed to coupling her neurosurgical practice with education and research.

Dr. Elwell has extensive teaching experience for undergraduate and post-graduate medical education. She is an instructor for the Advanced Trauma Life Support (ATLS) and Care of the Critically Ill Surgical Patient (CCrISP) courses.

She is an author of five medical textbooks, including *Neurosurgery: The Essential Guide to the Oral and Clinical Neurosurgical Examination* (CRC Press). She regularly teaches clinical and surgical skills to medical students, doctors, and surgical trainees.

Dr. Elwell's awards include the Swinford Edward Silver Medal Prize for her OSCE Examination; the Columbia University Research Fellowship at Columbia College of Physicians and Surgeons in New York; the Columbia University King's Crown Gold and Silver Medal Awards; the Kathrine Dulin Folger Cancer Research Fellowship; and the 'Who's Who of Young Scientists Prize'. In 2010, Dr. Elwell was a finalist for the BMA's Junior Doctor of the Year Award. She is noted in 'Who's Who in Science and Engineering' (2011–2012 and 2016–2017).

Jonathan M. Fishman, BA (Hons), MA (Cantab), BM BCh (Oxon), PhD, MRCS (Eng), DOHNS (RCS Eng), FHEA, FRCS (ORL-HNS) is an ENT Consultant, a Fellow of the Royal College of Surgeons of England, and senior editor for the *Journal of Laryngology & Otology* (Cambridge University Press). He graduated with a 'triple' First Class Honours degree in natural sciences from Sidney Sussex College, University of Cambridge, and completed his clinical training at St John's College, University of Oxford. He has held posts in accident and emergency, ENT, general surgery, and neurosurgery as part of the surgical rotation at St Mary's Hospital, Imperial College, London.

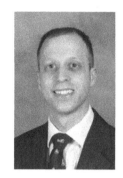

Dr. Fishman has extensive teaching experience and is the primary author of three undergraduate and three postgraduate medical textbooks, including the highly successful *History Taking in Medicine and Surgery* (Pastest Publishing), now in its third edition. He spent part of his medical training at both Harvard University and the NASA Space Center.

He was awarded the Royal Society of Medicine–Wesleyan Trainee of the Year Award in 2012 across all specialties and has been awarded the highly prestigious title of Lifelong Honorary Scholar by the University of Cambridge for academic excellence. He has been awarded a fellowship from the British Association of Plastic Surgeons for research at NASA, and from Cambridge University for research at Harvard University.

Dr. Fishman has received personal research fellowships from the Academy of Medical Sciences, the Medical Research Council, Sparks Children's Charity, the Royal College of Surgeons of England, the UCL–Berkeley Award Scheme, and the UCL–MRC Centenary Award Scheme. He was awarded a PhD from the University College London in 2013 and is currently Honorary Clinical Lecturer at UCL. He is committed to a career in academic ENT, with a strong emphasis on teaching, research, and career development.

Rajat Chowdhury, BSc (Hons), MA (Oxon), BM BCh (Oxon), MRCS, FRCR, FBIR, PGCME is a consultant musculoskel-etal radiologist at the Nuffield Orthopaedic Centre, Oxford University Hospitals. He was awarded an honours degree from University College London and completed his medi-cal studies at Oxford University, the Mayo Clinic, and Harvard University. He then trained on the surgical rota-tion at St Mary's Hospital, Imperial College, London, and held posts in accident and emergency, Orthopaedics and Trauma, Cardiothoracic Surgery, General Surgery, and Plastic Surgery.

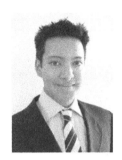

He has a diverse teaching record. He has taught clinical medicine to students and doctors in Oxford and London and has tutored biochemistry and genetics to under-graduate students at Oxford University. He was an anatomy demonstrator at the Imperial College School of Medicine, London, and was president of the Queen's College Medical Society, Oxford, as well as the Hugh Cairns Surgical Society. He was appointed as lecturer in anatomy at The Queen's College, University of Oxford in 2017.

Dr. Chowdhury's academic awards include Oxford University's Bristol Myers Squibb Prize in Cardiology, the Radcliffe Infirmary Prize for Surgery, the GlaxoSmithKline Medical Fellowship, the Warren Scholarship for Paediatric Studies at the University of Toronto, and the Exhibition Award to Harvard University. He is also the lead author of the undergraduate textbook, *Radiology at a Glance* (Wiley-Blackwell Publishing) amongst several other titles.

Introduction: The Insider's Guide to the MRCS Part A Examination

So, you want to be a surgeon?

Fantastic choice! The road to enlightenment begins with the first test – the Intercollegiate MRCS Part A Examination. This examination is designed to test knowledge at the level expected of all aspiring surgeons completing core surgical training in the UK.

The Part A Exam consists of two MCQ papers, taken on the same day. The papers cover generic surgical sciences and applied knowledge, and both papers consist of *single best answer* questions. Each question contains five possible answers, of which there is only one single best answer.

To achieve a 'pass', a minimum level of competence in each of the two papers is required in addition to achieving or exceeding the pass mark set for the combined total mark for the whole of the Part A Examination. There are equal marks for each question and there is no negative marking, so marks will not be deducted for a wrong answer.

Whilst preparing for an examination you are often faced with a vast range of revision sources from traditional textbooks to scientific journals. To accompany this book, we recommend *Bailey and Love's Short Practice of Surgery, 27th Edition*, which provides more detailed information on the selected topics. Inevitably, at some stage during the revision process, you will want to test yourself on examination-style questions, and this book aims to fulfil this need. The questions are designed as single best answers, as in the real examination, and the explanations have been separated into separate chapters so that you can attempt the questions under mock examination conditions or use each question as a syllabus guide.

As mentioned, each question will offer five possible answers. There may be more than one answer that could fit each question but there will always be one answer that is the best answer. Beware of absolute terms such as 'always' and 'never'. These are rarely ever the best answer! There is of course no obligation to answer the questions in the order they appear but you must keep a close check on those that you wish to revisit later. If you run out of time, it is well worth guessing any answer for the outstanding questions – you have nothing to lose and may well get lucky.

Finally, remember common things are common. The exam is testing your ability to diagnose and manage common and important conditions that are essential to being a safe and competent surgeon who is striving for excellence.

Happy studying and good luck!

SECTION 1: SINGLE BEST ANSWER QUESTIONS

1. **Concerning statistical analysis, which statement below is true?**
   A A Type I error accepts the false null hypothesis (e.g., false negative). A benefit is missed when it was there to be found.
   B A Type II error is the incorrect rejection of a true null hypothesis (e.g., false positive). A benefit is perceived when really there is none.
   C A Null hypothesis is a statement of no significant difference or effect.
   D Specificity (true negative rate) measures the proportion of positives that are correctly identified as such (e.g., the percentage of people with a disease who are correctly identified as having the disease).
   E Sensitivity (true positive rate) measures the proportion of negatives that are correctly identified as such (e.g., the percentage of healthy individuals who are correctly identified as not having the disease).

2. **With regard to hernias, which of the following is correct?**
   A A 28-year-old man presents with abdominal and groin pain following a rugby match. Diagnosis: Paraumbilical hernia.
   B A 73-year-old plumber presents with a painful groin. He has had the pain for years and it is associated with a swelling. He is able to reduce the lump with ease. Diagnosis: Lumbar hernia.
   C A 40-year-old woman presents with a painful groin. There is a small palpable mass, which is located in her right upper thigh. Diagnosis: Spigelean hernia.
   D A 53-year-old man presents with pain in the right iliac fossa with a palpable mass. His past surgical history includes an appendicectomy. Diagnosis: Umbilical hernia.
   E A 6-year-old boy had a reducible swelling around his umbilicus. Diagnosis: Paraumbilical hernia.

3. **Which nerve is damaged in the scenario below? A 65-year-old woman is referred with a loss of sensation over her thumb index and middle finger. Her radiograph confirms a distal radius fracture.**
   A Axillary nerve
   B Lateral pectoral nerve
   C Median nerve
   D Musculocutaneous nerve
   E Radial nerve

4. Which nerve is damaged in the scenario below? A 57-year-old man has follow off his ladder and presents with a wrist drop. His radiograph demonstrates a mid-shaft fracture.
   A Axillary nerve
   B Lateral pectoral nerve
   C Musculocutaneous nerve
   D Radial nerve
   E Suprascapular nerve

5. Which nerve is damaged in the scenario below? A 43-year-old man has a deep laceration to his right wrist following a fight. On examination, he has a loss of thumb adduction and loss of sensation over his little and ring fingers.
   A Median nerve
   B Musculocutaneous nerve
   C Radial nerve
   D Suprascapular nerve
   E Ulnar nerve

6. For each of the reflex described below, select the single best root values from the options listed. Biceps reflex.
   A C3/C4
   B C4/C5
   C C5/C6
   D C6/C7
   E C7/C8

7. Select the single best anatomical level in which the IVC is formed from the common iliac veins?
   A L1
   B L2
   C L3
   D L4
   E L5

8. Select the single best anatomical level in which the superior mesenteric artery comes off the aorta?
   A T12
   B L1
   C L2
   D L3
   E L4

9. For the equation described below, select the single best answer.
   [(2 × diastolic) + systolic]/3
   A Cardiac index
   B Cerebral blood flow
   C Cerebral perfusion pressure
   D Mean arterial pressure
   E Pulmonary vascular resistance

10. For the equations described below, select the single best answer. Cardiac output/heart rate (HR)
    A Cerebral blood flow
    B Cerebral perfusion pressure
    C Mean arterial pressure
    D Pulmonary vascular resistance
    E Stroke volume

11. For the equation described below, select the single best answer. (Mean pulmonary artery pressure – mean pulmonary capillary wedge pressure) × 80/cardiac output
    A Cardiac index
    B Cerebral blood flow
    C Cerebral perfusion pressure
    D Mean arterial pressure
    E Pulmonary vascular resistance

12. For the equation described below, select the single best answer. CPP/CVR
    A Cardiac index
    B Cerebral blood flow

C Cerebral perfusion pressure
D Mean arterial pressure
E Pulmonary vascular resistance

13. For the equation described below, select the single best answer. Cardiac output/body surface area
    A Cardiac index
    B Cerebral blood flow
    C Cerebral perfusion pressure
    D Mean arterial pressure
    E Pulmonary vascular resistance

14. For the equation described below, select the single best answer. MAP-ICP
    A Cardiac index
    B Cerebral blood flow
    C Cerebral perfusion pressure
    D Mean arterial pressure
    E Pulmonary vascular resistance

15. For the equation described below, select the single best answer. (Mean arterial pressure – mean right atrial pressure) × 80/cardiac output
    A Cardiac index
    B Cerebral blood flow
    C Mean arterial pressure
    D Pulmonary vascular resistance
    E Systemic vascular resistance

16. What carcinogen is associated with thyroid cancer?
    A Aniline dyes
    B Polyvinyl chloride
    C Asbestos
    D Ultraviolet radiation
    E Ionizing radiation

17. What carcinogen is associated with cancer of the nasal cavity?
    A Ultraviolet radiation
    B Ionizing radiation

C Chromium
D Benzene
E Nickel

18. What carcinogen is associated with transitional cell carcinoma of the urinary tract?
    A Aniline dyes
    B Polyvinyl chloride
    C Asbestos
    D Ultraviolet radiation
    E Ionizing radiation

19. What carcinogen is associated with hepatocellular carcinoma?
    A Aniline dyes
    B Polyvinyl chloride
    C Asbestos
    D Ultraviolet radiation
    E Ionizing radiation

20. A 63-year-old male patient presents with diarrhoea and fresh rectal bleeding for 1 month. He experiences occasional abdominal pain and loss of appetite. Select the single best diagnosis?
    A Diverticulitis
    B Rectal carcinoma
    C Colonic adenomata/polyps
    D Crohn's disease
    E Ulcerative colitis

21. A 28-year-old woman presents with central abdominal pains, bloodstained diarrhoea, and anaemia. She has no relevant past medical history. Select the single best diagnosis?
    A Diverticulitis
    B Rectal carcinoma
    C Colonic adenomata/polyps
    D Crohn's disease
    E Ulcerative colitis

22. A 69-year-old woman is awaiting surgery for a total hip replacement. She reports severe abdominal pain and nausea. She is currently taking nonsteroidal anti-inflammatory medication for pain relief. Select the single best diagnosis?
    - A Diverticulitis
    - B Rectal carcinoma
    - C Colonic adenomata/polyps
    - D Crohn's disease
    - E Ulcerative colitis

23. For each of the conditions described below, select the single best arterial blood gas result from the options listed below. Thiazide diuretics
    - A Metabolic acidosis
    - B Metabolic alkalosis
    - C Respiratory acidosis
    - D Respiratory alkalosis
    - E None of the above

24. For each of the conditions described below, select the single best arterial blood gas result from the options listed below. Chronic renal failure
    - A Metabolic acidosis
    - B Metabolic alkalosis
    - C Respiratory acidosis
    - D Respiratory alkalosis
    - E None of the above

25. For each of the conditions described below, select the single best arterial blood gas result from the options listed below. Guillain–Barré syndrome
    - A Metabolic acidosis
    - B Metabolic alkalosis
    - C Respiratory acidosis
    - D Respiratory alkalosis
    - E None of the above

26. At what single level does the thoracic duct pass through the diaphragm?
    - A T8 Level
    - B T9 Level
    - C T10 Level
    - D T11 Level
    - E T12 Level

27. At what single level does the oesophagus pass through the diaphragm?
    - A T8 Level
    - B T9 Level
    - C T10 Level
    - D T11 Level
    - E T12 Level

28. At what single level does the aorta pass through the diaphragm?
    - A T8 Level
    - B T9 Level
    - C T10 Level
    - D T11 Level
    - E T12 Level

29. The eustachian tube arises from what pharyngeal pouch?
    - A First pharyngeal pouch
    - B Second pharyngeal pouch
    - C Third pharyngeal pouch
    - D Fourth pharyngeal pouch
    - E Sixth pharyngeal pouch

30. The second pharyngeal pouch is innervated by which nerve?
    - A Trigeminal nerve (V)
    - B Abducent nerve (VI)
    - C Facial nerve (VII)
    - D Glossopharyngeal nerve (IX)
    - E Vagus nerve (X)

31. A 23-year-old is in a lower limb plaster following a complex tibial plateau fracture. He presents with a painful and swollen limb. A palpable distal pulse is detected. What is most appropriate intervention?
    A Commence low-molecular weight heparin
    B Venous duplex scan
    C Elevate the limb
    D Remove plaster
    E Fasciotomy

32. In regard to vascular supply, which artery is closely related to the greater splanchnic nerves?
    A Abdominal aorta
    B Aortic arch
    C Coeliac trunk
    D Superior mesenteric artery
    E Inferior mesenteric artery

33. A 72-year-old man presents with a cough and weight loss. His past medical history includes a recent history of prostate cancer. His chest radiograph demonstrates a cannonball lesion. Please select the best diagnosis?
    A Mesothelioma
    B Pancoast tumour
    C Small cell carcinoma
    D Secondary lung tumour
    E Squamous cell carcinoma

34. A 52-year-old woman presents with a rapidly worsening cough, haemoptysis, and shortness of breath at rest. Her chest radio-graph demonstrates mediastinal gland enlargement. Her blood tests reveal hypercalcaemia. Please select the best diagnosis?
    A Mesothelioma
    B Pancoast tumour
    C Small cell carcinoma
    D Secondary lung tumour
    E Squamous cell carcinoma

35. Select the appropriate hormone that the zona fasciculata of the adrenal cortex secretes?
    A Adrenaline
    B Aldosterone
    C Cortisol
    D Dehydroepiandrosterone (DHEA)
    E Renin

36. Select the best mediator associated with a Type I hypersensitivity reaction?
    A Helper T cells 4
    B Immunoglobulin A
    C Immunoglobulin D
    D Immunoglobulin E
    E Immunoglobulin G

37. Select the best mediator associated with a Type II hypersensitivity reaction?
    A Helper T cells 4
    B Immunoglobulin A
    C Immunoglobulin D
    D Immunoglobulin E
    E Immunoglobulin G

38. Select the best mediator associated with a Type III hypersensitivity reaction?
    A Helper T cells 4
    B Immunoglobulin A
    C Immunoglobulin D
    D Immunoglobulin E
    E Immunoglobulin G

39. Select the best mediator associated with a Type IV hypersensitivity reaction?
    A Helper T cells
    B Immunoglobulin A
    C Immunoglobulin D
    D Immunoglobulin E
    E Immunoglobulin G

40. Which structures comprise the roof of the inguinal canal?
    A External oblique and internal oblique (for the lateral 1/3)
    B Inguinal ligament
    C Internal oblique and transversus abdominis
    D Lacunar ligament
    E Transversalis fascia and conjoint tendon

41. Which structures comprise the lateral border of Hunter's (adductor's) canal?
    A Adductor muscles
    B Vastus medialis
    C Vastus lateralis
    D Rectus femoris
    E Sartorius

42. What is the single best treatment for the patients listed below?
    A A 35-year-old woman with blood group B RhD-negative following a left-sided nephrectomy is found to have a haemoglobin level of 6.5. Treatment: Group B RhD-positive.
    B A 66-year-old man with prostate carcinoma and blood group A RhD-positive is found to have a haemoglobin level of 7.1. Treatment: Group O RhD-negative.
    C A patient with blood group B RhD-positive following a right-sided hemicolectomy is found to have a haemoglobin level of 9.4. Treatment: Group B RhD-positive.
    D A 75-year-old man with metastatic colorectal carcinoma and blood group O RhD-negative is found to have a haemoglobin level of 7.3. Treatment: Group O RhD-positive.
    E A woman with blood group B RhD-negative and thyroid disease is found to have a haemoglobin level of 11.0 having just given birth to a baby with blood group B RhD-positive. Treatment: Anti-D immunoglobulin.

43. A 27-year-old man presents with a soft lump in the right scrotum. On examination there is a positive cough impulse and the doctor is unable to get above the lump. The patient is able to push the lump back, and when the doctor places his fingers over the right groin the lump does not reappear even when the patient coughs. Diagnosis?
    A Testicular cancer
    B Testicular torsion
    C Direct inguinal hernia
    D Indirect inguinal hernia
    E Varicocele

44. A 22-year-old man presents with a painless swelling in the right scrotum. On examination the swelling is non-tender but contains a firm mass which does not seem separate from the testicle. The scrotal swelling brightly transilluminates. Diagnosis?
    A Testicular cancer
    B Testicular torsion
    C Direct inguinal hernia
    D Indirect inguinal hernia
    E Varicocele

45. A 32-year-old man presents
    complaining of a 'dragging'
    sensation in the left scrotum.
    On examination, the doctor can
    palpate a soft mass which feels like
    a 'bag of worms' but only when the
    patient is standing. Diagnosis?
    A Testicular cancer
    B Testicular torsion
    C Direct inguinal hernia
    D Indirect inguinal hernia
    E Varicocele

46. A 34-year-old man presents with
    a firm lump in the right side of
    his neck just below the mandible.
    The lump measures 3 cm. The skin
    appears attached to the lump and
    there is a small punctum visible.
    Diagnosis?
    A Lymph node
    B Branchial cyst
    C Thyroglossal cyst
    D Cystic hygroma
    E Epidermal cyst

47. A 14-year-old girl presents with
    a 2 cm soft, fluctuant lump on
    the right side of her neck adjacent
    to the angle of the mandible. The
    lump transilluminates and is cys-
    tic on ultrasound. Diagnosis?
    A Lymph node
    B Branchial cyst
    C Thyroglossal cyst
    D Cystic hygroma

48. For the patients below, select
    the best pairing of their clinical
    presentation with the appropriate
    investigation:
    A A 65-year-old woman is referred
       with a 4-month history of weight
       loss and progressive jaundice.

Her CA19-9 is raised and her
ultrasound reveals dilated hepatic
ducts. ERCP was attempted but
was abandoned due to failure of
passage of the scope beyond the
distal common bile duct stricture.
Investigation: Magnetic resonance
cholangiopancreatogram (MRCP).

B A 43-year-old woman who is
   rather overweight presents with a
   3-day history of right upper quadrant pain, fevers, and vomiting.
   Her liver biochemistry is within
   normal limits but she does demonstrate a neutrophilia. Investigation:
   Contrast-enhanced CT.

C A 60-year-old woman with a
   previous history of gallstones
   presents with colicky abdominal
   pain and vomiting. Her abdomen is distended and bowel
   sounds are increased. She is often
   constipated but feels that this
   is different. Investigation: Plain
   abdominal X-ray (AXR).

D A 35-year-old man with a history
   of alcohol abuse presents to A&E
   with a 2-day history of epigastric
   pain. His amylase on admission is
   1200 and he is pyrexial. His liver
   biochemistry demonstrates an
   obstructive picture. Investigation:
   Pelvic X-ray.

E A 45-year-old woman presents
   with right upper quadrant pain
   and vomiting. Her bilirubin and
   alkaline phosphatase are raised.
   A stone is seen in the common
   bile duct on ultrasound and
   measures 1.2 cm. The common
   bile duct itself measures 1.3 cm.
   Investigation: Percutaneous
   transhepatic cholangiopancreatogram (PTC).

49. A 67-year-old woman suffers from rheumatoid arthritis which affects both hips. She falls when walking back from town. Her plain X-ray reveals an intracapsular fracture of the femoral neck. Select the operation you would recommend:
    A Dynamic hip screw
    B Cannulated screws
    C Uncemented hemiarthroplasty
    D Cemented hemiarthroplasty
    E Total hip replacement

50. A 35-year-old woman is hit by a car. The plain X-ray shows an intracapsular fracture of the right femoral neck. Select the operation you would recommend.
    A Traction
    B Dynamic hip screw
    C Cannulated screws
    D Intramedullary hip screw
    E Hemiarthroplasty

51. An 80-year-old man slips in the bathroom and presents to A&E with a shortened left leg. The plain X-ray demonstrates an extra-capsular fracture of the femoral neck. Select the operation that you would recommend.
    A Dynamic hip screw
    B Cannulated screws
    C Uncemented hemiarthroplasty
    D Cemented hemiarthroplasty
    E Total hip replacement

52. Extracellular fluid differs from intracellular fluid by which of the following?
    A Lower chloride concentration
    B Higher potassium concentration
    C Greater volume
    D Lower protein concentration
    E Lower pH

53. Which is a feature of metabolic acidosis?
    A There is negative base excess
    B Bicarbonate is the main intracel-lular buffer
    C Proteins and phosphates are the main extracellular buffer
    D Compensation occurs by a decrease in alveolar ventilation
    E Bicarbonate infusion is the main-stay of treatment

54. Which is a feature of the posterior third of the tongue?
    A Filiform papillae
    B Fungiform papillae
    C Sensory innervations from the internal laryngeal nerve
    D Sensory innervations from the chordae tympani
    E Villiform papillae

55. Which is a feature of the hepatic artery?
    A Supplies the same amount of blood to the liver as the portal vein
    B Provides the same amount of oxygen to the liver as the portal vein
    C Contains blood with the same oxygenation as the portal vein
    D Does not supply blood to hepatic metastases
    E Divides the liver into anatomical segments

56. Metabolic alkalosis is commonly seen in patients with which of the following?
    A Pancreatic fistula
    B Aspirin poisoning
    C Protracted vomiting
    D Hypoglycaemia
    E Hyperventilation

57. Osteomyelitis is most commonly caused by which microbe in adults?
   A *Staphylococcus aureus*
   B *Escherichia coli*
   C *Staphylococcus epidermidis*
   D *Pseudomonas*
   E *Streptococcus viridans*

58. Which is a feature of a keloid scar?
   A May respond to pressure dressing
   B Occurs within the limits of the surgical wound
   C Is most common on flexure surfaces of the limbs
   D Can be prevented by subcuticular sutures
   E May be re-excised with good results

59. Splenectomy patients are at particular risk of overwhelming sepsis from which organisms?
   A Anaerobic bacteria
   B *Bacteroides fragilis*
   C *Haemophilus influenzae*
   D Fungi
   E *Staphylococcus aureus*

60. A boy is found to have haemophilia B. What pathological problem does he have?
   A Deficiency of platelets
   B Deficiency of factor VIII
   C Deficiency of factor IX
   D Deficiency of factor X
   E Deficiency of factor XI

61. What features would you expect to find in a patient with haemorrhagic shock?
   A Decrease in catecholamine secretion
   B Oxygen–haemoglobin dissociation curve shifted to the right

   C Stimulation of aortic chemoreceptors
   D Increase in tidal ventilation
   E Decrease in antidiuretic hormone (ADH) secretion

62. Gastrointestinal consequences of major burns include which of the following?
   A Splanchnic vasodilation
   B Acute gastric dilatation
   C Cushing's ulcers
   D Terminal ileal hyperplasia
   E Mechanical bowel obstruction

63. When is nitrogen balance positive?
   A In sepsis
   B During the first 3 days following surgery
   C During growth
   D While adrenocorticotropic hormone (ACTH) levels are high
   E Following bone fractures

64. Hormones of the anterior pituitary include which of the following?
   A Prolactin
   B Oxytocin
   C Thyroxin
   D ADH
   E Vasopressin

65. Which is a feature of the scalenus anterior muscle?
   A Attaches into the anterior tubercles of the transverse processes of C1–C7 vertebrae
   B Attaches to the scalene tubercle of the 2nd rib
   C Has the subclavian vein passing posterior to it
   D Has the subclavian artery passing anterior to it
   E Lies deep to the prevertebral layer of the deep cervical fascia

66. What is the normal glomerular filtration rate?
    A 50 mL/min
    B 75 mL/min
    C 100 mL/min
    D 125 mL/min
    E 150 mL/min

67. What is the most common cancer in the UK?
    A Colorectal cancer
    B Lung cancer
    C Breast cancer
    D Melanoma
    E Leukaemia

68. Regarding enteral tube feeding, which statement is true?
    A Requires just as much monitoring as parental feeding
    B Continuous feeding with iso-osmolar fluids may cause diarrhoea
    C Elemental fluids require minimal digestion by the patient
    D Maintains the structural, but not the functional, integrity of the small bowel
    E Fluids should contain glucose rather than sucrose to lower the osmolality

69. What is a characteristic feature of the liver?
    A It weighs 750 g
    B It receives 60 per cent of the body's total cardiac output
    C It drains through hepatic veins into the superior vena cava
    D It receives its nerve supply from the right vagus via the superior mesenteric ganglia
    E It is attached to the diaphragm by the falciform ligament

70. Concerning bone tumours, which is true?
    A There is an association between osteosarcoma and Paget's disease of the bone
    B Chondosarcomas most commonly occur in young children
    C Chemotherapy has a limited role in overall management
    D Metastasis usually occurs via lymphatics
    E Pain is rarely a presenting feature

71. The posterior relations of the kidney include which structure?
    A Rectus abdominis muscle
    B Femoral nerve
    C Long thoracic nerve of Bell
    D Costodiaphragmatic recess of the pleura
    E Lumbar sympathetic trunk

72. Which statement is true of Meckel's diverticulum?
    A Is present in 20 per cent of the population
    B Arises from the mesenteric border of the jejunum
    C May contain heterotropic pancreas
    D Is present only in males
    E Is a diverticulum of the bladder

73. Which of the following is a recognized curative treatment option for localized carcinoma of the prostate?
    A Radiotherapy
    B Lithotripsy
    C Hormonal treatment
    D Cytotoxic therapy
    E Tamsulosin

74. Which of the following statements is true for a patient who has been maintained on haemodialysis for 10 years?
    A Will need a parathyroidectomy shortly after renal transplant
    B Will have vascular calcification, which will resolve after parathyroidectomy
    C Is no more likely to have secondary hyperparathyroidism than someone on continuous ambulatory peritoneal dialysis (CAPD) for the same period
    D Could have osteoporosis if has taken aluminium hydroxide over this time
    E Will need bisphosphonates after parathyroidectomy

75. Concerning statistical analysis of a population with a normal (Gaussian) distribution, which is true?
    A The population may be uniquely defined by its mean and its median values
    B About 95 per cent of the population lies within one standard deviation of the mean
    C It would be inappropriate to apply a chi-squared test because the distribution is not linear
    D Non-parametric tests could be used
    E Fewer than 5 out of 1000 of the population would be expected to be more than two standard deviations from the mode

76. Which of the following cells secrete intrinsic factor?
    A Goblet cells
    B Kupffer cells
    C Peptic cells
    D Chief (zymogenic) cells
    E Parietal cells

77. Splenectomy increases susceptibility to which of the following organisms?
    A Streptococcus pyogenes
    B Schistosoma haematobium
    C Bacteroides fragilis
    D Neisseria meningitidis
    E Staphylococcus aureus

78. Cardiac output is decreased under what circumstances?
    A During stimulation of sympathetic nerves to the heart
    B On cutting the vagus nerves to the heart
    C By increasing the end-diastolic volume of the heart
    D As a result of decreased pressure within the carotid sinus
    E Upon assuming the upright position

79. Which statement is true for flow through a vessel or lumen?
    A It is inversely proportional to the pressure head of flow
    B It is inversely proportional to the radius
    C It is directly proportional to the length of the tube
    D It is directly proportional to the viscosity of blood passing through the tube
    E It is directly proportional to the fourth power of the radius

80. You request preoperative lung function tests on a patient with long-standing emphysema. What is true of the functional residual capacity?
    A It is the sum of the tidal volume and residual volume
    B It is the sum of the inspiratory reserve volume, the expiratory reserve volume, and the tidal volume

C It can be measured directly by spirometry

D It is the sum of the residual volume and the expiratory reserve volume

E It is the volume of air that remains in the lung after forced expiration

81. Which statement is true of lung compliance?

A Is defined as the change in pressure per unit volume

B Is synonymous with elastance

C Is increased in emphysema

D Is equal in inflation and deflation

E Is reduced by the presence of surfactant

82. Which of the following hormones is secreted by the anterior pituitary gland?

A Testosterone

B Oxytocin

C Thyroid-stimulating hormone (TSH)

D Corticotropin-releasing hormone (CRH)

E ADH

83. The oxygen–haemoglobin dissociation curve is shifted to the left by what?

A An increase in pCO_2

B A fall in pH

C A rise in temperature

D An increase in 2,3-DPG

E Foetal haemoglobin

84. Which of the following cells are cytotoxic?

A CD4 T-cells

B CD8 T-cells

C B-cells

D TH1 cells

E TH2 cells

85. A 3-week-old baby exhibits projectile vomiting shortly after feeding, and failure to thrive. On examination, an olive-shaped mass is palpable in the right upper quadrant of the abdomen. A clinical diagnosis of pyloric stenosis is made. What biochemical laboratory features would support the diagnosis?

A Hypokalaemia, metabolic alkalosis, low urinary pH

B Hyperkalaemia, metabolic acidosis, high urinary pH

C Hypokalaemia, metabolic acidosis, high urinary pH

D Hyperkalaemia, metabolic alkalosis, low urinary pH

E Hypokalaemia, metabolic alkalosis, high urinary pH

86. Which antiarrhythmic drug acts by inhibiting potassium channels?

A Lignocaine

B Atenolol

C Amiodarone

D Verapamil

E Diltiazem

87. With regard to the branchial arches:

A Apart from the first cleft, the other branchial clefts are normally obliterated by overgrowth of the 2nd branchial arch

B Six pairs of branchial arches develop in humans

C The muscles of facial expression are 1st-arch derivatives

D All parathyroid glands originate from the same branchial arch

E The tongue principally develops from the 2nd branchial arch

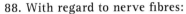

88. **With regard to nerve fibres:**
    A Impulses can travel in one direction only
    B They continue to conduct impulses when extracellular sodium is replaced by potassium
    C An action potential has an amplitude varying directly with the strength of the stimulus
    D The equilibrium potential for an ion species depends on the ratio of the concentrations of the ion outside to inside of the cell
    E Resting nerve cell membranes are more permeable to Na⁺ ions than to K⁺ ions

89. **The classic pathway of complement activation:**
    A Starts with the activation of the C3 component
    B Is activated by lipopolysaccharide cell-wall constituents
    C Is activated by IgA immune complexes
    D Is activated by IgM immune complexes
    E Is evolutionarily older than the alternative pathway

90. **The plateau stage of the cardiac action potential is caused by which one of the following mechanisms?**
    A Ingress of calcium ions
    B Ingress of potassium ions
    C Efflux of potassium ions
    D Ingress of sodium ions
    E Efflux of sodium ions

91. **With regard to development of the nervous system:**
    A Neural tube development requires signals from the underlying mesoderm
    B The nervous system is derived from endoderm
    C Neural tube defects originate during the final trimester of pregnancy
    D The notochord forms the spinal cord in adults
    E Neural tube defects result from the incomplete migration of neural crest cells

92. **With regard to smooth (visceral) muscle:**
    A Excitation depends more on the influx of extracellular calcium than release from internal stores
    B It contains no actin or myosin filaments
    C It classically relaxes when it is stretched
    D It contains an extensive T-tubular system
    E It is innervated through somatic motor nerve endings

93. **The incubation period for hepatitis A is:**
    A 2–10 days
    B 15–40 days
    C 40–60 days
    D 60–160 days
    E More than 160 days

94. **In the treatment of asthma, the drug salbutamol principally acts by which of the following mechanisms?**
    A α_1-adrenoceptor antagonism
    B β_1-adrenoceptor agonism
    C β_2-adrenoceptor agonism
    D β_2-adrenoceptor antagonism
    E Muscarinic antagonism

95. **A Meckel's diverticulum:**
    A Is a remnant of the urachus
    B Is found in 10 per cent of the population
    C Is most commonly situated immediately adjacent to the vermiform appendix

D Is completely asymptomatic and an incidental finding

E May contain ectopic tissue

96. With regard to the structure of cardiac muscle:

A The T-tubules are located at the junction of the A and I bands

B It has no visible striations in the cytoplasm

C It has an underdeveloped sarcoplasmic reticulum

D Specialized intercellular junctions exist between myocytes

E Muscle fibres are typically multinucleate with peripherally located nuclei

97. With regard to the acute-phase response:

A Bacterial endotoxin induces the acute-phase response

B Exogenous pyrogens act on the liver to release tumour necrosis factor (TNF)α

C The acute-phase response is mediated through interleukin-10

D Serum albumin levels increase during the acute-phase response

E TNFα decreases catabolic activity

98. Which one of the following cranial nerves carries parasympathetic fibres?

A V

B IV

C VI

D III

E II

99. With regard to properties of cardiac muscle:

A A fused tetanic response can be produced by repetitive stimulation

B The cardiac muscle action potential lasts approximately 2–3 ms

C Excitation–contraction coupling requires calcium-induced calcium release

D The force of contraction is independent of the length of the muscle fibre

E The plateau phase of the cardiac action potential is principally due to sodium influx

100. With regard to fever:

A It results from the direct action of microorganisms on the brain

B It depends on the action of prostaglandins within the hypothalamus

C It is always maladaptive and serves no purpose

D It only results from infectious causes

E The antipyretic action of aspirin results from boosting of the immune response

101. A patient presents with a torn medial collateral ligament of his left knee. Which of the following signs may be elicited on physical examination?

A Posterior displacement of the tibia

B Anterior displacement of the tibia

C Abnormal lateral rotation during extension

D Abnormal passive abduction of the extended knee

E Inability to lock knee on full extension

102. Which of the following is a technique used to identify specific sequences of DNA?

A Northern blotting

B Southern blotting

C Polymerase chain reaction (PCR)

D Western blotting

E Reverse-transcription PCR

103. **Which one of the following is true concerning the larynx?**
   A The posterior crico-arytenoids are the only muscles that separate the vocal cords
   B All the intrinsic muscles are supplied by the recurrent laryngeal nerve
   C The vocal cords are lined by pseudostratified columnar ciliated epithelium ('respiratory' epithelium)
   D The epiglottis is composed largely of hyaline cartilage
   E The cricoid cartilage and tracheal rings are all complete rings of cartilage

104. **With regard to chemical neurotransmitters:**
   A Noradrenaline is the predominant neurotransmitter found between first- and second-order sympathetic neurones
   B The nerve endings of second-order parasympathetic neurones release acetylcholine that acts on nicotinic cholinergic receptors
   C The neuromuscular junction releases acetylcholine that acts on muscarinic cholinergic receptors
   D The nucleus accumbens and substantia nigra are rich in dopamine
   E The locus coeruleus and periaqueductal grey are rich in acetylcholine

105. **Pathogenic bacteria enter the body by various routes, and entry mechanisms are critical for understanding the pathogenesis and transmission of each agent. Which pathogen is correctly linked with its mode of entry?**
   A *Neisseria meningitidis* – sexually transmitted entry
   B *Corynebacterium diphtheriae* – food-borne entry
   C *Clostridium tetani* – inhalation entry
   D *Borrelia burgdorferi* – arthropod vector-borne entry
   E *Rickettsia rickettsii* – contaminated wound with soil entry

106. **With regard to gene expression:**
   A Translation occurs in the nucleus of eukaryotes
   B Introns code for proteins
   C DNA polymerases manufacture DNA in a 3′-5′ direction
   D RNA polymerase II gives rise to protein encoding mRNA
   E Codons are formed from groups of three amino acids

107. **Concerning the thyroid gland, which one of the following is correct?**
   A Blood supply is through the internal carotid and subclavian arteries
   B Embryologically starts out at the foramen caecum of the tongue
   C Venous drainage is by way of the external jugular vein
   D Produces thyroid-stimulating hormone (TSH)
   E Is attached to the thyroid cartilage by Berry's ligament

108. **Opioids:**
   A Commonly cause diarrhoea
   B Act only centrally
   C Mediate most of their beneficial effects and side effects through ç-receptors
   D Lead to tolerance
   E Can be reversed by flumazenil

109. **Type I hypersensitivity:**
   A Is caused by antigen reacting with IgM antibodies

B   Results in mast-cell degranulation
C   Is characterized by the Arthus reaction
D   Takes 48–72 hours to develop
E   Is caused by the formation of antibody–antigen complexes

110. Which one of the following statements concerning referred pain is true?
A   Pain from the transverse colon is usually referred to the midline area below the umbilicus
B   Somatic pain is usually referred in a diffuse, poorly localized pattern
C   The mechanism of referred pain is well understood
D   Diaphragmatic pain is usually referred to the inguinal area
E   Pain from an inflamed appendix is referred to the medial thigh

111. With regard to cell division:
A   Transfer of genetic information between homologous chromosomes occurs in metaphase I of meiosis
B   Mitosis produces genetically identical daughter cells
C   It is controlled externally by cyclins
D   Cyclins are activated by dephosphorylation
E   p53 is an oncogene

112. With regard to the tongue:
A   All muscles of the tongue are innervated via the hypoglossal nerve
B   Special taste sensation on the anterior two-thirds of the tongue is through the mandibular division of the trigeminal nerve
C   It is composed of smooth musculature

D   Genioglossus muscle protrudes the tongue
E   Its epithelium is of the glandular columnar variety

113. With regard to the relationship of the electrocardiogram to the cardiac cycle:
A   The P-wave results from atrial repolarization
B   The QRS complex is due to ventricular repolarization
C   The Q-T interval gives a rough indication of the duration of ventricular systole
D   The first heart sound occurs at the same time as the P-wave
E   The second heart sound occurs at the same time as the QRS complex

114. Type III Hypersensitivity:
A   Is mediated by specifically sensitized T-lymphocytes
B   May cause allergic rhinitis
C   Is a feature of nickel sensitivity
D   May occur in systemic lupus erythematosus
E   Is cell mediated

115. With regard to DNA:
A   Adenine pairs only with thymine
B   Cytosine always pairs with guanine
C   The DNA double helix has 12 base pairs per turn
D   Uracil is an example of a purine base
E   All bases are paired by two non-covalent hydrogen bonds

116. A woman has warts caused by human papilloma virus (HPV). The infectious HPV is most likely to be found:
A   In terminally differentiated squamous cells

B In the basal layer of the warts
C In the surface cell layer of the
   warts
D In transformed cancer cells
E Throughout the warts

117. Hyperacute rejection:
    A Is a cell-mediated response
    B Occurs 48 hours after
       transplantation
    C Can occur in autografts
    D May be reversed by high-dose
       steroids
    E May be minimized by blood-
       group matching

118. A total of 100 hypertensive
     patients are followed over a
     4-week period for the effects
     of a diuretic drug on potassium
     concentrations. The statistical
     test used to compare the
     potassium serum levels before
     and after medication is most
     likely to be:
    A Discriminant analysis
    B Paired t-test
    C Regression analysis
    D Pearson correlation
    E Chi-squared test

119. Gene transcription is
     initiated by:
    A Exons
    B Promoters
    C Silencers
    D Introns
    E Enhancers

120. With regard to extra-ocular
     muscles:
    A Superior rectus is supplied by the
       trochlear nerve
    B Levator palpebrae superioris is
       supplied solely by the occulomo-
       tor nerve

C The superior oblique muscle is
   innervated by the occulomotor
   nerve
D Lateral rectus is supplied by the
   abducens nerve
E The inferior oblique muscle
   moves the eye inferiorly

121. Which of following substances is a
     vasodilator?
    A Angiotensin II
    B Nitric oxide
    C Noradrenaline
    D Vasopressin
    E Thromboxane A2

122. Hodgkin's lymphoma can be distin-
     guished from other forms of lym-
     phoma by the presence of:
    A Reed–Sternberg cells
    B Philadelphia chromosome
    C Auer rods
    D Decreased quantities of leukocyte
       alkaline phosphatase
    E Pappenheimer bodies

123. With regard to ABO blood
      grouping:
    A Blood group O is the universal
       recipient
    B The mode of inheritance is
       autosomal recessive
    C Blood group AB is the universal
       donor
    D Blood group O is recessive to A
       and B
    E Individuals of blood group O
       are resistant to *Plasmodium vivax*

124. With regard to the intercostal
     spaces:
    A The neurovascular bundle lies
       between the external intercos-
       tal and inner intercostal muscle
       layers

B The direction of fibres of the external intercostal muscle is downwards and medial

C The intercostal vein lies below the intercostal nerve

D The neurovascular bundle lies in a groove just above each rib

E The intercostals are the main muscles of respiration

125. With regard to chemoreceptors:
    A The carotid bodies have a blood flow per unit volume similar to that of the brain
    B The carotid bodies are stretch receptors in the walls of the carotid arteries
    C Central chemoreceptors are located in the aortic arch
    D Carotid bodies primarily respond to hypoxia
    E The response of the peripheral chemoreceptors to arterial pCO_2 is more important than that of the central chemoreceptors

126. With regard to malaria:
    A It is caused by a virus
    B It is transmitted by the Aedes mosquito vector
    C The most virulent strain is *Plasmodium malariae*
    D It may cause blackwater fever
    E It is effectively prevented by vaccination

127. The neurotransmitters adrenaline, noradrenaline, and dopamine are derived from which amino acid?
    A Tyrosine
    B Arginine
    C Aspargine
    D Phenylalanine
    E Tryptophan

128. Adult polycystic kidney disease:
    A Is inherited as an autosomal recessive condition
    B Affects only one kidney
    C Is associated with berry aneurysms of the circle of Willis
    D Commonly presents at birth
    E Is due to a mutation in polycystin-1 in all cases

129. With regard to the oesophagus:
    A It is a segmental muscular tube composed entirely of smooth muscle
    B Epithelium is always stratified squamous throughout its whole length
    C Blood supply is from the descending thoracic aorta along its entire length
    D It lacks a true serosal surface
    E It measures approximately 40 cm in length

130. With regard to carbon dioxide transport:
    A Carbon dioxide is mainly carried in the blood in its dissolved form
    B It is carried as carboxyhaemoglobin on the haemoglobin molecule
    C The Haldane effect describes changes in the affinity of the blood for CO_2 with variations in the PaO_2
    D Venous blood has a higher pH than arterial blood
    E Carbon dioxide is less soluble in plasma than is oxygen

131. With regard to the malaria life cycle:
    A Sporozoites invade erythrocytes
    B Parasites may remain dormant in the liver as hypnozoites
    C Trophozoites invade hepatocytes

D Schizonts are contained within the mosquito's salivary glands

E Fertilization and formation of a zygote occurs in humans

132. With regard to oesophageal constrictions:

A The lower oesophageal sphincter is a true anatomical sphincter

B They may be caused by the right principal bronchus

C The narrowest part of the oesophagus is at the level of cricopharyngeus

D They may be caused normally by the left atrium

E They may be caused by the descending thoracic aorta

133. Which one of the following is true of the haemoglobin oxygen/dissociation curve?

A It is a rectangular hyperbola

B It is shifted to the left by an increase in pCO_2

C Foetal haemoglobin shifts the curve to the right

D The Haldane effect describes the changes in affinity of the haemoglobin chain for oxygen following variations in pCO_2

E The shape of the curve is explained by the physico-chemical properties of haemoglobin

134. With regard to schistosomiasis:

A It is caused by a protozoan

B The intermediate host is the sandfly

C Schistosoma mansoni causes urinary schistosomiasis

D Disease results from the immune response to schistosome eggs

E It is treated with quinine

135. An 83-year-old man has chest pain, breathlessness, and ankle oedema. On clinical examination, cardiomegaly is identified and a subsequent diagnosis of viral myocarditis is made. Which of the following microorganisms is most likely responsible for this illness:

A Rhinovirus

B Mumps

C Coronavirus

D Adenovirus

E Coxsackie B

136. Which one of the following changes in disease patterns has occurred in Europe and North America over the past 50 years?

A The death rate from lung cancer in females has fallen

B The death rate from lung cancer in males has risen in recent years

C The numbers infected with the HIV virus has fallen

D The death rate from suicide has fallen

E The death rate from gastric carcinoma has fallen

137. With regard to the diaphragm:

A It is composed of smooth muscle

B It contracts with expiration

C It forms the main muscle of respiration at rest

D Motor innervation is through right and left phrenic nerves and lower intercostal nerves

E Sensation is via lower intercostals nerves only

138. At high altitude when the atmospheric pressure is halved, which one of the following changes occurs?

A Decreased pulmonary arterial pressure

B Decreased arterial pH
C Increased arterial P_{O_2}
D Decreased pulmonary ventilation
E Increased blood viscosity

139. Prions:
A Are infectious microorganisms
B Are destroyed by sterilization
C Contain nucleic acid
D Cause disease by inducing muta-
tions in the DNA of the host
E Are responsible for causing Kuru
in humans

140. Which of the following is the
best neutrophil and macrophage
chemotactant?
A C5a
B HLA-A
C HLA-B
D J-chain
E Variable region of heavy-chain
IgG

141. With regard to diaphragmatic
openings:
A The inferior vena cava passes
through the muscular part of the
diaphragm at T8
B The aortic opening lies at the T10
level
C The oesophageal opening transmits the right phrenic nerve
D The left phrenic nerve passes
with the oesophagus through the
oesophageal opening
E The sympathetic trunks pass
posterior to the medial arcuate
ligament

142. With regard to gas exchange:
A The rate of diffusion across the
alveolar wall is directly proportional to its thickness
B Under resting conditions, equilibration between alveoli P_{O_2} and

red blood cell P_{O_2} occurs one-
third of the way along the pulmonary capillary
C At rest, the red blood cell spends
approximately 5 seconds within
the pulmonary capillary
D The rate of diffusion across the
alveolar wall is inversely proportional to the surface area available for diffusion
E Chlorine is the gas of choice for
measuring the diffusion properties of the lung

143. Which of the following definitions
is correct?
A Hyperplasia is an increase in tissue growth through an increase
in cell size
B Dysplasia is a change from one
type of differentiated tissue to
another
C Carcinoma in situ is a carcinoma
with stromal invasion
D Anaplasia is almost a complete
lack of differentiation
E Metaplasia is the disordered
development of cells with loss of
organization

144. A 92-year-old man has died
secondary to lobar pneumonia. At
post-mortem he is diagnosed with
red hepatization. What pathological process within the lung was
responsible?
A Desquamation of tracheal and
bronchial epithelial cells
B Fibroblast proliferation
C Alcoholic toxic necrosis
D Leucocytes, erythrocytes, and
fibrin filling of the alveolar
spaces
E Pleural deposits of fibrin and low
molecular proteins

145. With regard to tumour suppressor genes:
   A They encode proteins that positively regulate growth
   B They behave in a dominant fashion
   C Gain-of-function of tumour suppressor genes results in neoplastic growth
   D p53 and Rb-1 are tumour suppressor genes
   E p53 normally functions as an anti-apoptotic factor

146. Which one of the following muscles is innervated by the facial nerve?
   A Temporalis
   B Anterior belly of digastric
   C Buccinator
   D Masseter
   E Lateral pterygoid

147. With regard to the transpyloric plane (of Addison):
   A It is halfway between the suprasternal notch and umbilicus
   B It lies at the level of T12
   C It lies at the origin of the inferior mesenteric artery
   D It lies level with the hilum of the kidneys
   E It is the point at which the aorta bifurcates

148. With regard to gastric acid secretion:
   A It is inhibited by gastrin
   B It is potentiated by histamine
   C It commences only when food enters the stomach
   D It is stimulated by the glossopharyngeal nerve
   E It is stimulated by somatostatin

149. With regard to the adrenal gland (suprarenal gland):
   A The suprarenal vein on each side drains into the corresponding renal vein
   B The adrenal gland is situated within the same fascial compartment as the kidney
   C The zona glomerulosa forms the innermost layer of the adrenal cortex
   D The anterior surface of the right adrenal gland is overlapped by the inferior vena cava
   E The adrenal medulla is derived from embryonic mesoderm

150. Which one of the following is true of gastrin?
   A It is secreted in the body of the stomach
   B It is stimulated by low pH
   C It stimulates gastric acid production
   D It inhibits gastric motility
   E Decreased secretion results in the Zollinger–Ellison syndrome

151. Lung carcinoma:
   A Is the third most common cause of death from neoplasia in the UK
   B Has rarely metastasized at the time of presentation
   C May produce paraneoplastic syndromes
   D Is most commonly due to small-cell (oat-cell) carcinoma
   E Is most commonly caused by asbestos exposure

152. Prokaryotes differ from eukaryotes in that prokaryotes have:
   A Peptidoglycan
   B Sterols in their membranes
   C 2–6 chromosomes

D An endoplasmic reticulum

E Larger 80S ribosomes

153. With regard to the vermiform appendix:

A It is most often situated in a pelvic position

B It receives blood via the right colic branch of the superior mesenteric artery

C It lies at McBurney's point (halfway between the anterior superior iliac spine and umbilicus)

D It is unimportant in humans

E It is a retroperitoneal structure

154. With regard to the exocrine pancreas:

A It secretes digestive juices with a pH of 4–5

B It develops from a single ventral pancreatic bud

C Secretion is inhibited by cholecystokinin

D The main stimulation for secretion occurs during the intestinal phase

E It produces secretin

155. A 17-year-old man attends his general practitioner surgery with a 7-day history of diarrhoea and vomiting and 3-day history of jaundice. He does not complain of any pain apart from mild abdominal discomfort. Examination of other systems were unremarkable. Blood tests show increased levels of unconjugated bilirubin. Which of the following is the most likely diagnosis?

A Crigler–Najjar syndrome

B Hereditary spherocytosis

C Autoimmune haemolytic anaemia

D Gilbert syndrome

E Rotor syndrome

156. Which of the following types of ulcers is associated with major burns?

A Cushing ulcer

B Curling ulcer

C Marjolin ulcer

D Venous ulcer

E Arterial ulcer

157. A 30-year-old man involved in a road traffic accident is brought into the resuscitation area of an accident and emergency department. He was in the passenger seat of a car that was hit from the side, causing the door to crush into his left side, which resulted in injury to the lateral aspect of his left knee. Radiographs show a fractured left neck of the fibula. Which one of the following would you most likely expect to find on examination?

A Loss of foot inversion

B Loss of ankle plantar flexion

C Loss of ankle dorsiflexion

D Paralysis of tibialis posterior

E Trendelenburg gait

158. Parasympathetic nervous supply for the parotid gland originates from which one of the following nerves?

A Vagus nerve

B Facial nerve

C Glossopharyngeal nerve

D Vestibulocochlear nerve

E Trigeminal nerve

159. Which of the following muscles act together to invert the foot?

A The peroneus brevis and peroneus longus

B   The peroneus brevis and peroneus tertius

C   The peroneus tertius and tibialis anterior

D   The peroneus longus and tibialis posterior

E   The tibialis anterior and tibialis posterior

160. Stratified squamous epithelium can be found in which of the following structures?
A   Epididymis
B   Colon
C   Trachea
D   Oesophagus
E   Uterus

161. A 22-year-old man is brought into the emergency department following a road traffic accident. He sustained an open fracture of the right tibia and fibula. His HR is 110 bpm, blood pressure (BP) 108/85, respiratory rate (RR) 28, urine output is 30 mL in the last hour. Which class of haemorrhagic shock does he fall into?
A   Class I
B   Class II
C   Class III
D   Class IV
E   Class V

162. Concerning pulse oximetry:
A   It measures arterial O_2 partial pressure
B   Readings are inaccurate in the presence of carbon monoxide
C   It gives a good indication of ventilation
D   Readings are usually reliable despite poor peripheral perfusion
E   It usually uses three wavelengths of light

163. Concerning the course of the phrenic nerve:
A   It arises from the posterior cervical rami of C3, 4, and 5
B   It travels anterior to the vagus nerve
C   The right passes through the central tendon of the diaphragm
D   It runs on scalenus medius in the neck
E   The left branch courses posterior to the left pulmonary artery in the mediastinum

164. A mother notices that her newborn baby boy is drooling excessively; on feeding him, he swallows normally, but moments later starts to cough and appears to choke on the milk, which is brought up through his nose. Which of the following is the most likely diagnosis?
A   Oesophageal atresia
B   Duodenal atresia
C   Small bowel atresia
D   Gastric outlet obstruction
E   Congenital diaphragmatic hernia

165. A newborn presents with profuse bilious vomiting at birth with fullness in the epigastric region. AXR shows the 'double bubble' sign. Which of the following pathologies is this associated with?
A   Oesophageal atresia
B   Congenital intestinal obstruction
C   Gastric outlet obstruction
D   Duodenal atresia
E   Meconium ileus

166. Within a few hours of being born a baby presents with bilious vomiting and abdominal distension. Which one of the following is the likely cause?
    A Hirschprung disease
    B Gastric outlet obstruction
    C Milk bolus obstruction
    D Gastritis
    E Meconium ileus

167. A 4-week-old baby presents with his mother with a 3-day history of absolute constipation. Examination reveals a diffusely tender abdomen with absent bowel sounds. Plain abdominal X-ray (AXR) shows a distended colon. A rectal biopsy is performed and demonstrates a lack of mural ganglionic cells. Which one of the following is the most likely diagnosis?
    A Rectal atresia
    B Pyloric stenosis
    C Hirschsprung's disease
    D Meconium ileus
    E Chagas disease

168. A 23-year-old male is diagnosed with a direct inguinal hernia. The surgical Registrar intraoperatively asks you to define Hesselbach's triangle. Hesselbach's triangle is bounded medially by which anatomical structure?
    A Lacunar ligament
    B Inferior epigastric artery
    C Femoral artery
    D Rectus abdominis
    E Inguinal ligament

169. A 45-year-old obese woman has an open cholecystectomy several weeks after an episode of acute cholecystitis. During the operation the surgeon correctly identifies Calot's triangle in order to locate the cystic artery. Which of the following anatomical structures form Calot's triangle?
    A Cystic duct, liver edge, and left hepatic duct
    B Portal vein, liver, and common bile duct
    C Common hepatic duct, cystic duct, and inferior border of the liver
    D Right hepatic artery, cystic duct, and common bile duct
    E Left hepatic duct and inferior border of liver and cystic duct

170. A 42-year-old woman undergoes right total mastectomy with axillary lymph node clearance for breast cancer. Two days postoperatively it was noted that she had winging of her right scapula. This is most likely caused by damage to which of the following nerves?
    A Musculocutaneous nerve
    B Axillary nerve
    C Long thoracic nerve
    D Pectoral nerve
    E Subscapular nerve

171. A 32-year-old male presents to the emergency department with a right-sided direct inguinal hernia. Past medical history includes an emergency appendicectomy. Iatrogenic injury at the time of the appendicectomy was thought to be the cause of the subsequent hernia. Which of the following structures was likely to have been damaged?
    A Genitofemoral nerve femoral branch

B Ilioinguinal nerve
C Obturator nerve
D Subcostal nerve
E Superior gluteal nerve

172. A 25-year-old female was involved in a road traffic accident and suffered a significant head injury. She is being monitored in the neurosurgical intensive care unit (ICU). Her BP is 100/70 and she has a HR) of 80 bpm. Her current intracranial pressure (ICP) is 10 mmHg. Which of the following is her cerebral perfusion pressure?
A 70 mmHg
B 170 mmHg
C 90 mmHg
D 180 mmHg
E 40 mmHg

173. A 52-year-old patient with known chronic obstructive pulmonary disease (COPD) and type 2 diabetes was admitted to the ICU after having an emergency Hartmann procedure for an obstructing colorectal carcinoma. He is currently ventilated on ICU as he, unfortunately, suffered a cardiac arrest postoperatively and needed ventilatory support. Five days postoperatively he has a temperature spike and his inflammatory markers have risen. Blood cultures are sent that are positive for Gram-negative bacilli. Based on this Gram stain, which of the following is the most likely causal organism that will be found/looked for?
A *Staphylococcus aureus*
B *Pseudomonas aeruginosa*

C *Actinomyces israelii*
D *Moraxella catarrhalis*
E *Listeria monocytogenes*

174. A 9-year-old boy was referred to orthopaedic outpatients with a 6-week history of left leg pain. X-rays revealed a large mass in the femur. Bone biopsy is performed and reveals small round blue cells. Which of the following is the most likely diagnosis?
A Osteosarcoma
B Chondrosarcoma
C Ewing sarcoma
D Malignant fibrous histiocytoma
E Myeloma

175. A 60-year-old male is scheduled to have a total gastrectomy for Zollinger–Ellison syndrome. He has been informed preoperatively that he will require lifelong intramuscular injections of vitamin B_{12}. Absence of which cell type is responsible for the vitamin replacement requirement?
A Goblet cells
B Mucous neck cells
C Parietal cells
D G-cells
E Chief cells

176. A 42-year-old woman has been diagnosed with thyroid cancer. A biopsy report demonstrates Orphan Annie nuclei. Which one of the following types of thyroid cancer does she have?
A Follicular
B Medullary
C Anaplastic
D Lymphoma
E Papillary

177. A 37-year-old male was admitted with a perforated duodenal ulcer. At laparotomy he was found to have a perforation at the posterior part of the first part of the duodenum. Which of the following anatomical structures lies just posterior to this?
A Splenic vein
B Inferior vena cava
C Gastroduodenal artery
D Coronary vein
E Superior mesenteric vein

178. A 35-year-old woman fell from the roof of her house. Paramedics on arrival report that she is opening her eyes to speech, moves in response to painful stimuli by withdrawing her arms and is using inappropriate words. Her vital signs are stable. What is her current Glasgow Coma Scale (GCS)?
A 4
B 10
C 9
D 7
E 3

179. A patient is having an emergency upper gastrointestinal endoscopy for a bleeding gastric ulcer. The ulcer is found to be in the lower greater curvature of the stomach. Which of the following arteries supplies this area?
A Left gastric artery
B Right gastric artery
C Superior pancreaticoduodenal artery
D Short gastric arteries
E Left gastroepiploic artery

180. A 50-year-old male is undergoing a total hip replacement. The operating surgeon takes a lateral approach to the joint. Which of the following anatomical structures does not attach to the greater trochanter?
A Obturator internus
B Gluteus minimus
C Iliacus
D Piriformis
E Obturator externus

181. A 24-year-old female is admitted as an emergency with appendicitis. While awaiting her procedure she is made nil by mouth (NBM) and is put on intravenous fluids. The first bag of fluids put up is 1 L of normal saline. How much sodium (Na+) is in this bag?
A 20 mM
B 44 mM
C 145 mM
D 154 mM
E 180 mM

182. As part of her triple assessment, a 55-year-old woman undergoes a fine-needle aspiration (FNA) of a breast lump. The cytology comes back as 'C3'. Which one of the following best describes C3?
A Insufficient (non-diagnostic) sample
B Breast cancer
C Equivocal
D Suspected breast cancer
E Benign

183. A 48-year-old woman undergoes a triple assessment for a left upper outer quadrant breast lump. The results of the clinical assessment show the lump to be 4.5 cm in diameter, with mobile lymph nodes on the same side and no evidence of distant metastases.

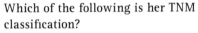

Which of the following is her TNM classification?

A T1N3M0

B T2N2M0

C T3N1M0

D T2N3M1

E T2N1M0

184. A 38-year-old female presents to your ear, nose, and throat (ENT) clinic complaining of a 1-month history of repeated attacks of vertigo, which are particularly severe when she turns over in bed. You conduct the Hallpike positional manoeuvre, which is positive. Which of the following is the most likely cause of her vertigo?

A Benign paroxysmal positional vertigo (BPPV)

B Acute labyrinthitis

C Ménière's disease

D Cervical spondylosis

E Labyrinthine fistula

185. The fundus of the stomach is supplied by which of the following arteries?

A Short gastric arteries

B Right gastric artery

C Left gastric artery

D Left and right gastroepiploic arteries

E Gastroduodenal artery

186. The pterion is the meeting of the squamous temporal bone, greater wing of the sphenoid, frontal bone, and which other bone?

A Lesser wing of the sphenoid

B Parietal

C Zygomatic

D Nasal

E Lacrimal

187. Which one of the following pigments is associated with ageing cells?

A Amyloid

B Melanin

C Eosin

D Lipofuscin

E Reticulin

188. Which one of the following is not a chemical mediator of inflammation?

A Histamine

B Prostaglandins

C Interleukins

D 5-Hydroxytryptamine (serotonin)

E Telomerase

189. Gas gangrene is most commonly caused by which of the following organisms?

A *Staphylococcus aureus*

B *Streptococcus pyogenes*

C *Clostridium tetani*

D *Clostridium perfringens*

E Mycobacteria

190. Which one of the following is a type of apoptosis?

A Histoplasmic

B Cytotoxic

C Morphogenetic

D Hypertrophic

E Kinetic

191. Metaplasia:

A Is a reversible transformation of one type of terminally differentiated cell into another fully differentiated cell type

B Is an irreversible transformation of one type of terminally differentiated cell into another fully differentiated cell type

C Is an increase in the size and number of cells

D Is an increase in the size of cells

E Is a decrease in the number of cells

192. Hamartomatous polyps of the gastrointestinal tract are commonly associated with which one of the following conditions?
    A   Turner syndrome
    B   Kartagener syndrome
    C   Kinefelter syndrome
    D   Peutz–Jeghers syndrome
    E   Di George syndrome

193. All of the following neoplasms are dependent on growth hormones except for which one?
    A   Thyroid carcinoma
    B   Endometrial carcinoma
    C   Osteosarcoma
    D   Prostate carcinoma
    E   Breast carcinoma

194. Which one of the following does not contribute to innate immunity?
    A   C-reactive protein
    B   Mucosal epithelium
    C   Lactoferrin
    D   Calcitonin
    E   Mannose-binding lectin

195. Which one of the following immunoglobulins is the first to be produced by B lymphocytes after primary encounter with antigen?
    A   Immunoglobulin A (IgA)
    B   Immunoglobulin D (IgD)
    C   Immunoglobulin E (IgE)
    D   Immunoglobulin G (IgG)
    E   Immunoglobulin M (IgM)

196. Immunoglobulin A (IgA) deficiency is associated with which of the following conditions?
    A   Scurvy
    B   Rickets
    C   Bleeding diathesis
    D   Mucosal infections
    E   Chondrocalcinosis

197. Patients with primary antibody deficiency are predisposed to which one of the following?
    A   Osteoporosis
    B   Salmonella osteomyelitis
    C   Mycoplasma arthritis
    D   Rheumatoid arthritis
    E   Psoriasis

198. Virus-laden cells are specifically killed by which of the following?
    A   T-cells
    B   Neutrophils
    C   Complement
    D   Natural killer cells
    E   Plasma cells

199. Psammoma bodies may be seen histologically in which malignancy?
    A   Follicular thyroid carcinoma
    B   Papillary thyroid carcinoma
    C   Medullary thyroid carcinoma
    D   Gliomas
    E   Breast carcinoma

200. Which of the following is an example of a malignant tumour of skeletal muscle (mesenchymal) origin?
    A   Osteoma
    B   Rhabdomyosarcoma
    C   Leiomyosarcoma
    D   Lipoma
    E   Adenoma

1. **C: A Null hypothesis is a statement of no significant difference or effect.**

   A Null hypothesis is a statement of no significant difference or effect. Sensitivity (true positive rate) measures the proportion of positives that are correctly identified as such (e.g., the percentage of people with a disease who are correctly identified as having the disease). Specificity (true negative rate) measures the proportion of negatives that are correctly identified as such (e.g., the percentage of healthy individuals who are correctly identified as not having the disease). Type I error is the incorrect rejection of a true null hypothesis (e.g., false positive). A benefit is perceived when really there is none. Type II error is accepting the false null hypothesis (e.g., False negative). A benefit is missed when it was there to be found (Table 1).

Table 1 Statistical table			
Disease			
		+	−
Test +		True positives (a)	False positives (b)	Positive predictive value (PPV) = a/(a+b)
	−	False negatives (c)	True negatives (d)	Negative predictive value (NPV) = d/(c+d)
		Sensitivity = a/(a+c)	Specificity = d/(b+d)	

2. **A: A 28-year-old man presents with abdominal and groin pain following a rugby match. Diagnosis: Gilmore's hernia**

   Gilmore's groin is a syndrome of groin disruption. Patients present with chronic pain, which is aggravated by sudden and twisting movements. Commonly known as the 'sportsman's hernia' or 'athletic pubalgia'. In general, there is no associated lump.

   In the case of the plumber, he has an inguinal hernia. An inguinal hernia is a protrusion of abdominal cavity contents through the inguinal canal. A direct inguinal hernia enters through a weak point in the fascia of the abdominal wall, and its sac is noted to be medial to the inferior epigastric vessels. Direct inguinal hernias are more common in males (10x). These hernias protrude through a weakened area in the transversalis fascia within the inguinal or Hesselbach's triangle. They are capable of protruding through the superficial inguinal ring and are not able to extend into the scrotum. Direct hernias tend to occur in the middle-aged and elderly. Additional risk factors include chronic constipation, overweight/obesity, chronic cough, and heavy lifting.

The 40-year-old woman with a painful groin suffers from a femoral hernia. Femoral hernias occur below the inguinal ligament when abdominal contents pass through the femoral canal. Anatomically, they are below and lateral to the pubic tubercle. Femoral hernias comprise 3 per cent of all hernias. They are more common in females due to a wider pelvis.

An incisional hernia occurs when the defect is a result of an incompletely healed surgical wound (e.g., appendicectomy). A scar associated with a mass is likely to be an incisional hernia.

The 6-year-old boy has a congenital umbilical hernia. In children, the gender ratio is roughly equal. Umbilical hernias in children are common with an incidence of 1 in 10. A typical umbilical hernia does not obliterate following birth. When the hernia's orifice is small (<2 cm), 90 per cent close by 5 years.

3. **C: Median nerve**

    Median nerve injury at the wrist causes sensory loss over the thumb, index finger, middle finger, and radial aspect of the ring finger. The muscles of the hand supplied by the median nerve can be remembered by using the mnemonic 'LOAF', Lumbricals 1 and 2, Opponens pollicis, Abductor pollicis, and Flexor pollicis brevis.

4. **D: Radial nerve**

    Damage to the radial nerve from mid-shaft humeral fracture can result in a wrist drop due to unopposed flexion at the wrist joint. Sensory loss occurs over the dorsal surface of the hand and the proximal ends of the lateral three and half fingers dorsally. It is commonly termed a 'Saturday night palsy'.

5. **E: Ulnar nerve**

    The ulnar nerve and its branches innervate the following muscles in the forearm and hand.

In the forearm (via the muscular branches of ulnar nerve)

    Flexor carpi ulnaris and Flexor digitorum profundus (medial half)

In the hand (via the deep branch of ulnar nerve):

    Hypothenar muscles: Opponens digiti minimi, Abductor digiti minimi, Flexor digiti minimi brevis

    Lumbrical muscles (3 and 4)

    Interossei (dorsal and palmar)

    Adductor pollicis

    Flexor pollicis brevis (deep head)

In the hand (via the superficial branch of ulnar nerve): Palmaris brevis

---

The ulnar nerve also provides sensory innervation to the fifth digit, the medial half of the fourth digit, and the corresponding part of the palm:

- *Palmar branch of ulnar nerve*: Supplies cutaneous innervation to the anterior skin and nails.
- *Dorsal cutaneous branch of ulnar nerve*: Supplies cutaneous innervation to the dorsal medial hand and the dorsum of the medial 1.5 fingers.

6. C: C5/C6

The biceps reflex is mediated by the C5 and C6 nerve roots, predominately by C5.

7. E: L5

At the L5 level, the IVC is formed from the common iliac vein. In addition, it is the site of the common iliac arteries bifurcation.

8. B: L1

At the L1 level, the superior mesenteric artery (SMA) comes off the aorta. This is an important anatomical level – the transpyloric plane of Addison (a horizontal line halfway between the suprasternal notch and pubic symphysis). The following structures are to be identified:

- Hilum of the kidneys
- Fundus of the gallbladder
- 2nd part of the duodenum
- Duodenojejunal flexure
- Neck of the pancreas
- Origin of the SMA
- Origin of the portal vein
- Pylorus of the stomach
- Attachment of transverse mesocolon
- Hilum of spleen (spleen on ribs 9, 10, 11)
- Tip of 9th costal cartilage
- Termination of the spinal cord
- Sphincter of Oddi
- L1 vertebral body

9. D: Mean arterial pressure

Mean arterial pressure (MAP) = [(2 × diastolic blood pressure) + systolic blood pressure]/3.

Diastole counts twice as much as systole because 2/3 of the cardiac cycle is spent in diastole. A MAP of 60 is required to perfuse the coronary arteries, brain, and kidneys. The reference range is 70–100 mmHg.

10. **E: Stroke volume**

    Stroke volume = cardiac output/heart rate.

    The reference range is 60–120 mL/beat.

11. **E: Pulmonary vascular resistance**

    Pulmonary vascular resistance = (mean pulmonary artery pressure – mean pulmonary capillary wedge pressure) × 80/cardiac output.

    The reference range is 125–250 dynes × sec/cm³.

12. **B: Cerebral blood flow**

    Cerebral blood flow (CBF) = cerebral perfusion pressure (CPP)/cerebral vascular resistance (CVR).

    - CBF is the amount of blood supply per unit area of cerebral tissue per unit time. In an adult, CBF is typically 750 mL/min or 15 per cent of the cardiac output. This equates to an average perfusion of 50–54 mL of blood per 100 g of brain tissue per minute.
    - It is directly proportional to volume of blood, but inversely related to CVR.

    > - Normal – 55 to 60 mL/100 g per minute
    > - Hyperaemia – CBF in excess of 55–60 mL/100 g per minute
    > - Ischemia – CBF below 18–20 mL/100 g per minute
    > - Tissue death – CBF below 8–10 mL/100 g per minute

13. **A: Cardiac index**

    Cardiac index = cardiac output/body surface area.

    The reference range is 2.5–4 L/min/m².

14. **C: Cerebral perfusion pressure**

    CPP = MAP – Intracranial pressure (ICP).

    Under normal circumstances of a MAP between 60 and 160 mmHg and ICP about 10 mmHg (CPP of 50–150 mmHg) sufficient blood flow can be maintained with autoregulation.

15. **E: Systemic vascular resistance**

    Systemic vascular resistance = (MAP – mean right atrial pressure) × 80/cardiac output.

    The reference range is 800–1200 dynes × sec/cm³.

16. **E: Ionizing radiation**

    The incidence of thyroid cancer is increasing. This may be attributed to improved detection and etiological factors including ionizing radiation. Ionizing radiation is a major known risk factor for thyroid cancer and particularly for papillary carcinoma. Both external radiation (X-ray and γ-radiation) and internal exposure to radioiodines through inhalation or ingestion carry an increased cancer risk. The well-documented examples include medical therapeutic external beam radiation and accidental exposure to γ-radiation and radioiodines as a result of nuclear weapon explosions or nuclear reactor accidents.

17. **E: Nickel**

Cancer of the nasal cavity is associated with many carcinogenic materials including nickel dust. Other carcinogens are listed in the following:

- Human papillomavirus (HPV)
- Specific inhalants including dust from the wood, textiles, or leather industries, flour dust, nickel dust, chromium dust, mustard gas, asbestos, fumes from rubbing alcohol (isopropyl alcohol), radium fumes, glue fumes, formaldehyde fumes, and solvent fumes used in furniture and shoe production
- Air pollution
- Marijuana use

18. **A: Aniline dyes**

Transitional cell carcinoma of the urinary tract is associated with cigarette smoking, which contributes to approximately one-half of the disease burden. Chemical exposure including petroleum, paints, and pigments (e.g., aniline dyes) is known to predispose to this disease. As with most epithelial cancers, physical irritation has also been associated with increased risk of malignant transformation (e.g., chronic urinary stones, chronic catheterization, and chronic infections).

19. **B: Polyvinyl chloride**

Hepatocellular carcinoma (HCC) is the most common type of liver cancer. Most cases of hepatocellular cancer are secondary to either a viral hepatitis (hepatitis B or C) or cirrhosis (alcoholism being the most common cause of liver cirrhosis). Known carcinogens include chronic viral infections (hepatitis B and C), toxins (alcohol, aflatoxin, iron overload), and metabolic diseases (nonalcoholic steatohepatitis and type 2 diabetes).

20. **B: Rectal carcinoma**

Common symptoms of colorectal cancer include change in bowel habits (persistent constipation or diarrhoea lasting more than 3 weeks), rectal bleeding (blood in the stool or in the toilet after having a bowel movement), dark or black stools, cramping or discomfort in the lower abdomen, decreased appetite, unintentional weight loss, and fatigue. Approximately 4.6 per cent of men (1 in 22) and 4.2 per cent of women (1 in 24) will be diagnosed with colon cancer in their lifetime. The risk of this cancer increases with age; the median age at diagnosis of rectal cancer is 63 years of age in both men and women.

21. **E: Ulcerative colitis**

Ulcerative colitis (UC) is characterised by inflammation and ulcers of the colon and rectum. The clinical presentation of UC depends on the extent of the disease process. With active disease, patients usually present with abdominal pain (with varying degrees) and diarrhoea mixed with blood and mucus. In addition, weight loss, fever, and anaemia may also occur. It is also associated with a general inflammatory process, which can result in extra-intestinal manifestations. The main differential diagnosis for this patient is Crohn's disease. There are similarities and differences with these two diseases. Both diseases often develop in teenagers and young adults although the disease can occur at any age. They affect men and women equally and their symptoms can be similar. However, whilst UC is limited to the colon, Crohn's disease can occur anywhere between the mouth and the anus. In Crohn's disease, there are skip lesions (normal intestine mixed in between inflamed areas). In UC, there is continuous inflammation of the colon. In this patient, her symptoms limited to the 'colon' and no mention of signs related the entire digestive tract (e.g., angular stomatitis, fistulas, fevers strictures); therefore, E is the best answer.

22. **A: Diverticulitis**

Diverticulitis is a condition in which the pouches within the large bowel wall become inflamed. These pouches are produced by the herniation of the colonic mucosa into the wall of the colon. Symptoms include severe lower abdominal pain, fever, nausea, and a change in bowel habit. Risk factors include obesity, lack of exercise, smoking, a family history of the disease, and the use of non-steroidal anti-inflammatory drugs (NSAIDs).

23. **B: Metabolic alkalosis**

Metabolic alkalosis is a metabolic condition in which there is an increased pH in the tissues. This is a result of decreased hydrogen ion concentration, leading to increased bicarbonate, or alternatively a direct result of increased bicarbonate concentrations. Thiazide diuretics inhibit the sodium-chloride transporter in the distal tubule. With diuretics, the increased hydrogen and potassium ion loss can lead to metabolic alkalosis.

24. **A: Metabolic acidosis**

Metabolic acidosis occurs when the body produces excessive quantities of acid or when the kidneys fail to remove enough acid from the body. If unchecked, metabolic acidosis leads to acidaemia, (pH less than 7.35) due to increased production of hydrogen ions by the body or the inability of the body to form bicarbonate (HCO_3^-) in the kidney.

MUDPILES is a useful mnemonic to remember the causes of metabolic acidosis:

- M – Methanol
- U – Uraemia (chronic kidney failure)
- D – Diabetic ketoacidosis
- P – Paraldehyde
- I – Infection, Iron, Isoniazid, Inborn errors of metabolism
- L – Lactic acidosis
- E – Ethylene glycol and Ethanol
- S – Salicylates (aspirin)

25. C: Respiratory acidosis

Respiratory acidosis occurs when there is a decreased ventilation (hypoventilation) which results in an increase concentration of carbon dioxide in the blood and a decrease in the blood pH. Alveolar hypoventilation results in an increased $PaCO_2$, which in turn decreases the $HCO_3^-/PaCO_2$ ratio and decreases the pH. Acute respiratory acidosis occurs when there is an abrupt failure of ventilation. This failure can be caused by depression of the central respiratory centre by central nervous/cerebral disease or drugs, inability to ventilate adequately due to neuromuscular disease (e.g., myasthenia gravis, amyotrophic lateral sclerosis, Guillain–Barré syndrome, muscular dystrophy), or airway obstruction (e.g., asthma). Moreover, chronic respiratory acidosis can occur with the following condition: (e.g., chronic obstructive pulmonary disorder), obesity hypoventilation syndrome (i.e., Pickwickian syndrome), neuromuscular disorders (e.g., amyotrophic lateral sclerosis) or related to severe restrictive ventilatory defects (e.g., interstitial lung disease and thoracic deformities).

26. E: T12 Level

The thoracic duct passes through the diaphragm at the aortic opening: T12 level.

27. C: T10 Level

The oesophagus passes through the diaphragm at the oesophageal opening: T10 level.

28. E: T12 Level

The aorta passes through the diaphragm at the aortic opening: T12 level (Table 2).

Table 2 Diaphragm opening (Questions 26–28, 141)	
Vena cava opening (T8)	Inferior vena cava
	Right phrenic nerve
Oesophageal opening (T10)	Oesophagus
	Left and right vagus nerves (RIP = right is posterior)
	Oesophageal branches of left gastric vessels
	Lymphatics from lower 1/3 oesophagus
Aortic opening (T12)	Aorta
	Azygous and hemiazygous veins
	Thoracic duct
Crura (T12)	Greater, lesser, and least splanchnic nerves
Behind medial arcuate ligament	Sympathetic trunks
Behind lateral arcuate ligament	Subcostal (T12) neurovascular bundle

29. **A: First pharyngeal pouch**

Eustachian tube arises from the first pharyngeal pouch.

> The following structures arise from each pharyngeal pouch:
>
> *First pouch*: Eustachian tube, middle ear, mastoid, and inner layer of the tympanic membrane
>
> *Second pouch*: Middle ear, palatine tonsils
>
> *Third pouch*: Inferior parathyroid glands, thymus
>
> *Fourth pouch*: Superior parathyroid glands, ultimobranchial body which forms the parafollicular C-cells of the thyroid gland, musculature, and cartilage of larynx (along with the sixth pharyngeal pouch)
>
> *Fifth pouch*: Rudimentary structure
>
> *Sixth pouch*: Along with the fourth pouch, contributes to the formation of the musculature and cartilage of the larynx

30. **C: Facial nerve (VII)**

- First pharyngeal pouch is innervated by the mandibular and maxillary branches of the trigeminal nerve (CN V).
- Second pharyngeal pouch is innervated by the facial nerve (CN VII).
- Third pharyngeal pouch is innervated by the glossopharyngeal nerve (CN IX).
- Fourth pharyngeal pouch is innervated by the superior laryngeal branch of the vagus nerve (CN X).
- Sixth pharyngeal pouch is innervated by the recurrent laryngeal branch of the vagus nerve (CN X).

31. **D: Remove plaster**

The patient has compartment syndrome related to external compression from his plaster. His immediate treatment is to remove the plaster and reassess the patient. The definitive treatment is a fasciotomy. Suspect compartment syndrome if:

> Pain is out of proportion to injury
>
> Pain on passive stretching of the individual compartment
>
> Paralysis and paraesthesia are late signs

32. **C: Coeliac trunk**

The coeliac trunk is closely related to the fibres of the greater splanchnic nerves (Figure 1).

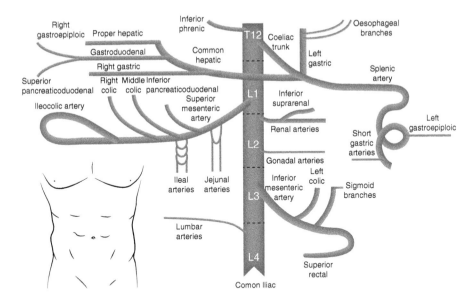

Figure 1   The abdominal aorta including the coeliac axis, SMA, and IMA.

33. D: Secondary lung tumour

Secondary lung tumours or metastatic tumours in the lungs are cancers that developed at other places in the body (or other parts of the lungs). They then spread through the bloodstream or lymphatics to the lungs. Cannonball metastases are large, well circumscribed, round pulmonary metastases. They are also termed 'envolée de ballons' which translates to 'balloons release'.

34. C: Small cell carcinoma

Small-cell carcinoma (also known as 'small-cell lung cancer', or 'oat-cell carcinoma') is a type of highly malignant cancer that most commonly arises within the lung. Compared to non-small cell carcinoma, small cell carcinoma has a more aggressive course: a shorter doubling time, higher growth fraction, and earlier development of metastases. These tumours are often associated with ectopic hormone production and paraneoplastic syndromes.

35. C: Cortisol

Zona fasciculata is responsible for producing glucocorticoids, including 11-deoxycorticosterone, corticosterone, and cortisol. Cortisol is the main glucocorticoid under normal conditions and its actions include mobilization of fats, proteins, and carbohydrates. Moreover, cortisol enhances the activity of other hormones including glucagon and catecholamines. The zona fasciculata secretes a basal level of cortisol but can also produce bursts of the hormone in response to adrenocorticotropic hormone (ACTH) release from the anterior pituitary gland.

36. **D: Immunoglobulin E**

    Type I Hypersensitivity (or immediate hypersensitivity) is an allergic reaction provoked by re-exposure to a specific type of antigen referred to as an allergen. In Type 1 hypersensitivity, B-cells are stimulated (by CD4+TH2 cells) to produce IgE antibodies specific to an antigen. Examples include allergic asthma and anaphylaxis.

37. **E: Immunoglobulin G**

    In Type II hypersensitivity reaction (or tissue-specific, or cytotoxic hypersensitivity), the antibodies produced by the immune response bind to antigens on the patient's own cell surfaces. IgG and IgM antibodies bind to these antigens to form complexes that activate the classical pathway of complement activation to eliminate cells presenting foreign antigens. Examples include ABO blood incompatibility and autoimmune haemolytic anaemia.

38. **E: Immunoglobulin G**

    Type III hypersensitivity reaction occurs when there is accumulation of immune complexes (antigen-antibody complexes) that have not been adequately cleared by innate immune cells, giving rise to an inflammatory response and activation of leukocytes. Such reactions result in immune complex diseases. Antibody (IgG) binds to soluble antigen, forming a circulating immune complex. Examples include systemic lupus erythematosus (SLE) and rheumatoid arthritis (RA).

39. **A: Helper T cells 4**

    Type IV hypersensitivity (or delayed type hypersensitivity) is a reaction that takes several days to develop. Unlike the other types, it is not antibody-mediated but rather is a type of cell-mediated response. CD4+ T_h1 helper T cells recognize antigen in a complex with the MHC class II major histocompatibility complex on the surface of antigen-presenting cells. Examples include the Mantoux test and chronic transplant rejection.

40. **C: Internal oblique and transversus abdominis**

    - Roof of the inguinal canal is composed of the arching fibres of internal oblique and transversus abdominis.
    - Anterior wall of the inguinal canal is composed of external oblique and internal oblique (for the lateral 1/3).
    - Posterior wall of the inguinal canalis is composed of transversalis fascia and conjoint tendon.
    - Floor of the inguinal canal is composed of the inguinal canal.

41. **B: Vastus medialis**

    The adductor canal is an aponeurotic tunnel in the middle third of the thigh, extending from the apex of the femoral triangle to the opening in the adductor magnus, the adductor hiatus.

- Lateral border of Hunter's canal is composed of vastus medialis.
- Medial border of Hunter's canal is composed of adductor longus superiorly and adductor magnus inferiorly.
- Roof of Hunter's canal is sartorius, fascia, subsartorial plexus (contributed to by the anterior branch of obturator, medial cutaneous nerve of the thigh and saphenous nerve).

> Hunter's canal contains the femoral artery, femoral vein, saphenous nerve, and nerve to vastus medialis. It transmits a small branch of the posterior division of the obturator nerve to the knee joint.

42. **E: A woman with blood group B RhD-negative and thyroid disease is found to have a haemoglobin level of 11.0 having just given birth to a baby with blood group B RhD-positive. Treatment: Anti-D immunoglobulin.**

- Patient A: Group A RhD-negative

A patient with group B blood has anti-A antibodies and therefore cannot receive group A blood. This patient is also RhD-negative and so cannot receive RhD-positive blood. The patient could take iron sulphate tablets but, with a haemoglobin level of 6.0, a blood transfusion is a better option.

- Patient B: Group A RhD-negative

A patient with group A blood has anti-B antibodies and therefore cannot receive group B blood. This patient is also RhD-positive and so can receive RhD-positive or negative blood. The patient could take iron sulphate tablets but, with a haemoglobin level of 6.0, a blood transfusion is a better option.

- Patient C: Iron sulphate tablets

The haemoglobin level is not very low and so a gradual normalization with iron sulphate tablets is a better option compared with the risks associated with blood transfusion. Blood transfusion is usually considered when the haemoglobin level drops below 8 g/dL.

- Patient D: Group O RhD-negative

A patient with group O blood has anti-A and anti-B antibodies and can only therefore receive group O blood. This patient is also RhD-negative and so cannot receive RhD-positive blood.

- Patient E: Anti-D immunoglobulin

A woman who is RhD-negative but exposed to the RhD-antigen via childbirth or transfusion will go on to develop antibodies that would attack a subsequent RhD-positive baby *in utero*. Anti-D immunoglobulin will reduce her immune response and therefore reduce the risk of developing antibodies.

43. **D: Indirect inguinal hernia**

There is a positive cough impulse suggestive of bowel herniation. The doctor cannot get above the lump, suggesting that it arises from the inguinal canal.

The hernia can be reduced back along the inguinal canal from the scrotum and upon occlusion of the deep inguinal ring the hernia is controlled. This is pathognomonic for an indirect inguinal hernia.

44. **A: Testicular cancer**

Any firm scrotal mass is cancer until proven otherwise. Testicular cancer may often be associated with a hydrocele.

45. **E: Varicocele**

This is a classic description of a varicocele. These are more common on the left as the left testicular vein drains into the left renal vein whereas the right testicular vein drains directly into the IVC.

46. **E: Epidermal cyst**

Epidermal cysts originate in the skin and have a characteristic punctum. They commonly occur in the head and neck region.

47. **D: Cystic hygroma**

A cystic hygroma is a lymphangioma which usually presents in childhood. Cystic hygromas typically occur in the neck and transilluminate.

48. **C: A 60-year-old woman with a previous history of gallstones presents with colicky abdominal pain and vomiting. Her abdomen is distended and bowel sounds are increased. She is often constipated but feels that this is different. Investigation: Plain abdominal X-ray (AXR)**

- Patient A: Percutaneous transhepatic cholangiopancreatogram (PTC)

This woman has a tumour at the head of the pancreas. If retrograde stenting via ERCP is not possible, then anterograde stenting via a percutaneous approach (PTC) is the next step to relieve jaundice.

- Patient B: Ultrasound scan

This is a classic story of acute cholecystitis which can be diagnosed on ultrasound, which can also detect gallstones.

- Patient C: Plain abdominal X-ray

This is a story of bowel obstruction which may be due to gallstone ileus. Dilated loops of bowel may be seen and perhaps the gallstone itself.

- Patient D: Ultrasound scan

This man has acute pancreatitis. The most common causes include alcohol excess and gallstones. There is an obstructive picture, so ultrasound can confirm and may detect the obstructing gallstone. CT is used to detect pancreatic necrosis several days later.

- Patient E: Endoscopic retrograde cholangiopancreatogram (ERCP)

There is a gallstone obstructing the common bile duct. It can be removed by ERCP.

49. **E: Total hip replacement**

   In elderly patients, hemiarthroplasty is indicated for intracapsular fractures unless there is a diseased acetabulum, when a total hip replacement is preferred.

50. **C: Cannulated screws**

   Cannulated screws are preferred in younger patients with intracapsular fractures and thereby preserving the head of the femur. This is because femoral head prostheses have a limited lifespan.

51. **A: Dynamic hip screw**

   Dynamic hip screws are preferred for extracapsular femoral fractures.

52. **D: Lower protein concentration**

   Intracellular fluid contains a higher concentration of potassium, phosphate, protein, and magnesium, but extracellular fluid contains a higher concentration of sodium, calcium chloride, and bicarbonate (Figure 2). Roughly two-thirds of the total body water content is intracellular and one-third is extracellular. The intracellular compartment is more acidic (lower pH; higher hydrogen ion concentration) due to nucleic acids (DNA and RNA) present within cells. The protein content inside cells is higher than the extracellular compartment; osmotic shock (cell lysis) is prevented by the $3Na^+/2K^+$-ATPase pump.

EXTRACELLULAR			INTRACELLULAR	
Na^+	143 mM	>	10 mM	Na^+
K^+	4 mM	<	140 mM	K^+
Ca^{2+}	1.5 mM	>	0.1 µM	Ca^{2+}
Mg^{2+}	1.0 mM	<	58 mM	Mg^{2+}
Cl^-	118 mM	>	10 mM	Cl^-
HCO_3^-	24 mM	<	10 mM	HCO_3^-
pH	7.4	>	7.0	pH

Figure 2   The ionic composition of intracellular and extracellular spaces.

53. **A: There is negative base excess**

   In metabolic acidosis, there is a negative base excess. Bicarbonate is the main extracellular buffer, not intracellular. The main intracellular buffers are phosphate and proteins. Compensation in metabolic acidosis occurs through hyperventilation (an increase in alveolar ventilation) and blowing off of CO_2. The mainstay of treatment is to treat the underlying cause (e.g., treatment of hypoxia, shock, hypovolaemia, sepsis). Bicarbonate infusions are used as a last resort since they shift the oxygen–haemoglobin dissociation curve to the left.

54. **C: Sensory innervations from the internal laryngeal nerve**

The posterior one-third of the tongue is innervated (light touch and special taste sensation) by branches of the glossopharyngeal (IX) and vagus (X) nerves. The chorda tympani supplies special taste sensation to the anterior two-thirds of the tongue, and light touch to the anterior two-thirds of the tongue is supplied by the lingual nerve.

Filiform (for gripping food) and fungiform (for sweet/salty taste) papillae are found on the anterior aspect of the tongue. Valate papillae are found further back but still on the anterior two-thirds of the tongue and are concerned with bitter taste. Foliate papillae are found on the sides of the tongue and are concerned with sour taste. The mucous membrane covering the posterior one-third of the tongue is devoid of papillae but has a nodular irregular surface caused by the presence of underlying lymphoid tissue, the lingual tonsil.

55. **B: Provides the same amount of oxygen to the liver as the portal vein**

The liver has a rich blood supply derived from two sources: two-thirds from the portal vein, the remaining one-third from the hepatic artery. Portal vein blood is rich in nutrients absorbed from the intestine but has a relatively low oxygen tension. Hepatic arterial blood contains few nutrients but is rich in oxygen. The hepatic artery supplies roughly 50 per cent of the oxygen delivered to the liver and the portal vein the other 50 per cent of hepatic oxygen supply. The liver is divided into segments by planes defined by the main hepatic veins (Couinaud classification). Purposeful embolization of hepatic arterial branches may be used to treat hepatic metastases.

56. **C: Protracted vomiting**

Metabolic alkalosis is commonly seen in protracted vomiting where there is a loss of hydrochloric acid. Aspirin (salicylic acid) poisoning will lead to a metabolic acidosis with a raised anion gap. A pancreatic fistula will lead to loss of bicarbonate-rich (alkaline-rich) digestive juices, resulting in a metabolic acidosis (normal anion gap). Hyperventilation will cause a respiratory, rather than a metabolic, alkalosis. Hypoglycaemia will lead to a metabolic acidosis secondary to lactic acidosis and the production of ketone bodies.

57. **A: *Staphylococcus aureus***

Osteomyelitis is most commonly caused by *S. aureus* in all age groups.

58. **A: May respond to pressure dressing**

Keloid scars extend beyond the margins of the wound (unlike hypertrophic scars which are confined to the wound margins). Keloid scars are most common on the sternum and deltoid area. Re-excision will usually lead to recurrence. Steroid injections (e.g., triamcinolone) may reduce keloid scar formation around the time of surgery. Pressure dressings also help. The use of subcuticular sutures will not reduce keloid formation.

59. **C: Haemophilus influenzae**

Splenectomised patients are at high risk of postsplenectomy sepsis, especially from encapsulated organisms such as:

- Haemophilus influenzae
- Neisseria meningitidis (*meningococcus*)
- Streptococcus pneumoniae (*pneumococcus*)

They are prevented by administering the relevant vaccinations and giving prophylactic penicillin. Patients are also at risk of malaria (especially *Plasmodium falciparum*).

60. **C: Deficiency of factor IX**

Haemophilia B (also known as Christmas disease) is less common than haemophilia A and is due to a deficiency in factor IX. Haemophilia A is due to a deficiency in factor VIII.

61. **D: Increase in tidal ventilation**

During haemorrhagic shock, catecholamine levels increase as a result of secretion by the adrenal medulla during the 'fright, fight, or flight' (stress) response. A hypovolaemic state stimulates antidiuretic hormone (ADH) secretion. Hypoxia as a result of haemorrhage stimulates chemoreceptors, resulting in increased ventilation (tidal ventilation). The carotid body peripheral chemoreceptors are most sensitive. There is also stimulation of baroreceptors located in the carotid sinus and aortic arch that act to maintain blood pressure. Haemorrhagic shock leads to hypothermia and a reduction in pCO_2 (secondary to hyperventilation) and consequently a shift in the oxygen–haemoglobin dissociation curve to the left, thereby increasing the affinity of haemoglobin for oxygen.

62. **B: Acute gastric dilatation**

Major burns are associated with splanchnic vasoconstriction on both the arteriolar and venous sides of the circulation. Curling's ulcers are stress ulcers related to major burns, not to be confused with Cushing's ulcers which occur in the setting of head injury. They were once a common complication of major burns and commonly resulted in perforation and haemorrhage, more often than other forms of intestinal ulceration, with correspondingly high mortality rates. Major burns are associated with paralytic ileus, rather than mechanical bowel obstruction.

63. **C: During growth**

Following trauma, sepsis, surgery or any other catabolic state, nitrogen balance is negative. Metabolic rate increases and protein from muscle stores is mobilized for repair and energy, which results in increased urea production and a net nitrogen loss. This may be prolonged for many weeks if sepsis or multiorgan failure occurs. ACTH stimulates cortisol secretion, leading to a catabolic state and a negative nitrogen balance. During growth there is a positive nitrogen balance as protein synthesis occurs.

64. A: Prolactin

The anterior pituitary gland (adenohypophysis or pars distalis) synthesizes and secretes the following six hormones: follicle-stimulating hormone (FSH), luteinizing hormone (LH), growth hormone, prolactin, ACTH, and thyroid-stimulating hormone (TSH). The posterior pituitary gland (neurohypophysis) produces only two hormones: ADH (also known as vasopressin) and oxytocin. These hormones are synthesized by the hypothalamus and then stored and secreted by the posterior pituitary gland into the bloodstream.

65. E: Lies deep to the prevertebral layer of the deep cervical fascia

Scalenus anterior arises from the anterior tubercles of the transverse processes of the 3rd, 4th, 5th, and 6th cervical vertebrae and descends almost vertically to insert into the scalene tubercle on the inner border of the 1st rib and into the ridge on the upper surface of the rib in front of the subclavian grove. It lies deep to the prevertebral layer of the deep cervical fascia in the posterior triangle of the neck. The important anterior relations include the phrenic nerve and subclavian vein. Important posterior relations include the second part of the subclavian artery and the roots of the brachial plexus (anterior rami of lower cervical and first thoracic nerves).

66. D: 125 mL/min

The normal glomerular filtration rate (GFR) in humans is 125 mL/min. After the age of 40, GFR decreases progressively by about 0.4–1.2 mL/min per year.

67. B: Lung cancer

The three most common cancers in the female population in the UK in descending order of frequency are lung, breast, and colorectal. In the male population, the three most common in descending order of frequency are lung, prostate, and colorectal.

68. C: Elemental fluids require minimal digestion by the patient

Enteral tube feeding may be administered in the presence of a functional gastrointestinal tract and may be achieved by a nasogastric tube, gastrostomy, or enterostomy. Most patients will tolerate a non-lactose, iso-osmolar non-elemental feed, but those suffering from intestinal fistulae, short bowel syndrome or inflammatory bowel disease benefit from an elemental diet which requires minimal digestion. Diarrhoea is a possible complication, but less likely if feeds are given continuously rather than in bolus and if iso-osmolar rather than hyperosmolar fluid administration. Osmolality is increased when the feed contains glucose and is lowered when the feed contains sucrose or glucose polymers as the carbohydrate source. Enteral feeding is more cost-effective, safer, and requires less monitoring than parental feeding. Moreover, the enteral route allows maintenance of the structural and functional integrity of the intestine.

69. E: Is attached to the diaphragm by the falciform ligament

The liver weighs 1500 g and is the largest organ in the body. It receives 30 per cent of the body's total cardiac output (1500 mL blood flow/min). The liver is drained by the hepatic veins into the inferior vena cava. The nerve supply of the liver is by the right vagus nerve via the celiac ganglia and left vagus, which is supplied directly into the porta hepatis. Sympathetic innervation is carried on vessels. The liver is attached to the diaphragm by the falciform ligament.

70. **A: There is an association between osteosarcoma and Paget's disease of the bone**

    Bone tumours are rare. The three predominant malignant tumours are the osteosarcomas, chondrosarcomas, and Ewing's sarcoma. Chondrosarcomas commonly occur in the middle-aged and elderly. Chemotherapy is now given routinely for osteosarcomas and Ewing's sarcoma, but has a limited role for chondrosarcomas. Metastasis usually occurs via the bloodstream. Pain and swelling are the two most common features.

71. **D: Costodiaphragmatic recess of the pleura**

    The posterior relations of the kidney include:

    - Diaphragm and costodiaphragmatic recess of the pleura
    - Psoas muscle
    - Quadratus lumborum muscle
    - 12th rib
    - Subcostal neurovascular bundle (vein, artery, and nerve)
    - Iliohypogastric and ilio-inguinal nerves

72. **C: May contain heterotropic pancreas**

    Meckel's diverticulum is the anatomical remnant of the vitello-intestinal duct. In the developing fetus, the vitello-intestinal duct connects the primitive midgut to the yolk sac and plays a part in intestinal rotation. It is present in 2 per cent of the population. It is often observed as a 5 cm intestinal diverticulum projecting from the antimesenteric wall of the ileum and about 60 cm from the ileocaecal valve. Its blind end may contain ectopic tissue, namely gastric mucosa (10 per cent of cases), liver, pancreatic, carcinoid, or lymphoid tissue. It is about twice as common in males.

73. **A: Radiotherapy**

    Recognized curative treatment for localized carcinoma of the prostate includes primarily surgery, radiation therapy, and proton therapy. Alternative treatments (hormonal therapy, chemotherapy, cryosurgery, and high-intensity focused ultrasound (HIFU)) can halt the progression of disease but not provide a cure. Tamsulosin is an α_{1a}-selective alpha-blocker used in the symptomatic treatment of benign prostatic hyperplasia (BPH).

74. **C: Is no more likely to have secondary hyperparathyroidism than someone on CAPD for the same period**

    Patients with end-stage renal failure, whether they are on haemodialysis or continuous ambulatory peritoneal dialysis (CAPD), are at an increased risk of secondary hyperparathyroidism – an increase in parathyroid hormone as a physi-ological response to hypocalcaemia as a result of low levels of activated vitamin D in chronic renal failure. Many years after renal transplantation, a condition known as tertiary hyperparathyroidism may develop where the parathyroid glands begin to function autonomously and complications may ensue. In such situations a parathyroidectomy may be indicated. Bisphosphonates following surgery would be counterproductive as they would lower calcium even further (bisphosphonates inhibit osteoclasts and thereby decrease calcium). Vascular calcification causes hardening and sclerosis of the blood vessels and is irreversible. Patients on haemo-dialysis who have taken aluminium hydroxide (to control high levels of phosphate) over long periods are at increased risk of osteomalacia (not osteoporosis).

75. **D: Non-parametric tests could be used**

A normal distribution is shown to be a symmetrical bell-shaped curve on a graph. A population is defined in terms of its mean and its standard deviation. The mean, median, and mode have the same value. A chi-squared test can be applied to a normally distributed population, whereas non-parametric tests can be applied whether a population is distributed normally or otherwise. One standard deviation from the mean contains 68 per cent of the population, two standard deviations include 95 per cent, and three standard deviations include 99.7 per cent. Twenty-five out of 1000 individuals (2.5 per cent) would be expected to be more than two standard deviations from the mode.

76. **E: Parietal cells**

Goblet cells are mucus-secreting cells, widely distributed throughout epithelial sur-faces, but especially dense in the gastrointestinal and respiratory tracts. Kupffer cells have phagocytic properties and are found in the liver; they participate in the removal of ageing erythrocytes and other particulate debris. The gastric mucosa contains many cell subtypes, including acid-secreting cells (also known as parietal or oxyntic cells), pepsin-secreting cells (also known as peptic, chief, or zymogenic cells) and G-cells (gastrin-secreting cells). Peptic cells synthesize and secrete the proteolytic enzyme, pepsin. Parietal cells actively secrete hydrochloric acid into the gastric lumen, accounting for the acidic environment encountered in the stomach. However, parietal cells are also involved in the secretion of the glycoprotein, intrinsic factor.

Intrinsic factor plays a pivotal role in the absorption of vitamin B_{12} from the terminal ileum. Autoimmune damage to parietal cells leads to a lack of intrinsic factor and hydrochloric acid, leading to vitamin B_{12} deficiency and achlorhydria. This is known as pernicious anaemia. Pernicious anaemia is associated with a threefold increase in gastric cancer risk.

77. **D: *Neisseria meningitidis***

The spleen plays an important role in the removal of dead and dying erythrocytes and in the defence against microbes. Removal of the spleen (splenectomy) leaves the host susceptible to a wide array of pathogens, but especially to encapsulated organisms.

Certain bacteria have evolved ways of evading the human immune system. One way is through the production of a 'slimy' capsule on the outside of the bacterial cell wall. Such a capsule resists phagocytosis and ingestion by macrophages and neutrophils. This allows them not only to escape direct destruction by phagocytes, but also to avoid stimulating T-cell responses through the presentation of bacterial peptides by macrophages. The only way that such organisms can be defeated is by making them more 'palatable' by coating their capsular polysaccharide surfaces in opsonizing antibody.

The production of antibody against capsular polysaccharide primarily occurs through mechanisms that are independent of T-cells. The spleen plays a central role in both the initiation of the antibody response and the phagocytosis of opsonized encapsulated bacteria from the bloodstream. This helps to explain why the asplenic individuals are most susceptible to infection from encapsulated organisms, notably *Streptococcus pneumoniae* (pneumococcus), *Neisseria meningitidis* (meningococcus), and *Haemophilus influenzae*.

The risk of acquiring these infections is reduced by immunizing individuals against such organisms and by placing patients on prophylactic penicillin, in most cases for the rest of their life. In addition, asplenic individuals should be advised to wear a MedicAlert bracelet to warn other healthcare professionals of their condition.

78. **E: Upon assuming the upright position**

Stimulation of the sympathetic nervous system results in a rise in heart rate and stroke volume and therefore cardiac output increases. Cutting the vagus nerves to the heart results in an increase in heart rate because of the abolition of vagal tone and therefore cardiac output increases.

If the end-diastolic volume of the heart (preload) is increased, under normal physiological circumstances, cardiac output is increased by the Frank–Starling mechanism. The exception is in the failing heart where the law of LaPlace becomes more important and cardiac output actually falls.

Arterial blood pressure is homeostatically regulated through the action of baroreceptors, principally located in the carotid sinus and the wall of the aortic arch. If the carotid sinus pressure is reduced, the baroreceptors become inactive and lose their inhibitory effect on the vasomotor centre in the brainstem. The result is activation of the sympathetic nervous system. This produces a rise in heart rate, stroke volume, mean systemic filling pressure, and venous return, leading to an increase in cardiac output and return of the mean arterial blood pressure (MAP) to its original value.

Cardiac output falls when one stands up owing to the pooling of blood on the venous side of the circulation, which has a large capacitance. Stepping out of a hot bath exacerbates this pooling effect because superficial cutaneous veins dilate in response to heat, increasing their capacitance even further. Under normal circumstances, activation of the baroreceptor reflex compensates to some degree, preventing syncope. However, in the elderly, or in patients on antihypertensives, inadequate compensation from the baroreceptor reflex may result in a vasovagal syncope, or orthostatic hypotension.

79. **E: It is directly proportional to the fourth power of the radius**

The Hagen–Poiseuille law states that the flow through a vessel is:

- *Directly* proportional to the *pressure* head of flow
- *Directly* proportional to the *fourth power* of the radius
- *Inversely* proportional to the *viscosity*
- *Inversely* proportional to the *length* of the tube

The radius of the tube is therefore the most important determinant of flow through a blood vessel. Thus, doubling the radius of the tube will lead to a 16-fold increase in flow at a constant pressure gradient. The implications of this are several fold.

First, owing to the fourth-power effect on resistance and flow, active changes in radius constitute an extremely powerful mechanism for regulating both the local blood flow to a tissue and central arterial pressure. The arterioles are the main resistance vessels of the circulation and their radius can be actively controlled by the tension of smooth muscle within its wall.

Second, in terms of intravenous fluid replacement in hospital, flow is greater through a peripheral cannula than through central lines. The reason is that peripheral lines are short and wide (and therefore of lower resistance and higher flow) compared to central lines, which are long and possess a narrow lumen. A peripheral line is therefore preferential to a central line when urgent fluid resuscitation, or blood, is required.

80. **D: The sum of the residual volume and the expiratory reserve volume**

Spirometry traces are easy to understand if you remember the following 2 rules:

1. There are 4 lung volumes and 5 capacities that you need to remember.
2. A capacity is made up of 2 or more lung volumes.

The *4 lung volumes* are:

- *Tidal volume* = volume of air inspired or expired with each normal breath in quiet breathing; approximately 500 mL
- *Residual volume* = volume of air that remains in the lung after forced expiration
- *Inspiratory reserve volume* = extra volume of air that can be inspired over and above the normal tidal volume
- *Expiratory reserve volume* = extra volume of air that can be expired by forceful expiration after the end of a normal tidal expiration

The *5 lung capacities* are:

- *Functional residual capacity* = volume of air that remains in the lung at the end of quiet expiration, equal to the sum of the residual volume and the expiratory reserve volume
- *Inspiratory capacity* = inspiratory reserve volume + tidal volume
- *Expiratory capacity* = expiratory reserve volume + tidal volume
- *Vital capacity* = inspiratory reserve volume + tidal volume + expiratory reserve volume (or total lung capacity – residual volume)
- *Total lung capacity* = vital capacity + residual volume

The residual volume (and therefore functional residual capacity and total lung capacity) cannot be measured directly by spirometry. They are measured by either whole-body plethysmography or by using the helium dilution or nitrogen washout techniques.

81. **C: Is increased in emphysema**

Compliance is expressed as volume change per unit change in pressure. Elastance is the reciprocal of compliance. The pressure–volume curve of the lung is nonlinear with the lungs becoming stiffer at high volumes. The curves which the lung follows in inflation and deflation are different; this behaviour is known as 'hysteresis'. The lung volume at any given pressure during deflation is larger than during inflation. This behaviour depends on structural proteins (collagen, elastin), surface tension, and the properties of surfactant.

Surfactant is formed in, and secreted by, type II pneumocytes. The active ingredient is dipalmitoyl phosphatidylcholine. It helps prevent alveolar collapse by lowering the surface tension between water molecules in the surface layer. In this way it helps to reduce the work of breathing (makes the lungs more compliant) and permits the lung to be more easily inflated.

Various disease states are associated with either a decrease or an increase in the lung compliance. Fibrosis, atelectasis, and pulmonary oedema all result in a decrease in lung compliance (stiffer lungs). An increased lung compliance occurs in emphysema where an alteration in elastic tissue is probably responsible (secondary to the long-term effects of smoking). The lung effectively behaves like a 'soggy bag' so that a given pressure change results in a large change in volume (i.e., the lungs are more compliant). However, during expiration the airways are less readily supported and collapse at higher lung volumes, resulting in gas-trapping and hyperinflation.

82. **C: Thyroid-stimulating hormone (TSH)**

The pituitary gland (hypophysis) is the conductor of the endocrine orchestra. It is divided into an anterior part and a posterior part. The *anterior pituitary* (adenohypophysis or pars distalis) secretes 6 hormones, namely:

- *FSH/LH*: Reproduction
- *ACTH*: Stress response

- *TSH*: Basal metabolic rate
- *GH*: Growth
- *Prolactin*: Lactation

The *posterior pituitary* (neurohypophysis or pars nervosa) secretes only 2 hormones:

- *ADH (vasopressin)*: Osmotic regulation
- *Oxytocin*: Milk ejection and labour

Testosterone is produced from Leydig cells in the testes and from the adrenal glands. CRH is produced by the median eminence of the hypothalamus.

83. **E: Fetal haemoglobin**

The haemoglobin oxygen dissociation curve is sigmoidal in shape, which reflects the underlying biochemical properties of haemoglobin. The significance of the sigmoidal curve is that haemoglobin becomes highly saturated at high oxygen partial pressures (and is therefore highly efficient at collecting oxygen) and releases a significant amount of oxygen at pressures that are fairly low, but not extremely so (with the result that haemoglobin is highly effective at supplying oxygen where it is needed).

The effect of things that shift the curve to the right (raised CO_2, lowered pH, increased temperature, increase in 2,3-DPG) is to increase oxygen availability in the tissues. The effect of CO_2/H^+ on O_2 carriage is known as the Bohr shift or effect. This is exactly what is needed in metabolizing tissues; release of acids or CO_2 thus liberates O_2 to fulfil the metabolic needs of the tissue. Do not confuse this with the effect of changes in O_2 on CO_2 carriage, which is called the Haldane effect.

A shift of the oxygen dissociation curve to the left is characteristic of foetal haemoglobin. When compared with adult haemoglobin, it is composed of two alpha and two gamma chains, instead of the usual two alpha and two beta chains of adult haemoglobin. This arrangement assists in the transfer of oxygen across the placenta from the maternal to the foetal circulation. The corollary of this is that foetal tissue oxygen levels have to be low to permit the release of oxygen from the haemoglobin (Figure 3).

84. **B: CD8 T-cells**

Lymphocytes can be divided into 2 main subtypes: T-cells and B-cells. B-cells (or plasma cells) secrete antibodies. T-cells can be divided into two further subtypes: CD4 T-cells and CD8 T-cells. CD4 (helper) T-cells can recognize antigen only in the context of MHC Class II, whereas CD8 (cytotoxic) T-cells recognize cell-bound antigens only in association with Class I MHC. This is known as MHC restriction.

CD4 and CD8 T-cells perform distinct but somewhat overlapping functions. The CD4 helper T-cell can be viewed as a master regulator. By secreting cytokines (soluble factors that mediate communication between cells), CD4 helper T-cells influence the function of virtually all other cells of the immune system including other T-cells,

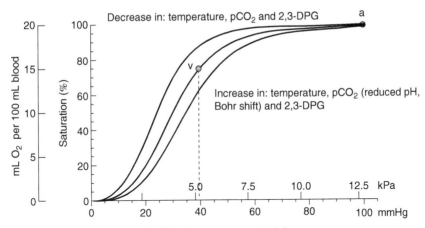

Figure 3 The carriage of oxygen by blood. v, venous; a, arterial.

B-cells, macrophages, and natural killer (NK) cells. The central role of CD4 cells is tragically illustrated by the HIV virus, which cripples the immune system by selective destruction of this T-cell subset. In recent years two functionally different populations of CD4 helper T-cells have been recognized – TH1 cells and TH2 cells –each characterized by the cytokines that they produce. In general, TH1 cells facilitate cell-mediated immunity, whereas TH2 cells promote humoral-mediated immunity.

CD8 cytotoxic T-cells mediate their functions primarily by acting as cytotoxic cells (i.e., they are T-cells that kill other cells). They are important in the host defence against cytosolic pathogens. Two principal mechanisms of cytotoxicity have been discovered: perforin–granzyme-dependent killing and Fas–Fas ligand-dependent killing.

85. **A: Hypokalaemia, metabolic alkalosis, low urinary pH**

Following a diagnosis of pyloric stenosis, the first concern is to correct the metabolic abnormalities that invariably coexist with the condition. The serum electrolytes and capillary gases should be measured and corrected prior to surgery.

With prolonged vomiting, the infant becomes dehydrated, with a hypochloraemic metabolic alkalosis. The alkalosis is a result of loss of unbuffered hydrogen ions in gastric juice with concomitant retention of bicarbonate.

Fluid loss stimulates renal sodium reabsorption, but sodium can be reabsorbed only either with chloride, or in exchange for hydrogen and potassium ions (to maintain electroneutrality). Gastric juice has a high concentration of chloride and patients losing gastric secretions become hypochloraemic. This means that less sodium than normal can be reabsorbed with chloride.

However, it appears that the defence of extracellular fluid volume takes precedence over acid–base homeostasis and further sodium reabsorption occurs in exchange for hydrogen ions (perpetuating the alkalosis) and potassium ions (leading to potassium depletion). This explains the apparently paradoxical finding of acidic urine in patients with pyloric stenosis. Potassium is also lost in the gastric juice and thus patients frequently become potassium-depleted and yet are losing potassium in their urine.

86. **C: Amiodarone**

This question requires knowledge of the Vaughan Williams classification of antiarrhythmic drugs. Lignocaine is a class 1B drug and blocks sodium channels.

All class I drugs have membrane stabilizing properties. Procainamide, a class 1A drug, and flecainide, a class 1C drug, also block sodium channels.

All class I drugs have membrane stabilizing properties.

Class II drugs comprise the beta-blockers. They are believed to work by blocking the pro-arrhythmic effects of catecholamines and the sympathetic nervous system.

Class III drugs (e.g., amiodarone, sotalol) act through the blockade of potassium channels. They work by prolonging the action potential, thereby increasing the refractory period and hence suppressing ectopic and re-entrant activity. Note that sotalol has both class II and class III actions.

Class IV includes drugs such as verapamil and diltiazem which act by blocking calcium channels.

87. **A: Apart from the first cleft, the other branchial clefts are normally obliterated by overgrowth of the 2nd branchial arch**

The pharyngeal, or branchial arches, are the mammalian equivalent of the gill arches in fish. In humans, there are five pairs of branchial arches that develop in a craniocaudal sequence (equivalent to gill arches 1, 2, 3, 4, 6). Note that the 5th branchial arch never forms in humans, or forms as a short-lived rudiment and promptly regresses. Each arch contains a central cartilaginous element, striated muscle, cranial nerve, and aortic arch artery, surrounded by ectoderm on the outside and lined by endoderm. The arches are separated externally by ectodermally lined branchial clefts and internally by endodermally lined branchial pouches.

- The 1st arch gives rise to the muscles of mastication
- The 2nd arch gives rise to the muscles of facial expression
- The 3rd and 4th arches gives rise to the muscles of vocalization and deglutition
- The 6th arch gives rise to the intrinsic muscles of the larynx

Certain key features concerning the branchial arches are worth remembering. First, the superior parathyroid glands develop from the fourth branchial pouch; the inferior parathyroids, along with the thymus, are third-pouch derivatives. Consequently, the inferior parathyroids may migrate with the thymus down into the mediastinum, hence its liability to end up in unusual positions.

The tongue is derived from several sources. The anterior two-thirds of the tongue mucosa is a 1st-arch derivative, whereas the posterior one-third is contributed to by the 3rd and 4th arches. The tongue muscles, in contrast, are formed from occipital somite mesoderm. For this reason, the motor and sensory nerve fibres of the tongue are carried by separate sets of cranial nerves.

The thyroid gland arises from between the 1st and 2nd arches as a diverticulum (thyroglossal duct) which grows downwards leaving the foramen caecum at its origin. Incomplete thyroid descent may give rise to a lingual thyroid, or a thyroglossal cyst.

Apart from the first branchial cleft (which forms the external ear), the other clefts are normally obliterated by overgrowth of the 2nd pharyngeal arch, enclosing the remaining clefts in a transient, ectoderm-lined, lateral cervical sinus. This space normally disappears rapidly and completely. It may persist in adulthood as a branchial cyst or fistula.

88. **D: The equilibrium potential for an ion species depends on the ratio of the ion concentrations outside to inside of the cell**

In axons, impulses can travel in both directions (orthodromic and antidromic) from a point of electrical stimulation. Antidromic activity explains certain clinical phenomena such as how infection of a dorsal root by herpes zoster virus causes the segmental cutaneous hyperaemia characteristic of shingles. The amplitude of the action potential generated by an excitatory stimulus is independent of the stimulus strength; this is known as the 'all or nothing' law. This means stimulus intensity is coded for by frequency rather than through the amplitude of action potential.

The resting membrane potential is dependent on the electrogenic sodium–potassium ATPase pump and the relative intracellular and extracellular concentrations of ions on each side of the nerve cell membrane, as well as their relative permeabilities across the membrane. This establishes both a concentration (chemical) gradient and an electrical gradient across the nerve cell membrane – an electrochemical gradient. The equilibrium potential for a given ion species depends on the ratio of the concentrations of the ion outside to that inside the cell (the Nernst potential or equation). The Goldman constant-field (or Goldman–Hodgkin–Katz) equation is a more general form of the Nernst equation which allows for different permeabilities. Resting nerve cell membranes are about 100 times more permeable to K^+ ions than to Na^+ ions.

If extracellular sodium is replaced by potassium it would follow from the Nernst equation that this would depolarize the fibres completely. The resulting depolarization inactivates sodium channels and blocks the propagation of impulses down nerves. This is why hyperkalaemia is so dangerous. Cardiac muscle is especially sensitive to small changes in extracellular potassium concentrations and death often ensues from cardiac standstill.

89. **D: Is activated by IgM immune complexes**

The complement system consists of a large number of distinct plasma proteins, triggering a cascade of reactions where the activation of one complement component results in the activation of another. This amplifies the effector molecules of the complement system. The main consequences of complement activation are opsonization of pathogens, the recruitment of inflammatory cells and direct killing of pathogens. There are two principal pathways of complement activation, the alternative and classical. The alternative pathway is the evolutionary older of the two pathways but the classical pathway was discovered first, hence the term classical pathway.

The alternative pathway is activated by the lipopolysaccharide (LPS) of cell wall constituents, whereas the classical pathway is activated by IgM or IgG (but not IgA) which has bound to its specific antigen. Thus, in a transfusion reaction IgM from the recipient's blood binds to the incompatible donor red cells leading to complement activation, haemolysis, and acute renal failure. The alternative pathway begins with the activation of the C3 component, but the classical pathway starts with the activation of the C1 component.

90. **A: Ingress of calcium ions**

The cardiac action potential is divided into a number of phases (Figure 4):

- 0 – rapid depolarization (caused by the rapid influx of sodium ions)
- 1 – early repolarization (caused by the inactivation of sodium channels and the outward passage of potassium ions)
- 2 – plateau phase (caused predominantly by the ingress of calcium ions and the efflux of potassium ions)
- 3 – late repolarization (caused predominantly by the efflux of potassium ions)
- 4 – diastolic phase

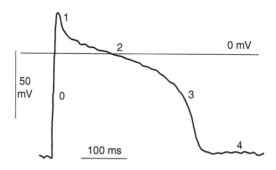

Figure 4   The cardiac plateau. 0 – rapid depolarization, 1 – early repolarization, 2 – plateau phase, 3 – late repolarization, 4 – diastolic phase.

91. **A: Neural tube development requires signals from the underlying mesoderm**

The nervous system arises from a special type of ectoderm that has been neurally induced to form neuroectoderm. The first stage in neurulation (i.e., development of the nervous system) is the establishment in the ectoderm of a region of cells that acquire neural competence (neural induction). The second stage is the morphogenetic process of neurulation that transforms the neuroepithelial sheet into the neural tube.

Neurulation involves communication between the mesoderm and the overlying ectoderm. The mesoderm primarily involved is the notochord, a dense rod of axial mesoderm that is very important in patterning the embryo early in development, but forms only the nucleus pulposus in the adult (in the centre of the intervertebral disc) and the apical ligament of the dens. Signals (specialized secreted proteins) are secreted by the notochord and induce the specialization of the overlying ectoderm cells to form the floor of the neural tube.

Closure of the neural tube proceeds bidirectionally, ending with closure of the cranial and caudal openings (neuropores). The cranial neuropore finally closes on day 24 and the caudal neuropore closes on day 26 of development. Closure of the neural tube is susceptible and a common cause of birth defects.

The neural crest, a migratory cell population, begins to emigrate from the dorsal half of the neural tube around the time of neural tube closure. They have a diverse and complex fate that includes cartilage in the head, melanocytes, the medullary cells of the adrenal gland, glial Schwann cells, and neurones of both the peripheral and autonomic nervous systems. Aberrant neural crest migration may result in Hirschsprung's disease of the bowel (congenital megacolon or aganglionosis), but not neural tube defects.

A variety of malformations result from failure of part of the neural tube and overlying skeleton to close, usually at the cranial or caudal end of the nervous system. Such neural tube defects originate during the third week of development and are the most common group of neurological malformations encountered in humans, occurring in 1 in 300 to 1 in 5000 births, depending on the geographical region. In spina bifida, the vertebral arch is defective dorsally, usually caudally in the lumbosacral region (spina bifida occulta), and in severe cases the meninges protrudes from the vertebral canal (meningocele), sometimes including neural tissue (myelomeningocele) with associated neural impairment. Rarely, failure of cranial neural tube closure results in anencephaly where the forebrain is in contact with the amniotic fluid and degenerates (it is fatal). Approximately 50 per cent of neural tube defects may be prevented by women taking folic acid, even in the babies of mothers who have previously given birth to infants with neural tube defects. However, it must be taken during the first few weeks of pregnancy since this is when the neural tube is closing and hence susceptible to perturbations.

92. **A: Excitation depends more on the influx of extracellular calcium than release from internal stores**

In smooth muscle, actin and myosin filaments occur but are less obvious on microscopy, giving it a non-striated appearance. Most smooth muscle has extensive electrically conducting gap junctions between cells which allows propagation of waves of electrical excitation through the tissue. Smooth muscle is usually under autonomic (involuntary nervous) or hormonal control, unlike skeletal muscle which is under somatic control. Unlike skeletal muscle, smooth muscle can generate active tension in the absence of any neural activity (latch bridge mechanism).

There is a vesicular sarcoplasmic reticulum close to the membrane (caveolae), but no T-tubular system. This is because the slow speed of smooth muscle does not require an elaborate mechanism for intracellular calcium release. For this reason, and because of the higher surface area to volume ratio of smooth muscle cells, excitation depends more on the influx of extracellular calcium than release from internal stores since smooth muscle has a less well-developed sarcoplasmic reticulum.

The intrinsic myogenic response in smooth muscle opposes stretch. The result is that contraction may be generated by mechanical stretch of muscle fibres, for example in blood vessel walls. This is partly the basis for autoregulation of blood flow in the cerebral, coronary, and renal vascular beds. It also plays a role in the peristaltic movements of material in the intestine.

93. **B: 15–40 days**

Hepatitis A has a short incubation period of between 15 and 40 days. The infection is transmitted by the faecal–oral route and takes hold very quickly. The virus replicates in the gastrointestinal tract and is shed in the faeces during both the incubation and acute phases of the disease.

94. **C: β_2-adrenoceptor agonism**

Asthma is an inflammatory (reactive) disorder of the airways characterized by reversible airway obstruction (or bronchospasm). It results from a Type I hypersensitivity reaction, where the IgE-mediated degranulation of mast cells and release of inflammatory mediators is central to the pathogenesis.

Bronchial smooth muscle contains β_2-adrenoceptors. Throughout the body, β_2-adrenoceptors act to relax smooth muscle. Salbutamol stimulates these receptors (i.e., it is a selective β_2-adrenoceptor agonist), thereby relaxing the smooth muscle in the airways and increasing their calibre. Longer-acting β_2-adrenoceptor agonists (such as salmeterol) play a role in more severe asthma.

Bronchial smooth muscle also contains muscarinic receptors. Stimulating these receptors causes smooth muscle contraction. Therefore, muscarinic antagonists (such as ipratropium) are useful adjuncts in the management of asthma.

Other drugs used in the management of asthma include steroids (oral or inhaled), leukotriene receptor antagonists (e.g., Montelukast), xanthines (e.g., theophylline), and sodium cromoglycate.

95. **E: May contain ectopic tissue**

A Meckel's diverticulum is the anatomical remnant of the vitello-intestinal duct. In the developing fetus the vitello-intestinal duct connects the primitive midgut vto the yolk sac and also plays a part in intestinal rotation. The urachus (a derivative of the allantois) is different and connects the bladder to the umbilicus in the fetus. After birth the urachus becomes known as the median umbilical ligament.

The vitello-intestinal duct normally regresses between the fifth and eighth weeks of development, but in 2 per cent of individuals it persists as a remnant of variable length and location, known as a Meckel's diverticulum in honour of J. F. Meckel, who first discussed the embryological basis of this anomaly in the nineteenth century. Most often it is observed as a 2 inches (5 cm) intestinal diverticulum projecting from the antimesenteric wall of the ileum, about 2 feet (60 cm) from the ileocaecal valve. It is about twice as common in males as in females. However, this useful mnemonic ('the rule of 2s') holds true in only two-thirds of cases; the length of the diverticulum is variable and its site may be more proximal.

It is estimated that 15–30 per cent of individuals with a Meckel's diverticulum develop symptoms from intestinal obstruction, gastrointestinal bleeding, acute inflammation (diverticulitis), or perforation. Its blind end may contain ectopic tissue, namely gastric mucosa (in 10 per cent of cases), liver, pancreatic, carcinoid, or lymphoid tissue. This is important because gastric mucosa bears HCl-secreting parietal cells and can therefore ulcerate within the diverticulum (like a stomach ulcer), causing bleeding. Bowel obstruction may be caused by the trapping of part of the small bowel by a fibrous band (that represents a remnant of the vitelline vessels) connecting the diverticulum to the umbilicus. Symptoms may closely mimic appendicitis. Therefore, if a normal-looking appendix is found at laparoscopy, or during an open appendicectomy, it is important to exclude Meckel's diverticulum as a cause of the patient's symptoms. Mortality in untreated cases is estimated to be 2.5–15 per cent.

96. D: Specialized intercellular junctions exist between myocytes

The structure of cardiac muscle correlates beautifully with its function. Certain features concerning cardiac myocytes are worth remembering:

- They are shorter than skeletal muscle cells
- They are branched
- Cardiac myocytes typically contain a single, centrally placed nucleus (unlike skeletal muscle fibres that are multinucleate, with peripherally located nuclei)
- Intercalated discs with gap junctions results in a syncytium where adjacent cardiac cells are mechanically and electrically coupled to one another, optimizing cardiac contractility
- They are rich in mitochondria
- There is sarcoplasmic reticulum

- There are transverse tubules at the Z-line. Note that in skeletal muscle the T-tubules are located at the junction of the A and I bands
- There are unstable resting membrane potentials of pacemaker cells
- Cardiac muscle contracts spontaneously (myogenic)

A property shared by skeletal and cardiac muscle is their striated microscopic appearance from the highly organized arrangement of actin and myosin filaments.

97. A: Bacterial endotoxin induces the acute-phase response

The acute-phase response is part of the innate (natural) immune system. Macrophages are exquisitely sensitive to the LPS present in certain bacteria. They respond by producing cytokines, notably TNFα, IL-1 and IL-6 (but not IL-10 which can generally be thought of as an inhibitory cytokine). The aforementioned cytokines act on the liver to increase the concentration of many key serum proteins to aid the host defence response (such as C-reactive protein [CRP], serum amyloid protein, mannose binding protein, fibrinogen, complement). CRP concentrations form a useful marker for detecting the presence (or confirming the absence) of inflammation or infection; this is a readily available laboratory test in the hospital setting. In addition, monitoring the trend in CRP values (as opposed to one-off values) provides the clinician with extremely valuable information as to whether the patient is getting better or worse.

Activation of the acute-phase response is responsible for a number of different effects. First, it is responsible for the fever that may accompany a variety of different inflammatory and infectious states, through the action of IL-1 on the thermosensory centres in the anterior hypothalamus. Second, hepatic protein synthesis is diminished and the level of serum albumin decreases. This is an attempt by the body to conserve protein and is responsible for the hypoalbuminaemia that often accompanies many disease states. Third, TNFα (cachectin) and IL-1 have catabolic effects and are responsible for the cachexia and anorexia seen in a variety of chronic inflammatory and infectious conditions. TNFα is also believed to be responsible for the cachexia seen in malignancy (cancer cachexia). In the latter, TNFα is produced by macrophages in response to the tumour, or by the tumour cells themselves. Finally, activation of the acute-phase response is central to the pathogenesis of septic shock where excessive activation of the acute-phase response leads to an overproduction of cytotoxic cytokines, resulting in a massive inflammatory reaction that may culminate in multiple organ failure and death.

98. D: III

There are 12 pairs of cranial nerves and 31 pairs of spinal nerves. The central nervous system comprises the brain and spinal cord. A peripheral nerve is a mixed nerve containing motor, sensory, and autonomic (parasympathetic, sympathetic) elements. Parasympathetic outflow arises from the 'craniosacral' region; that is, from certain cranial nerves and sacral roots S2–4. Cranial nerves III (occulomotor), VII (facial), IX (glossopharyngeal), and X (vagus) carry parasympathetic fibres whose function is primarily secretomotor (e.g., salivary secretions in the case of cranial nerve VII) and ciliary motor (pupillary reflexes and accommodation in the case of cranial nerve III), while cranial nerves IX and X play an integral role in blood pressure regulation. Sympathetic outflow is principally 'thoracolumbar' (i.e., from spinal segments T1 through to L2). The sympathetic nervous system serves vasomotor (vascular tone), sudomotor (sweating), and pilomotor functions, in addition to controlling smooth muscle and sphincter tone and playing a key role in cardiovascular homeostasis.

Understanding the anatomy and function makes it easy to predict the outcome of particular lesions in certain clinical settings. Take an occulomotor (3rd) cranial nerve palsy, for instance. Interruption of the parasympathetic fibres to the constrictor pupillae muscle results in a unilaterally dilated pupil (mydriasis) as an important hallmark of a 3rd-nerve palsy. This can thus easily be distinguished from a Horner's syndrome (sympathetic chain disruption), which causes a unilaterally constricted pupil (miosis).

99. **C: Excitation–contraction coupling requires calcium-induced calcium release**

The most important source of activator calcium in cardiac muscle remains its release from the sarcoplasmic reticulum. Calcium, however, also enters from the extracellular space during the plateau phase of the action potential. This calcium entry provides the stimulus that induces calcium release from the sarcoplasmic reticulum (calcium-induced calcium release). The result is that tension generated in cardiac, but not in skeletal, muscle is profoundly influenced both by extracellular calcium levels and factors that affect the magnitude of the inward calcium current. This is of practical value in two key clinical situations: in heart failure where digoxin is used to increase cardiac contractility (by increasing the intracellular calcium concentration) and in hyperkalaemia where calcium gluconate is used to stabilize the myocardium.

The force of contraction of cardiac muscle is heavily dependent on its stretched fibre length. This is the basis of the Frank–Starling mechanism that adjusts the energy of cardiac contraction in response to diastolic stretch (filling). This auto-regulatory mechanism makes the heart a self-regulating pump with respect both to demands from the peripheral circulation and in balancing the pumping by the right and left sides of the heart.

The plateau phase of the action potential in cardiac muscle (principally due to calcium influx) maintains the membrane at a depolarized potential for as long as 500 ms. The result is that the cell membrane is refractory throughout most of the mechanical response, largely due to the inactivation of fast sodium channels. This prevents tetany upon repetitive stimulation which would be detrimental to cardiac output. Furthermore, the prolonged refractory period in cardiac muscle allows the impulse that originates in the sinoatrial node to propagate throughout the entire myocardium just once, thereby preventing re-entry arrhythmias.

100. **B: It depends on the action of prostaglandins within the hypothalamus**

Fever is brought about by toxins from microorganisms which act on cells of the immune system to produce cytokines (including IL-1, IL-6, and TNFα). It is the body's immune response to the invading microorganism, rather than a direct result of the microorganism *per se* that results in fever. The cytokines produced by the immune system act as endogenous pyrogens and act on the hypothalamus to generate fever, via the production of prostaglandins. Aspirin works as an antipyretic by blocking the enzyme (cyclo-oxygenase) that generates prostaglandins.

Fever also results from a variety of non-infectious causes, in addition to the infectious ones. Examples are various inflammatory conditions, connective tissue diseases, drug reactions, and malignancies.

Fever is evolutionarily advantageous; it inhibits the growth of some microorganisms (most organisms only grow well in narrow temperature range), increases the rate of production of antibodies, improves the efficiency of leukocyte killing, and decreases the mobility of the host (thereby aiding recovery of the host and preventing spread of infection to other individuals). However, in some situations fever becomes maladaptive resulting in hyperpyrexia, dehydration, and death.

101. **D: Abnormal passive abduction of the extended knee**

The medial collateral ligament of the knee prevents abduction of the leg at the knee. It extends from the medial femoral epicondyle to the shaft of the tibia. The oblique popliteal ligament resists lateral rotation during the final degree of extension. The posterior cruciate ligament prevents posterior displacement of the tibia. The anterior ligament helps lock the knee joint on full extension.

102. **B: Southern blotting**

The polymerase chain reaction (PCR) is an amplification process used to amplify small amounts of DNA in order to perform analysis. It does not identify specific sequences. The DNA can then be analysed using Southern blotting. PCR involves synthesizing two oligonucleotide primers, that is short segments of RNA, that will bind to the DNA and when added to denatured DNA will bind to the DNA and amplify the DNA. The cycle is continually repeated 20–30 times, resulting in an exponential increase in the quantity of DNA. Reverse transcription PCR uses RNA. RNA is too unstable to be used for PCR, so it must be converted to a complementary copy of DNA using reverse transcriptase. PCR is then performed.

- Southern blotting involves digestion of DNA and are denatured in alkali making them single-stranded. A permanent copy of the single strands is made by placing the DNA on a nitrocellulose filter – that is, the Southern blot. A target radioactively labelled DNA fragment is then added and will bind to its homologous DNA fragment (if present). The DNA is then washed to remove any unbound DNA. The hybridized DNA can then be visualized as a band using autoradiography.

- Northern blotting is similar to Southern blotting but uses mRNA as the target nucleic acid, rather than DNA. The mRNA can be hybridized to a radiolabelled DNA probe.
- Western blotting is used to analyse proteins that are separated by electrophoresis, transferred to nitrocellulose, and reacted with antibody for detection.

103. **A: The posterior crico-arytenoids are the only muscles that separate the vocal cords**

The posterior crico-arytenoid muscles are perhaps the most important muscles in the body as they are the only intrinsic muscles of the larynx that open up the airway by separating the vocal cords. Without them asphyxiation would quickly ensue.

All the intrinsic muscles of the larynx are supplied by the recurrent laryngeal nerve of the vagus, with the exception of the important cricothyroid muscle, which is supplied by the external branch of the superior laryngeal nerve. Cricothyroid is the muscle which is principally concerned with altering voice pitch by altering the length of the vocal cords. Damage to the superior laryngeal or recurrent laryngeal nerves can occur during thyroid, oesophageal, or aortic arch surgery, leading to changes in the character of the voice and even airway compromise (Semon's law).

The true vocal cords form the superior border of the cricothyroid membrane and are lined by stratified squamous mucosa, not the typical respiratory epithelium that lines the rest of the respiratory tract. This confers protective properties on the vocal cords, which are subject to 'wear and tear' from vocalization. The same is true of the epiglottis which is also lined by 'protective' stratified squamous epithelium. The epiglottis is largely composed of elastic cartilage, rather than hyaline cartilage.

The cricoid cartilage is the only complete ring of cartilage within the human body, in contrast to the tracheal rings which are C-shaped rings of hyaline cartilage which provide support to the trachea but are deficient posteriorly.

104. **D: The nucleus accumbens and substantia nigra are rich in dopamine**

The nervous system can be arbitrarily divided into the somatic (or 'voluntary') and autonomic (or 'involuntary') parts. The autonomic nervous system consists of two arms, namely the sympathetic and parasympathetic nervous systems. Both sympathetic and parasympathetic fibres consist of two neurones (first-order or preganglionic, and second-order or postganglionic) and two synapses (the synaptic cleft between the first- and second-order neurones and the synaptic cleft between the second-order neurone and the organ or effector). There are key differences between both the neurones and the synapses of the sympathetic and parasympathetic nervous systems.

First-order (preganglionic) sympathetic and parasympathetic neurones are myelinated, whereas second-order (postganglionic) sympathetic and parasympathetic neurones are small, unmyelinated fibres. In both the sympathetic and parasympathetic nervous systems, preganglionic neurones release acetylcholine which acts on postsynaptic nicotinic cholinergic receptors. However, they differ at the second synapse (between second-order neurones and the effector) where noradrenaline is the principal chemical neurotransmitter used within the sympathetic nervous system (although this is not entirely true because the postganglionic sympathetic nerve fibres to the sweat glands, the piloerector muscles and a few blood vessels are cholinergic), but acetylcholine is the principal neurotransmitter used within the parasympathetic nervous system (but this time acting on muscarinic cholinergic receptors).

The neuromuscular junction (the synapse between somatic motor neurones and skeletal muscle) operates by way of acetylcholine acting through nicotinic acetylcholine receptors. The substantia nigra is a dense area of dopaminergic neurones which forms part of the basal ganglia; degeneration leads to Parkinson's disease. The periaqueductal grey is a region rich in endogenous opioids which is believed to play a pivotal role in attenuation of painful stimuli through descending inhibition from higher centres. The noradrenergic-rich locus coeruleus is believed to play a key role in attention. The nucleus accumbens is dopamine-rich and plays an important role in addiction and reward. The adrenal medulla is an endocrine gland but is effectively a specialized second-order (postganglionic) sympathetic nerve terminal that secretes approximately 70 per cent adrenaline, 30 per cent noradrenaline. Excess catecholamines are secreted by the adrenal medulla in a condition known as a phaeochromocytoma, which is a rare tumour of the adrenal gland. A thorough grounding of the aforementioned chemical neurotransmitters is imperative if one is to understand certain disease states and how particular drugs act within the nervous system.

105. D: *Borrelia burgorferi* – arthropod vector-borne entry

Borrelia burgorferi is spread by ticks and is caused by Lyme disease. *Rickettsia rickettsii* is also usually spread by ticks. *Clostridium tetani* enters the body through wounds. *Neisseria meningitidis* and *Corynebacterium diphtheriae* both enter via the respiratory tract.

106. D: RNA polymerase II gives rise to protein encoding mRNA

In prokaryotes, both transcription and translation occur in the cytoplasm; whereas in eukaryotes, transcription occurs in the nucleus and translation in the cytoplasm. Transcription is the process of synthesizing messenger RNA (mRNA) from DNA; it is catalysed by the enzyme RNA polymerase II. RNA and DNA are always synthesized in a $5' \rightarrow 3'$ direction.

The production of mature mRNA is a result of gene splicing. The introns which are non-coding sequences of DNA are removed and intervening exons are joined together. The exons are then coded into proteins during translation.

Amino acids are coded for by groups of three bases and these three bases together make up a codon. As there are four types of base, there is a potential for 4^3 (or 64) amino acids. Only 20 amino acids are used in protein synthesis, so in fact, 44 codons are considered redundant.

107. **B: Embryologically starts out at the foramen caecum of the tongue**

The thyroid gland is an endocrine gland that sits as the base of the neck like a bow-tie. It consists of two lateral lobes and an isthmus which is attached via Berry's ligament to the second to fourth tracheal rings (it is not attached to the thyroid cartilage but sits lower down in the neck). The fact that the thyroid gland is attached to the trachea by Berry's ligament and also the fact that it is invested within pretracheal fascia explains why the thyroid gland moves up with swallowing. This is important clinically as it defines a swelling within the neck as being of thyroid origin.

The embryology is important. The thyroid gland descends from the foramen caecum between the anterior two-thirds and posterior one-third of the tongue via the thyroglossal duct. If the embryology is faulty it can lead to problems in later adult life. An incompletely descended thyroid gland may persist in adult life as a lingual thyroid or a thyroglossal cyst.

The blood supply to the thyroid is by way of the superior thyroid artery (which is a branch of the external thyroid artery), the inferior thyroid artery (which is a branch of the thyrocervical trunk of the first part of the subclavian artery) and, rarely, the small thyroidea ima which arises from the aorta to supply the isthmus. Venous drainage is through the superior and middle thyroid veins to the internal jugular veins and via the inferior thyroid veins to the brachiocephalic veins (usually on the left). The arterial supply and venous drainage is important to know about when considering thyroid surgery.

The thyroid gland is stimulated by TSH (which is produced from the anterior lobe of the pituitary gland) to produce T3 and T4 – hormones that play an important role in basal metabolic rate.

108. **D: Lead to tolerance**

Opioids are mainly used in the hospital setting for their analgesic properties. They are now believed to act both peripherally (outside the central nervous system) and within the CNS itself. Unfortunately, opioids exert most of their beneficial effects and side effects through the same opioid receptor (μ-receptors). It is therefore unlikely that we will ever be able to develop a synthetic opioid agent that has the analgesic properties of other opioids without their unpleasant side effects.

Opioids induce side effects through both excitatory and inhibitory mechanisms. Excitatory effects are:

- Pinpoint pupils (direct effect of opioids on the Edinger–Westphal nucleus)
- Nausea and vomiting (direct effect on the area postrema)
- Pruritus (due to mast-cell degranulation and histamine release)
- Dysphoria and euphoria (direct effect on the CNS)

Inhibitory effects are:

- Cardiorespiratory depression
- Sedation
- Relaxation of smooth muscles – constipation, urinary retention

Constipation and nausea/vomiting are common side effects of opioids. It is therefore always a good idea to prescribe laxatives and antiemetics whenever an opioid is prescribed.

Opioids cause tolerance, dependence, and withdrawal with increasing use. Tolerance means increasing dosages of the drug needed to be used in order to obtain the same effect.

It is important to know how to reverse the effects of opioids because opioid overdose may be fatal. Specific opioid antagonists include naloxone and naltrexone. Flumazenil antagonizes the effects of benzodiazepines.

109. **B: Results in mast-cell degranulation**

Hypersensitivity is a condition in which undesirable tissue damage follows the development of humoral or cell-mediated immunity. Gell and Coombs classified hypersensitivity reactions into four types. However, some also include a fifth type, as shown in the following.

Gell and Coombs' classification of hypersensitivity reactions

- *Type I*: Mast-cell degranulation mediated by pre-formed IgE bound to mast cells. Immediate (within minutes). Anaphylaxis, atopic allergies.
- *Type II*: Antibodies directed towards antigens present on the surface of cells or tissue components. Humoral antibodies participate directly in injuring cells by predisposing them to phagocytosis or lysis. Initiates within several hours. Good examples are transfusion reactions, autoimmune haemolytic anaemia, and Goodpasture's syndrome.
- *Type III*: Formation of antibody–antigen complexes (immune complex mediated). Initiates within several hours. Good examples are the Arthus reaction, serum sickness, and SLE.
- *Type IV*: Delayed type of hypersensitivity. Cell-mediated. T-lymphocytes involved. Granulomatous conditions. Initiation time is 24–72 hours. Contact dermatitis.
- *Type V*: Due to the formation of stimulatory autoantibodies in autoimmune conditions such as Graves' disease.

110. **A: Pain from the transverse colon is usually referred to the midline area below the umbilicus**

Referred pain is not well understood. Somatic referred pain is very well localized and intense. Visceral pain is the opposite and conveyed by automatic fibres.

Diaphragmatic pain is usually referred to the shoulder. Appendix pain is usually referred to the umbilicus.

111. **B: Mitosis produces genetically identical daughter cells**

Mitosis is the process of cell division in somatic cells and produces two genetically identical diploid cells. Meiosis occurs in gamete formation and differs from mitosis in two important respects: each daughter cell contains half the genetic information (haploid) and the resultant cells differ in their genetic material. There are two separate phases (or divisions) in meiosis. In the first division, two genetically different haploid cells are formed, and in the second each of the haploid cells divides.

The exchange of genetic material occurs in Prophase I. The cell cycle is controlled internally by gene products called cyclins which vary in concentration throughout the cell cycle. Cyclin-dependent kinases control the activity of cyclins by switching on cyclins through phosphorylation. p53 is an example of a tumour suppressor gene. It normally functions to inhibit the cell cycle. p53 is the most common mutated gene in cancers. It encodes a transcription factor which downregulates the cell cycle preventing the cell from undergoing mitosis. Oncogenes control cell growth and differentiation, examples of which include growth factors, growth factor receptors, and nuclear transcription factors.

112. **D: Genioglossus muscle protrudes the tongue**

The tongue is composed of striated, voluntary, or skeletal muscle, not smooth muscle. The tongue assists in the formation of a food bolus and propagation towards the back of the mouth and thence into the oesophagus. The tongue also plays a key role in the suckling reflex in neonates, in the articulation of speech and the special sense of taste. Its epithelium is composed of stratified squamous (protective) epithelium as, like the skin, it is subject to 'wear and tear'. Tumours arising from the tongue are therefore typically squamous cell carcinomas.

Special taste sensation is by way of the chorda tympani division of the facial nerve for the anterior two-thirds of the tongue and the glossopharyngeal nerve for the posterior one-third. Taste sensation on the anterior two-thirds of the tongue is therefore commonly lost in a facial nerve (or Bell's) palsy. Somatic sensation is by way of the mandibular division of the trigeminal nerve for the anterior two-thirds of the tongue (lingual nerve) and the glossopharyngeal nerve for the posterior one-third.

All the muscles of the tongue are supplied by the hypoglossal or 12th cranial nerve, with the exception of the palatoglossus muscle which is supplied by the pharyngeal plexus of nerves (IX, X, and sympathetics). The hypoglossal nerve may be injured in a carotid endarterectomy or submandibular gland procedures. The most important muscle to know about is the genioglossus muscle, which serves to protrude the tongue. When genioglossal muscle tone is lost, as in someone with a decreased level of consciousness, or a fractured mandible (where the genioglossus muscle arises), the tongue falls back and obstructs the airway, rapidly resulting in hypoxia and death if basic life support measures are not quickly instigated.

113. **C: The Q-T interval gives a rough indication of the duration of ventricular systole**

The nature of the electrocardiogram (ECG) is important to understand. As a junior doctor you will be reading and interpreting ECGs every day at work.

- P-wave = atrial depolarization
- QRS complex = ventricular depolarization
- T-wave = ventricular repolarization

(Electrical activity resulting from atrial repolarization is 'hidden' within the QRS complex.)

The Q-T interval gives a rough indication of the duration of ventricular systole. The first heart sound results from closure of the atrioventricular valves and occurs as the ventricles contract. It therefore coincides with the QRS complex. The second heart sound is due to closure of the aortic and pulmonary valves, respectively, and occurs at about the same time as the T-wave.

114. **D: May occur in systemic lupus erythematosus**

Type III hypersensitivity reactions are mediated by antibodies. SLE is a type III hypersensitivity reaction where large amounts of immune complexes form between nuclear antigens and antibodies. Allergic rhinitis is a type I hypersensitivity reaction. Type IV reactions are cell-mediated through specifically sensitized T-lymphocytes. Nickel sensitivity is a Type IV hypersensitivity reaction.

Allergic rhinitis is a Type I hypersensitivity reaction. SLE is a Type III hypersensitivity reaction where large amounts of immune complexes form between nuclear antigens and antibodies.

Latex allergies can be one of three types:

- Irritant contact dermatitis (non-immune)
- Allergic contact dermatitis (Type IV hypersensitivity reaction)
- Immediate hypersensitivity (Type I hypersensitivity reaction or anaphylaxis) – what everyone worries about!

115. **B: Cytosine always pairs with guanine**

DNA consists of a right-handed double helix with 10 bases per turn. Adenine and guanine are purine bases; cytosine, thymine (and uracil) are pyrimidine bases (remembered by the 'y' in pyrimidine, thymine, cytosine). Adenine pairs with thymine in DNA via two hydrogen bonds. Adenine pairs with uracil in RNA. Guanine pairs with cytosine in DNA via three hydrogen bonds.

116. **A: In terminally differentiated squamous cells**

Warts, caused by papilloma virus, are non-malignant tumours of squamous cells. Infectious papilloma viruses are most likely to be found in terminally differentiated squamous cells and are not found in the basal cells, in the surface layers of warts, in transformed cancer cells, or throughout the warts.

117. **E: May be minimized by blood-group matching**

Hyperacute rejection is due to the formation of preformed antibodies against the donor organ. It occurs within minutes of transplantation so the surgeon can usually see the changes taking place as the anastomoses are completed.

The antibodies are usually directed against blood group antigens and it can therefore be minimized by blood-group matching. The blood groups and HLA antigens of autografts (tissue from the same individual) will be identical, so hyperacute rejection will never occur in such circumstances.

No drug treatment can reverse hyperacute rejection; the main treatment is removal of the transplanted organ.

Transplant rejections can be classified into the following types:

- *Hyperacute*: Preformed antibodies (minutes to hours)
- *Accelerated acute*: Reactivation of sensitized T-cells and secondary antibody response (days)
- *Acute*: Cytotoxic T-cell mediated with primary activation of T-cells (days to weeks)
- *Chronic*: Antibody-mediated vascular damage (months to years, controversial)

118. **B: Paired t-test**

A paired t-test allows a comparison of mean potassium values before and after treatment by comparing each patient's initial serum level with his or her repeat value.

119. **B: Promoters**

Transcription of genes is initiated by promoters. Enhancers and silencers are proteins that bind to the promoter region on the DNA and will influence gene transcription. Exons carry the coding sequences of DNA.

120. **D: Lateral rectus is supplied by the abducens nerve**

The extra-ocular muscles are innervated by the 3rd (occulomotor), 4th (trochlear), and 6th (abducens) cranial nerves. The trochlear nerve supplies only one muscle and that is the superior oblique muscle. The abducens nerve also supplies only one muscle and that is the lateral rectus muscle. This may be remembered by 'SO4, LR6'. All the remaining muscles are supplied by the occulomotor nerve – that is, the superior rectus, inferior rectus, inferior oblique, and medial rectus are all supplied by the occulomotor, or 3rd, cranial nerve. Injury to any of these cranial nerves (3rd, 4th, or 6th) may result in ophthalmoplegia and double vision (diplopia).

The recti muscles are easily understood as they move the eyeball in the respective directions indicated by their name. The superior and inferior obliques are more difficult to understand. The superior oblique muscle moves the cornea downwards and outwards, whereas the inferior oblique muscle moves the cornea

upwards and inwards. The reason for this is that the oblique muscles pass posteriorly to attach behind the axis of movement and therefore impart movement
opposite to their suggested names. Weakness of the extra-ocular muscles may
occur in the autoimmune condition, myasthenia gravis.

The levator palpebrae superioris is the exception to the earlier. It elevates the eyelid
but has a dual innervation from both the occulomotor nerve and sympathetic
fibres. The latter innervate a small smooth muscle portion of the levator muscle
known as Muller's muscle. The clinical significance of this dual innervation
is that a 3rd cranial nerve (occulomotor) palsy, or sympathetic interruption
(Horner's syndrome), may result in a droopy eyelid (ptosis). To distinguish the
two, it is essential to lift up the eyelid and inspect the pupil to see if it is enlarged
(mydriasis, in an occulomotor nerve palsy) or constricted (miosis, in a Horner's
syndrome). Furthermore, in an occulomotor palsy the eyeball points downwards
and outwards from the unopposed action of superior oblique and lateral rectus,
supplied by the 4th and 6th cranial nerves. Horner's syndrome is associated with
hemifacial anhidrosis (absent sweating of the ipsilateral face), flushing symptoms
(the so-called Harlequin syndrome or effect) and enophthalmos (a sunken eyeball),
in addition to ptosis and miosis.

121. **B: Nitric oxide**

The importance of endothelium in vascular responses was first noted when it
was discovered that removing the endothelium from perfused arteries prevented
the vasodilator action of acetylcholine on those vessels. The endothelium-
derived relaxing factor has since been recognized as nitric oxide (a vasodilator).
Vasopressin, angiotensin II, thromboxane A2, and noradrenaline are all
vasoconstrictors.

Since its discovery, nitric oxide has been implicated in a diverse array of
different biological processes, both physiological and pathological, besides
vasodilatation, including:

- Acting as a neurotransmitter
- The killing of microorganisms by phagocytes
- Long-term potentiation (memory)
- Male erection (Viagra enhances the effect of nitric oxide)
- Sepsis
- Excitotoxicity

In addition, nitric oxide explains how glyceryl trinitrate exerts its beneficial effect
in angina. More and more is being discovered about nitric oxide all the time.

122. **A: Reed–Sternberg cells**

Reed–Sternberg cells are diagnostic for Hodgkin's lymphoma. The Philadelphia
chromosome and decreased quantities of leucocytes alkaline phosphatase are

commonly observed in chronic myelogenous leukaemia. Auer rods are most often seen in increased numbers in acute myelogenous or myelomonocytic leukaemia. Pappenheimer bodies are abnormal iron granules found inside red blood cells. They are associated with sideroblastic anaemia, haemolytic anaemia, and sickle cell disease.

123. **D: Blood group O is recessive to A and B**

ABO blood groups are inherited in the following manner. Blood group O is recessive to both A and B, but A and B exhibit co-dominance. Thus, AO or AA = blood group A; BO or BB = blood group B; OO = blood group O; AB = blood group AB. Blood group O is the most common blood group in the UK population. There is no known evolutionary advantage of being one ABO blood group over another, although people with blood group O are more susceptible to duodenal ulceration than other blood groups, and patients with blood group A are at higher risk of developing gastric carcinoma. Duffy blood group–negative individuals are resistant to *Plasmodium vivax*, since the Duffy antigen acts as a receptor for invasion by the human parasite.

Since individuals with blood group AB have no antibodies present in their serum it follows that they are universal recipients. However, they can only donate to other AB individuals. Individuals of blood group O have antibodies present in their serum against blood groups A and B. It follows that they can only receive from other group O individuals. However, they are universal donors since the antibodies are rapidly diluted in the recipient's blood. Since blood group O is the universal donor it is used in emergency situations where there is not enough time to determine the exact blood grouping of the patient.

124. **B: The direction of fibres of the external intercostal muscle is downwards and medial**

The intercostal neurovascular bundle lies in a groove on the undersurface of each rib, running in the plane between the internal and innermost intercostal muscles.

The vein, artery, and nerve lie in that order, from above downwards, under cover of the lower border of the rib. This may be remembered by VAN:

- V = Vein
- A = Artery
- N = Nerve

Thus, a needle or trocar for drainage, or aspiration, of fluid from the pleural cavity is inserted just above the rib in order to avoid the main vessels and nerves.

The fibres of the external intercostal muscle pass obliquely downwards and forwards from the sharp lower border of the rib above to the smooth upper border of the rib below. This may be remembered because it follows the same direction as having one's hands in pockets. Although important for the mechanics of respiration, the diaphragm is the main muscle of respiration.

125. D: Carotid bodies primarily respond to hypoxia

A chemoreceptor is a receptor that responds to a change in the chemical composition of the blood. They are the most important receptors involved in the minute-to-minute control of ventilation. There are both central and peripheral chemoreceptors.

Central chemoreceptors lie within the medulla of the brainstem. They primarily respond to hypercapnia by increasing the ventilatory rate and depth of ventilation.

Peripheral chemoreceptors lie in the carotid bodies (at the origin of the internal carotid artery) and in the aortic arch. Carotid bodies are not to be confused with the nearby carotid sinus baroreceptors which comprise stretch receptors in the wall of internal carotid arteries. Carotid bodies primarily respond to hypoxia by increasing the ventilatory rate and depth of ventilation.

Eighty per cent of the hypercapnic response driving ventilation arises from the central chemoreceptors; 20 per cent arises from the peripheral chemoreceptors. The response of the central chemoreceptors to arterial pCO_2 is therefore more important than that of the peripheral chemoreceptors. The hypoxic response driving ventilation almost all comes from the peripheral chemoreceptors.

Each carotid body is only a few millimetres in size and has the distinction of having the highest blood flow per tissue weight of any organ in the body (20 mL/g per minute). This high flow is consistent with the prompt physiological reflex functions of the carotid body. Carotid bodies sample the partial pressure of oxygen in the blood, not its oxygen content. Anaemia, when the oxygen content is low but the pCO_2 is normal, does not stimulate them.

126. D: It may cause blackwater fever

Malaria is a worldwide infection that affects 500 million people and kills 3 million people (mostly children) per year; it is therefore the major parasitic cause of death and is the deadliest vector-borne disease in the world. Malaria is caused by protozoan parasites of the genus *Plasmodium*. There are 4 main strains that infect humans: *P. falciparum, vivax, malariae,* and *ovale.*

Of these, *P. falciparum* is the most virulent, most widespread, and most drug-resistant and causes the most morbidity and mortality through its ability to cause cerebral malaria, severe anaemia, hypoglycaemia, lactic acidosis, renal failure, pulmonary oedema, and shock ('algid malaria'). Blackwater fever is characterized by intravascular haemolysis, haemoglobinuria, and kidney failure.

P. falciparum is the most pathogenic strain for 2 principal reasons:

- It can develop in red cells of all ages; the other less pathogenic species are limited to growing in subpopulations of cells – either very young or very mature cells. *P. falciparum* can therefore cause higher levels of parasitaemia.
- The distinctive behaviour of *P. falciparum*-infected red cells – namely cytoadherence to vascular endothelium and sequestration – minimizes removal of infected erythrocytes by the spleen.

Plasmodia is transmitted to humans by more than a dozen species of female *Anopheles* mosquito which require a blood meal before they can breed (the *Aedes* mosquito acts as a vector for yellow fever and Dengue fever, not malaria). The male mosquitoes feed harmlessly on plant sap. The *Anopheles* mosquito vector is also the definitive host in which sexual reproduction occurs; thus, fertilization occurs in the insect, not in the human!

Malaria is treated with supportive management and chemotherapy. Preventative strategies include chemoprophylaxis (which is by no means 100 per cent effective!), vector control (such as insecticides), and bite prevention (insect repellents, mosquito nets, covering up exposed areas especially at dawn and dusk). Unfortunately, at present no effective vaccination exists for the prevention of malaria. The quest to develop a malaria vaccine is currently an active area of research.

127. **A: Tyrosine**

Tyrosine is the precursor of each of these neurotransmitters. Tyrosine hydroxylase converts tyrosine to DOPA, which is in turn converted to dopamine, then to noradrenaline and finally adrenaline.

128. **C: Is associated with berry aneurysms of the circle of Willis**

Adult polycystic kidney disease is one of the most common inherited disorders in humans, affecting approximately 1 in 1000 individuals and accounting for 10 per cent of cases of end-stage renal failure. It is inherited as an autosomal dominant condition with a late-onset mode of presentation. Eighty-five per cent of cases have been localized to a gene on the short arm of chromosome 16 (*PKD1* gene). A second gene (*PKD2*), responsible for around 15 per cent of cases, has been localized to the long arm of chromosome 4. The corresponding gene products have been named polycystin-1 and polycystin-2, although their exact function is unknown.

Both kidneys are progressively replaced by enlarging cysts which compress and replace the functioning renal parenchyma, leading to renal failure. The condition usually presents in adult life (typically around 40 years of age). When renal failure occurs it usually progresses to end-stage renal failure at between 40–60 years of age.

Adult polycystic kidney disease is associated with cerebral berry aneurysms (so that death may occur due to subarachnoid haemorrhage). Other extrarenal manifestations include liver, pancreatic, and splenic cysts.

129. **D: It lacks a true serosal surface**

The oesophagus is a segmental muscular tube running from the cricoid ring, at the level of C6, to the cardia of the stomach. It is 25 cm long (with the distance from the upper incisor teeth to the lower oesophageal sphincter being approximately 40 cm). These distances are useful to learn for the purposes of endoscopy. The upper third of the oesophagus consists of skeletal muscle (voluntary muscle which initiates swallowing) but then there is a progressive change to smooth muscle, such that the lower third of the oesophagus consists only of smooth muscle.

Blood supply and lymphatic drainage is segmental. The upper third of the oesophagus is supplied by the inferior thyroid artery and lymphatics drain to the deep cervical group of lymph nodes. The middle third of the oesophagus is supplied directly by branches from the descending thoracic aorta and lymphatics drain to the pre-aortic and para-aortic lymph nodes. The lower third of the oesophagus is supplied by the left gastric artery and lymphatics drain to the coeliac group of lymph nodes. However, within the oesophageal walls there are lymphatic channels which enable lymph to pass for long distances within the viscus so that drainage from any given area does not strictly follow the previous pattern.

The surface epithelium is largely non-keratinizing stratified squamous epithelium. This is normally replaced by columnar epithelium at the gastro-oesophageal junction, but columnar epithelium may line the lower oesophagus. An oesophagus that has the squamocolumnar junction 3 cm or more above the gastro-oesophageal junction is abnormal and called Barrett's oesophagus. This is a metaplastic change taking place in response to acid reflux and is a premalignant condition.

Except for the short intra-abdominal segment of the oesophagus there is no serosal surface. This is important to know about for two reasons. First, it makes the oesophagus vulnerable to anastomotic leakage in the postoperative period. Second, because the oesophagus lacks a serosal covering, oesophageal carcinoma encounters few anatomic barriers to local invasion.

130. **C: The Haldane effect describes changes in the affinity of the blood for CO_2 with variations in the PaO_2**

Carbon dioxide is transported in the blood in 3 ways:

- Bicarbonate accounts for about 80–90 per cent of the total CO_2 in the blood
- Carbamino compounds (5–10 per cent)
- Physically dissolved in solution (only 5 per cent)

Carbon dioxide is carried on the haemoglobin molecule as carbamino-haemoglobin; carboxyhaemoglobin is the combination of haemoglobin with carbon monoxide.

Venous blood contains a higher pCO_2 than arterial blood and is therefore more acidic (through the formation of carbonic acid), with a lower pH.

Carbon dioxide is approximately 20 times more soluble in plasma than is O_2. This means that CO_2 diffuses about 20 times more rapidly than does O_2. This rapid diffusion of CO_2 through aqueous solutions means that the elimination of CO_2 is much less of a problem than is O_2 delivery, so O_2 is likely to be the factor affected first in disorders of respiration.

Binding of oxygen with haemoglobin tends to displace carbon dioxide from the blood; this is known as the Haldane effect. In the capillaries, the Haldane effect causes increased pick up of CO_2 because of O_2 removed from the haemoglobin, while in the lungs it causes increased release of CO_2 because of O_2 pick up by the haemoglobin.

131. **B: Parasites may remain dormant in the liver as hypnozoites**

The malaria parasite has a complex life cycle. In their definitive host (the mosquito), the parasites undergo a cycle of sexual and asexual development. In their intermediate host (the human), the parasites undergo two cycles of asexual development (in the liver and in red blood cells). In addition, there are alternating and extracellular stages. The genetic recombination allowed by the sexual stage is one element in the remarkable antigenic diversity seen within malaria parasite populations that enables it to evade the immune response. The malaria life cycle is easiest to understand if it is broken down into three stages.

The intermediate host (humans) – Hepatic stage: Human infection begins when sporozoites are introduced into an individual's bloodstream as an infected mosquito takes a blood meal. Within 30 minutes, they disappear from the blood as they infect hepatocytes. Here they undergo the first round of asexual reproduction (exoerythrocytic schizogony) and develop into exoerythrocytic schizonts. These exoerythrocytic schizonts may contain many thousands of merozoites. On invasion of the hepatocyte by *Plasmodium vivax* and *P. ovale,* the development of the schizont is retarded, and a 'dormant' stage of the parasite, the hypnozoite, is formed. This is responsible for disease relapse months to years after supposed chemotherapeutic cure and clearance of bloodstream forms of the parasite.

The intermediate host (humans) – Erythrocytic stage: The released merozoites infect red cells where they undergo another round of asexual reproduction (erythrocytic schizogony) changing from merozoite, to trophozoite (feeding stage), to schizont. Eventually, the cell ruptures and releases new merozoites (usually between 8 and 32), which go on to infect more red cells. Generally, the parasite's life cycle stages are highly synchronized, such that at any one time all the parasites are at the trophozoite stage, or all are at the schizont stage. Fever in malaria is either tertian (every 48 hours in *Plasmodium falciparum, vivax*, and *ovale*) or quartan (every 72 hours in *P. malariae*) and is due to the synchronized release of merozoites from red cells. Malignant tertian fever is due to *P. falciparum*. In addition, on infection of new blood cells, instead of forming trophozoites the parasites may grow into the immature gametocytes. These are not released from the red cell until taken up by a feeding mosquito.

The determinate host (mosquito): The female *Anopheles* mosquitoes ingest blood as part of their life cycle. Here the normal asexually dividing bloodstream forms die, but the gametocytes are stimulated to mature to microgametes (male) and macrogametes (female). Fertilization occurs in the mosquito midgut resulting in the formation of a zygote. This then goes on to produce a wormlike form, the ookinete, which penetrates the midgut wall of the mosquito, forming an oocyst, located between the epithelium and the basement membrane. Note that the zygote is the sole diploid stage of malaria parasites; the only meiosis event during this life cycle occurs within a few hours of zygote formation. Within the oocyst a cycle of asexual reproduction (sporogeny) then takes place, with the formation of numerous sporozoites. When mature, the oocyst bursts open releasing these sporozoites, which then migrate to the insect's salivary glands. From here they may enter the bloodstream of a new host, thus completing the parasite's life cycle.

132. **C: The narrowest part of the oesophagus is at the level of cricopharyngeus**

There are 4 classical points along the oesophagus where constrictions take place:

- *Point 1*: Cricopharyngeus sphincter, 15 cm from the incisor teeth, which is the narrowest part of the oesophagus. Its function is to prevent air entering the oesophagus and stomach. The cricopharyngeus sphincter relaxes with the swallowing reflex

- *Point 2*: Where the oesophagus is crossed by the aortic arch, 22 cm from the incisor teeth

- *Point 3*: Where the oesophagus is crossed by the left principal bronchus, 27 cm from the incisor teeth

- *Point 4*: Where the oesophagus passes through the opening in the diaphragm, 38 cm from the incisor teeth

Although the left atrium is in front of the lower part of the oesophagus below the left bronchus, it is only when enlarged (e.g., in mitral valve disease) that the left atrium causes an indentation in the oesophagus, resulting in difficulty swallowing, or dysphagia.

These constrictions are of considerable clinical importance since they are sites where swallowed foreign bodies can lodge, or through which it may be difficult to pass an oesophagoscope. Since a slight delay in the passage of food or fluid occurs at these levels, strictures commonly develop here following the drinking of caustic fluids. These constrictions are also common sites of carcinoma of the oesophagus.

The lower oesophageal sphincter is not a true anatomical sphincter, but rather a functional one. Maintenance of the lower oesophageal sphincter is largely brought about through the following features:

- The effect of the right crus of the diaphragm forming a 'sling' around the lower oesophagus

- The oblique angle the oesophagus takes on entering the gastric cardia (Angle of His) acting as a flap-valve mechanism

- Greater intra-abdominal pressure than intra-gastric pressure acting to compress the abdominal part of the oesophagus

- Mucosal rosette (prominent folds at the gastro-oesophageal junction)

- Phrenico-oesophageal ligament (fold of connective tissue)
- The effect of gastrin in increasing lower oesophageal sphincter tone
- Unidirectional peristalsis

A problematic lower oesophageal sphincter may lead to problems, such as gastro-oesophageal reflux disease, hiatus hernia, or a condition known as achalasia.

133. **E: The shape of the curve is explained by the physico-chemical properties of haemoglobin**

The haemoglobin oxygen dissociation curve is sigmoidal in shape. The sigmoid response reflects the underlying biochemical properties of haemoglobin and results from cooperativity. That is, the protein cannot be considered in terms of four independently oxygen-binding subunits. As haemoglobin binds successive oxygens, the oxygen affinity of the subunits increases. Hyperbolic curves are exhibited by monomeric molecules such as myoglobin. The significance of the sigmoidal curve is that it means that haemoglobin becomes highly saturated at high oxygen partial pressures (and is therefore highly efficient at collecting oxygen) and releases a significant amount of oxygen at pressures which are fairly low, but not extremely so (with the result that haemoglobin is highly effective at supplying oxygen where it is needed).

The effect of things that shift the curve to the right (raised CO_2, lowered pH, increased temperature, increase in 2,3-DPG) is to increase oxygen availability in the tissues. The effect of CO_2/H^+ on O_2 carriage is known as the Bohr shift or effect. This is exactly what is needed in metabolizing tissues; release of acids or CO_2 thus liberates O_2 to fulfil the metabolic needs of the tissue. Do not confuse this with the effect of changes in O_2 on CO_2 carriage, which is called the Haldane effect.

A shift of the oxygen dissociation curve to the left is characteristic of foetal haemoglobin. When compared with adult haemoglobin, it is composed of two alpha and two gamma chains, instead of the usual two alpha and two beta chains of adult haemoglobin. This arrangement assists in the transfer of oxygen across the placenta from the maternal to the foetal circulation. The corollary of this is that foetal tissue oxygen levels have to be low to permit the release of oxygen from the haemoglobin.

134. **D: Disease results from the immune response to schistosome eggs**

Parasitic infections may be caused by protozoa or metazoa. Parasitic protozoa (e.g., *Plasmodium falciparum*) are single-celled nucleate organisms that possess all processes necessary for reproduction. A metazoon is a multicellular organism. Examples of infective metazoa include helminths (parasitic worms) which can be subdivided into three classes: nematodes (roundworms), cestodes (flatworms), and trematodes (flukes). Schistosomiasis is the most important helminth disease infecting 200 million people worldwide. Three major species of schistosome parasite can infect humans: *Schistosoma mansoni, japonicum,* and *haematobium.* All are trematodes (flukes).

The life cycle of the flatworm that causes human schistosomiasis involves a sexual stage in the human (the definitive host) and an asexual stage in the freshwater snail host, which acts as a vector or intermediate host. Schistosome eggs excreted in the faeces or urine hatch out in fresh water and release miracidia that invade snails; free-swimming cercaria are released from the snail and invade human skin, losing their tails and becoming known as schistosomulae. The larvae migrate through the bloodstream via the lungs and liver to the veins of the bladder (*Schistosoma haematobium*) or bowel (*Schistosoma mansoni* and *japonicum*) where they develop into adult males and females. The adults lay eggs, which are excreted by the host, thus completing the cycle.

The pathophysiology of schistosomiasis is mainly due to the immune response against the schistosome eggs. In the liver this may result in granuloma formation, extensive fibrosis (pipe-stem portal fibrosis), and portal hypertension (hepatosplenic schistosomiasis). *Schistosoma haematobium* is responsible for urinary schistosomiasis, where granulomatous inflammation and fibrosis in the bladder may result in haematuria, obstructive uropathy, and squamous cell carcinoma of the bladder.

Schistosomiasis is treated with praziquantel which removes the flukes, but in advanced cases the pathology is irreversible. Intense inflammatory reactions are provoked when the worms killed by treatment are carried back into the liver.

135. **E: Coxsackie B**

Myocarditis is most commonly caused by Coxsackie group B virus and may be preceded by gastrointestinal or respiratory symptoms. Rhinoviruses, coronaviruses, and adenoviruses are associated with the common cold, influenza-like illnesses, and gastrointestinal disturbances. Mumps causes orchitis and parotitis/parotidomegaly.

136. **E: The death rate from gastric carcinoma has fallen**

The death rate from lung cancer in women has shown a steep rise since 1955 with no decline in the rate of increase. This may be attributable to the increasing smoking habits of women in modern society. In males the death rate from lung cancer peaked in the mid-1980s and has shown a slight fall since then. Suicide rates in all countries fall during wartime and was low in the 1950s. Since then it has shown a steady increase in both sexes.

In the 1980's, the terms HIV and AIDS did not even exist. However, as of January 2006, just over 25 years after its recognition, the World Health Organization has estimated that 38.6 million people worldwide are HIV-positive and more than 25 million people have died of AIDS-related deaths since its recognition, making it one of the most destructive pandemics in recorded history.

Much more mysterious is the downward trend in deaths from stomach carcinoma over the past 50 years. Such trends provide us with valuable information regarding the aetiology of stomach cancer. This downward trend may be due to a decrease in some dietary carcinogens. However, the more recent decline may in part be due to *Helicobacter pylori* eradication therapy since it is now believed that *H. pylori* plays a pivotal role in the development of gastric carcinoma.

137. **C: It forms the main muscle of respiration at rest**

The diaphragm is a musculo-tendinous structure composed of outer skeletal muscle fibres and a central tendinous region. It partitions the thoracic from the abdominal cavity and is the main muscle of respiration at rest (accounting for 70 per cent of inspiration at rest). Upon inspiration, the diaphragm contracts, which lowers the diaphragm. This decreases pressure within the thoracic cavity and air moves into the lungs, resulting in lung inflation. Upon expiration, the diaphragm relaxes and the diaphragm moves up.

The diaphragm receives motor innervation from the phrenic nerve (C3, C4, C5). ('C3, C4, C5, keeps the diaphragm alive!'). The diaphragm has no other motor supply other than the phrenic nerve. This is why cervical spine injuries with injury to the cervical spinal cord can be so disastrous – and hence the importance of proper cervical spine immobilization in trauma victims.

The phrenic nerve is two-thirds motor and one-third sensory. The sensory nerve supply to the diaphragmatic parietal pleura and diaphragmatic peritoneum covering the central surfaces of the diaphragm is from the phrenic nerve. The sensory supply to the periphery of the diaphragm is from the lower six intercostal nerves.

138. **E: Increased blood viscosity**

At high altitude, a decreased atmospheric pressure results in decreased ambient oxygen concentrations and therefore a decrease in arterial Po_2. In the short term, an increase in pulmonary ventilation occurs due to stimulation of peripheral chemoreceptors by an oxygen lack. Hyperventilation causes a respiratory alkalosis (rise in arterial pH) by blowing off CO_2. This inhibits the central chemoreceptors and thereby opposes the effect of low Po_2 to stimulate the peripheral chemoreceptors (braking effect). Hypoxia leads to pulmonary vasoconstriction and pulmonary hypertension.

Acclimatization (i.e., adaptive responses to sustained and gradually increasing hypoxia) occurs in the longer term through a variety of different mechanisms:

- Removal of the braking effect – By changes in the composition of the cerebrospinal fluid (a reduction in the bicarbonate concentration of the cerebrospinal fluid) and increasing the renal excretion of bicarbonate – results in increased pulmonary ventilation

- Erythropoiesis – Through the effect of hypoxia stimulating erythropoietin secretion from the kidney – increases the oxygen carrying capacity of the blood, but in doing so raises blood haematocrit and blood viscosity, the effects of which can be deleterious
- There is increased cardiac output
- There is increased capillarity (increased number of capillaries in tissues)
- An increase in the concentration of 2,3-DPG causes a rightward shift of the oxygen dissociation curve that results in better unloading of oxygen
- There is cellular acclimatization – Changes occur in the mitochondria and oxidative enzymes inside cells

If a person ascends to a high altitude too quickly (without giving enough time for these acclimatization mechanisms to develop), or remains at high altitude for too long, high-altitude or mountain sickness may result. There is only one treatment for high-altitude sickness and that is immediate descent from the mountain.

139. **E: Are responsible for causing Kuru in humans**

Prions are a novel, infectious agent composed of protein only. They differ from all known pathogens. They lack nucleic acid and cannot be considered microorganisms. They are highly resistant to decontamination methods such as standard autoclaving (heat), disinfectants (chemicals), and ionizing radiation.

If abnormal prion protein is inoculated into a normal host, conformational changes are induced in the normal host prions resulting in their conversion to abnormal host prions. These abnormal host proteins then induce further conformational changes in remaining normal host prions. Thus, the original inoculated protein is able to catalyse a chain reaction in which host proteins become conformationally abnormal. This is unaccompanied by inflammation, immune reaction, or cytokine release.

Well-known prion diseases include Kuru, scrapie, bovine spongiform encephalopathy (BSE), and Creutzfeldt–Jakob disease (CJD). Kuru is probably one of the most fascinating stories to have emerged from any epidemiological investigation. It occurred in villages occupied by the Fore tribes in the highlands of New Guinea who practised ritual cannibalism as a rite of mourning for their dead. The first cases occurred in the 1950s and involved progressive loss of voluntary control, followed by death within a year of the onset of symptoms. Interestingly, Kuru occurred only in individuals who participated in cannibalistic feasts. Such cannibalism was believed to be responsible for the transmission of prions in Kuru.

There is still much work to be done in determining the exact modes of transmission of prions and in enhancing our understanding of the molecular biology of prions. In addition, the exact interrelations between the different prion-related diseases (e.g., BSE and a new-variant CJD) needs to be clarified.

140. **A: C5a**

C5a is a component of complement. Activation of complement by endotoxin or antigen-antibody complexes produces C5a, which is a neutrophil and macrophage chemotactant. *HLA-A* and *HLA-B* are genes for the human leucocyte antigens and they control the synthesis of class I major histocompatibility complex. The J-chain of IgM and IgA does not possess chemotactant properties. The variable region of the heavy chain of IgG is not known as a best neutrophil or macrophage chemotactant.

141. **E: The sympathetic trunks pass posterior to the medial arcuate ligament.**

See Table 3. The left phrenic nerve pierces the muscle of the left dome of the diaphragm.

Table 3 Diaphragm openings	
Vena cava opening (T8)	Inferior vena cava
	Right phrenic nerve
Oesophageal opening (T10)	Oesophagus
	Left and right vagus nerves (RIP = right is posterior)
	Oesophageal branches of left gastric vessels
	Lymphatics from lower 1/3 oesophagus
Aortic opening (T12)	Aorta
	Azygous and hemiazygous veins
	Thoracic duct
Crura (T12)	Greater, lesser, and least splanchnic nerves
Behind medial arcuate ligament	Sympathetic trunks
Behind lateral arcuate ligament	Subcostal (T12) neurovascular bundle

The inferior vena cava passes through the central tendinous portion of the diaphragm and not the muscular portion of the diaphragm at the T8 level. The reason for this is clear: if the vena cava passed through the muscular part of the diaphragm, each time the diaphragm contracted with respiration it would obstruct venous return, causing syncope.

142. **B: Under resting conditions, equilibration between alveoli Po_2 and red blood cell Po_2 occurs one-third of the way along the pulmonary capillary**

Gas exchange within the lung takes place at the level of the alveoli. It obeys Fick's law, which states that the rate of transfer of a gas through a sheet of tissue is directly proportional to the tissue surface area and the difference in partial pressure between the two sides and inversely proportional to the tissue thickness. The area of the blood gas barrier in the lung is enormous (50–100 m², about the size of a tennis court) and the thickness is only 0.3 μm in some places, so the dimensions of the barrier are ideal for diffusion.

Any disruption to the factors that affect the rate of gas transfer through the respiratory membrane may result in disease states. For example, the thickness of the respiratory membrane increases significantly in interstitial fibrosis, pulmonary oedema, and pneumonia, interfering with the normal respiratory exchange of gases. Likewise, the surface area may be greatly decreased in emphysema, to name just a few examples.

The capillaries form a dense network in the walls of the alveoli. The diameter of a capillary is just large enough for a red blood cell; this further increases the efficacy of gaseous exchange by reducing the distance required for diffusion to take place. At rest, each red blood cell spends, on average, about 0.75 seconds in the capillary network, and during this time probably traverses two or three alveoli. Under typical resting conditions, the capillary Po_2 virtually reaches that of the alveolar gas (i.e., equilibration occurs) when the red cell is about one-third of the way along the capillary. This acts as a safety factor so that, during exercise, when the time spent in the capillary by the red cell decreases, it does not compromise oxygenation.

Carbon monoxide (rather than chlorine gas), is the gas of choice for measuring the transfer factor (i.e., the effectiveness of the diffusing surface). Carbon monoxide is used in the test because its great avidity for haemoglobin means that its concentration in the blood can be assumed zero and does not need to be measured.

143. **D: Anaplasia is almost a complete lack of differentiation**

There are certain definitions regarding tumours that need to be remembered and understood:

- *Tumour* simply means 'swelling', which can be benign or malignant
- *Neoplasm* simply means a 'new growth'. It is synonymous with tumour and can be benign or malignant. Malignant neoplasms can be primary or secondary. The latter are also known as metastases
- *Hypertrophy* is an increase in tissue growth through an increase in cell size
- *Hyperplasia* is an increase in tissue growth through an increase in cell numbers
- *Metaplasia* is an adaptive response resulting in the replacement of one differentiated cell type with another
- *Dysplasia* literally means 'disordered growth'. It is the disordered development of cells resulting in an alteration in their size, shape, and organization

- *Carcinoma in situ* is an epithelial tumour with features of malignancy but it has not invaded through the basement membrane
- *Carcinoma* is a malignant tumour of epithelial derivation. By definition, because it is malignant, the basement membrane has been breached
- *Anaplasia* is the almost complete lack of differentiation (i.e., poorly differentiated)

A more formal definition of a neoplasm is 'an abnormal mass of tissue, the growth of which exceeds and is uncoordinated with that of the normal tissues and persists in the same excessive manner after cessation of the stimuli which evoked the change'. The latter part of this definition is to distinguish a true neoplasm from the endometrial growth that normally accompanies the menstrual cycle; endometrial tissue is normally responsive to sex hormones and regresses upon its cessation; a true neoplasm would persist.

144. **D: Leucocytes, erythrocytes, and fibrin filling of the alveolar spaces**

Lobar pneumonia may progress through 4 stages:

- Congestion (in the first 24 hours) – inflammatory exudate
- Red hepatization
- Grey hepatization
- Resolution (complete recovery)

Red hepatization is characterized by a firm consistency to the lung due to filling of the alveolar spaces by extravasated erythrocytes, fibrin, and leucocytes. A fibrin meshwork and degenerating erythrocytes defines grey hepatization.

145. **D: p53 and Rb-1 are tumour suppressor genes**

Tumour suppressor genes encode proteins that negatively regulate cell proliferation and thus suppress tumour growth. p53 and Rb-1 are good examples located on chromosomes 17 and 13, respectively. Normal p53 is the so-called 'guardian of the genome' and triggers apoptosis and cell-cycle arrest in genetically damaged cells (i.e., it is pro-apoptotic). Mutations in p53 therefore result in the propagation of genetically damaged cells and tumourigenesis. Indeed, approximately 50 per cent of human tumours contain mutations in the p53 gene. p53-related cancers are more aggressive and have a poorer prognosis.

In contrast to oncogenes, tumours caused by tumour suppressor genes are generally caused by mutations that result in a loss of function of the gene product; neoplastic growth resulting from the loss of the protective role of tumour suppressor genes. Loss of tumour suppressor function usually requires the inactivation of both alleles of the gene, so that all of the protective effect of tumour suppressor genes is lost. That is, tumour suppressor genes are generally deemed to behave in a recessive manner.

Cellular proliferation is therefore tightly regulated by two sets of opposing functioning genes: the growth-promoting genes (proto-oncogenes) and the negative cell-cycle regulators (tumour suppressor genes). Abnormal activation of proto-oncogenes and/or loss of function of tumour suppressor genes leads to the transformation of a normal cell into a cancer cell.

146. **C: Buccinator**

Buccinator is a muscle of facial expression and is therefore innervated by the facial nerve. The lateral pterygoid, masseter, anterior belly of digastric, and temporalis are all muscles of mastication and therefore innervated by the mandibular division of the trigeminal nerve (Vc).

147. **D: It lies level with the hilum of the kidneys**

The transpyloric plane (of Addison) is an important landmark. It lies halfway between the suprasternal notch and the symphysis pubis at the level of L1. It coincides with the following:

- L1 vertebra
- Fundus of gallbladder
- Hilum of kidneys
- Hilum of spleen
- Pylorus of the stomach (hence the name transpyloric)
- Termination of the spinal cord in adults
- Neck of pancreas
- Origin of the portal vein
- Origin of the superior (not inferior) mesenteric artery
- Duodenojejunal flexure
- Attachment of transverse mesocolon
- Tip of 9th costal cartilage

The aorta bifurcates at the level of L4, not L1.

148. **B: It is potentiated by histamine**

There are 3 classic phases of gastric acid secretion:

- *Cephalic* (preparatory) phase [significant]. This results in the production of gastric acid before food actually enters the stomach. It is triggered by the sight, smell, thought, and taste of food acting via the vagus nerve
- *Gastric* phase [most significant]. This is initiated by the presence of food in the stomach, particularly protein-rich food
- *Intestinal* phase [least significant]. The presence of amino acids and food in the duodenum stimulate acid production

Gastric acid is *stimulated* by three factors:

- *Acetylcholine*: From parasympathetic neurones of the vagus nerve that innervate parietal cells directly
- *Gastrin*: Produced by pyloric G-cells
- *Histamine*: Produced by mast cells

Histamine stimulates the parietal cells directly and also potentiates parietal cell stimulation by gastrin and neuronal stimulation. H_2 blockers such as ranitidine are therefore an effective way of reducing acid secretion.

Gastric acid is *inhibited* by 3 factors:

- Somatostatin
- Secretin
- Cholecystokinin

149. **D: The anterior surface of the right adrenal gland is overlapped by the inferior vena cava**

The adrenal glands lie anterosuperior to the upper part of each kidney. They weigh approximately 5 grams each and measure 50 mm vertically, 30 mm across, and 10 mm thick. They are somewhat asymmetrical, with the right adrenal being pyramidal in shape and left adrenal being crescentic, and lie within their own compartment of (Gerota's) renal fascia. A fascial septum separates the adrenal gland from the kidney, which explains why in nephrectomy (removal of the kidney) the latter gland is not usually displaced (or even seen).

Each gland, although only weighing a few grams, has three arteries supplying it: a direct branch from the aorta, a branch from the renal artery, and a branch from the inferior phrenic artery. This reflects the high metabolic demands of the tissue. The single main suprarenal vein drains into the nearest available vessel: on the right it drains into the inferior vena cava and on the left directly into the renal vein. The right adrenal gland is tucked medially behind the inferior vena cava. In addition, the right suprarenal vein is particularly short and stubby. Both these features make the inferior vena cava vulnerable to damage in a right adrenalectomy.

The adrenal gland comprises an outer cortex and an inner medulla, which represent two developmentally and functionally independent endocrine glands within the same anatomical structure. The medulla is derived from the neural crest (ectoderm). It receives preganglionic sympathetic fibres from the greater splanchnic nerve and secretes adrenaline (70 per cent) and noradrenaline (30 per cent). The cortex is derived from mesoderm and consists of three layers, or zones. The layers from the surface inwards may be remembered by the mnemonic GFR:

- G = zona Glomerulosa (secretes aldosterone)
- F = zona Fasciculata (secretes cortisol and sex steroids)
- R = zona Reticularis (secretes cortisol and sex steroids)

150. **C: It stimulates gastric acid production**

Gastrin is secreted by gastrin-secreting cells (G-cells) found in two locations: the pyloric region of the stomach and the upper half of the small intestine.

Gastrin is released by:

- Vagal stimulation
- Distension of the pyloric antrum
- Proteins (especially partially digested proteins) in the food

Gastrin is inhibited by:

- A low pH in the lumen of the pyloric antrum (negative feedback loop)
- Somatostatin

Gastrin has 3 main actions:

- It stimulates gastric acid secretion
- It stimulates gastric motility
- It stimulates exocrine pancreatic secretions

Overproduction of gastrin leads to excessive gastric acid secretion and the formation of multiple peptic ulcers. This is known as the Zollinger–Ellison syndrome and is often due to a gastrin-secreting tumour (gastrinoma).

151. **C: May produce paraneoplastic syndromes**

Currently lung cancer is the most common cause of death from cancer in both men and women. It is estimated that some 50 per cent of bronchial carcinomas have metastasized by the time of clinical presentation. Lung carcinoma is most commonly due to squamous cell carcinoma as a result of squamous cell metaplasia from smoking. Tobacco smoking is believed to account for 80–90 per cent cases of lung carcinoma; the remainder are associated with radon gas and asbestos exposure.

The pathological effects of any tumour may be local or distant; distant effects may be metastatic or non-metastatic (paraneoplastic). Applying this to lung carcinoma we have:

Local effects

- *Pulmonary involvement*: Cough (infection distal to airway blocked by tumour caused by disruption of the mucociliary escalator), haemoptysis (ulceration/necrosis of tumour), breathlessness (local extension of tumour), chest pain (involvement of pleura and/or chest wall), and wheeze (narrowing of airways)
- *Local invasion*: Hoarseness (recurrent laryngeal nerve infiltration), Horner's syndrome (infiltration of the ipsilateral sympathetic chain), wasting of the intrinsic hand muscles (brachial plexus infiltration), diaphragmatic paralysis (phrenic nerve invasion), pleural effusions (tumour spread into pleura), pericarditis (pericardial involvement), superior vena cava obstruction (direct compression by tumour)

Distant effects

- *Metastatic*: Pathological fractures (bone metastases), neurological symptoms (brain metastases), hepatomegaly, or jaundice (liver metastases)
- *Non-metastatic (paraneoplastic) effects*: Ectopic hormone production (ADH, ACTH, PTHrP, serotonin, etc.), common generalized symptoms (weight loss, anorexia, lassitude) from the acute-phase response (IL-1, IL-6, TNFα)

Paraneoplastic syndromes are symptoms and signs associated with a malignant tumour that are not due to direct local effects of the tumour or the development of metastases.

152. **A: Peptidoglycan**

Prokaryotes have peptidoglycan in their cell walls, which makes them susceptible to penicillin. Sterol and endoplasmic reticulum are features of eukaryotic cells. Bacteria generally contain single, circular chromosomes (plasmids). Prokaryotes contain 70S, rather than 80S ribosomes which are characteristic of eukaryotes.

153. **D: It is unimportant in humans**

The vermiform (worm-shaped) appendix is a blind-ending tube varying in length (commonly 6–9 cm) which opens into the posteromedial wall of the caecum, where the taeniae coli converge. The appendix is an intraperitoneal structure and therefore has its own short mesentery, the mesoappendix. Within the mesentery lies the appendicular artery, a branch of the ileocolic artery which arises from the SMA.

The surface marking of the base of the appendix is situated one-third of the way up the line joining the anterior superior iliac spine to the umbilicus (McBurney's point). This is an important landmark when making an appendicectomy (McBurney's or Gridiron) incision. The position of the free end of the appendix, however, is very variable. The most common, as found at operation, is the retro-caecal or retrocolic position (75 per cent of cases), with the subcaecal or pelvic position next in order of frequency (20 per cent of cases). Less commonly, in 5 per cent of cases it lies in the pre-ileal or retro-ileal positions, in front of the caecum, or in the right paracolic gutter.

The appendix has no known physiological function in man and can therefore be removed without any consequences. It probably represents a degenerated portion of the caecum that, in ancestral forms, aided in cellulose digestion. In the other animals, the appendix is much larger and provides a pouch off the main intestinal tract, in which cellulose can be trapped and be sub-jected to prolonged digestion. The abundance of lymphoid tissue within the submucosa of the appendix has prompted the concept that the appendix is the human equivalent of the avian bursa of Fabricius as a site of matura-tion of thymus-independent lymphocytes. While no discernible change in immune function results from appendicectomy, the prominence of lymphatic tissue in the appendix of young adults seems important in the aetiology of appendicitis.

154. **D: The main stimulation for secretion occurs during the intestinal phase**

The pancreas is a mixed endocrine (ductless) and exocrine gland that forms embryologically from the fusion of separate dorsal and ventral pancreatic buds (endodermal outgrowths from the primitive foregut). The embryology helps to explain how aberrations of development lead to the formation of an annular pancreas, or pancreas divisum, either of which may lead to problems in later life.

The exocrine component of the pancreas consists of closely packed secre-tory acini which drain into a highly branched duct system. Approximately 1500 mL of pancreatic juice is secreted each day into the duodenum via the pancreatic duct. The alkaline pH of the pancreatic secretion (approximately 8.0) is due to a high content of bicarbonate ions and serves to neutralize the acidic chyme as it enters the duodenum from the stomach.

With regard to the secretion of gastric acid, it is possible to distinguish cephalic, gastric, and intestinal phases in the pattern of secretion. The weak cephalic phase contributes only 15 per cent of the total response, an enzyme-rich secretion caused by vagal efferents. The weak gastric phase also contrib-utes only 15 per cent of the total response and is again enzyme-rich, caused by vaso-vagal reflexes originating in the stomach and gastrin secretion. The main stimulation (70 per cent of the total response) is the intestinal phase caused by food entering the duodenum from the stomach. Secretin, a hormone released by endocrine cells scattered in the duodenal mucosa, promotes the secretion of copious watery fluid rich in bicarbonate. The major stimulus for the release of secretin is acid. Cholecystokinin, also derived from duodenal endocrine cells, stimulates the secretion of enzyme-rich pancreatic fluid. Secretin and cholecystokinin act synergistically.

155. **D: Gilbert syndrome**

Gilbert syndrome is an autosomal recessive inherited metabolic disorder (although occasionally inherited in an autosomal dominant fashion depending on the type of mutation), causing increased levels of unconjugated bilirubin in the blood. It is a common hereditary cause of hyperbilirubinaemia. There is decreased activity of the enzyme glucuronyltransferase, which conjugates bilirubin in the liver. Bilirubin is excreted from the body only in the conjugated form. Typical presentation is painless jaundice during an intercurrent illness.

156. **B: Curling ulcer**

Curling ulcer is an acute peptic ulcer associated with major burns. Reduced plasma levels lead to hypovolaemic shock, which causes sloughing of the gastric mucosa secondary to ischaemia. It may result in perforation and haemorrhage and have a high mortality rate. Cushing's ulcers are associated with head injuries and raised ICP. One possible explanation for Cushing's ulcers is that stimulation of vagal nuclei due to raised ICP leads to increased gastric acid production. A Marjolin ulcer is a squamous cell carcinoma (SCC) that develops within a chronic venous ulcer.

157. **C: Loss of ankle dorsiflexion**

In a neck of fibula fracture, the common peroneal nerve is most likely to be damaged as it surrounds the neck as part of its course. The common peroneal nerve supplies muscles in the lateral and anterior compartment of the leg, allowing ankle dorsiflexion and foot eversion. If damaged, the patient is unable to dorsiflex or evert the foot, causing a foot drop and a high-stepping gait.

158. **C: Glossopharyngeal nerve**

Parasympathetic supply is limited to viscera and glands of the body, sparing skin, and skeletal muscles. The majority of the supply arises from the cranial nerves. Cranial nerve (CN) III (oculomotor) supplies the sphincter pupillae and ciliary muscles of the eye. CN VII (facial) supplies the lacrimal, submandibular and sublingual glands, mucosa of the palate, and glands in the nose. CN IX (glossopharyngeal) supplies the parotid gland through the lesser petrosal nerve, otic ganglion, and auriculotemporal nerves. CN X (vagus) supplies the thoracic and abdominal viscera up to two-thirds of the way along the transverse colon.

159. **E: The tibialis anterior and tibialis posterior**

Foot inversion occurs when the foot turns medially at the subtalar joint. The muscles responsible for this movement are tibialis anterior and posterior. When acting independently, the tibialis anterior dorsiflexes the foot and the tibialis posterior plantarflexes the foot. The tibialis anterior is innervated by the deep peroneal nerve whereas the tibialis posterior is innervated by the tibial nerve.

160. **D: Oesophagus**

Stratified squamous epithelium consists of several layers of epithelial cells arranged upon a layer of basement membrane. The layers can be sloughed off and replaced constantly; hence it is suited for areas with constant insults and abrasions. Stratified squamous epithelium can be divided into keratinised and non-keratinised types, depending on the presence of keratin on its surface. Examples of keratinised types include the skin, tongue, and outer lips. Examples of non-keratinised types are cornea, oesophagus, rectum, and vagina. The epididymis and trachea have pseudo-stratified columnar epithelium, whereas the colon and uterus are lined by simple columnar epithelium.

161. **B: Class II**

The Advanced Trauma Life Support (ATLS) classification of haemorrhage is based on the percentage of acute blood loss and the physiological manifestations of haemorrhagic shock. Class I haemorrhage is when less than 15 per cent of circulating volume is lost (<750 mL). There may be a mild increase in heart rate but no other physiological changes. It is exemplified by the condition of a person who has given 1 unit of blood for donation. Class II haemorrhage is when 15–30 per cent of the circulating volume is lost (approximately 0.75–1.5 L). There is tachypnoea (20–30 bpm), tachycardia (>100 bpm), reduced urine output (20–30 mL/h), and narrowed pulse pressure (owing to an increase in diastolic pressure because of catecholamine release). However, systolic blood pressure remains normal. Class III haemorrhage is when 30–40 per cent of the circulating volume is lost (approximately 1.5–2 L). There is tachypnoea (30–40 bpm), tachycardia (>120 bpm), a drop in blood pressure, and reduced urine output (5–15 mL/h). These patients may require blood replacement along with fluid resuscitation. Class IV haemorrhage is when more than 40 per cent of the circulating volume is lost (>2 L). This can be considered a pre-terminal event unless aggressive measures are taken. There is tachypnoea (>35 bpm), tachycardia (>140 bpm), very low blood pressure and pulse pressure, anuria, and possibly unconsciousness.

For an average 70 kg man	Class I	Class II	Class III	Class IV
Blood loss (mL)	<750	750–1500	1500–2000	>2000
Blood loss (%)	<15%	15%–30%	30%–40%	>40%
Pulse rate	<100	>100	>120	>140
Blood pressure (mmHg)	Normal or increased	Narrow pulse pressure	Decreased	Decreased
Respiratory rate	14–20	20–30	30–40	>40
Urine output (mL/hour)	>30	20–30	5–15	Negligible (anuric)
Mental status	Slightly anxious	Mildly anxious	Anxious/ confused	Confused/ lethargic

162. **B: Readings are inaccurate in the presence of carbon monoxide**

Pulse oximetry measures arterial oxygen saturation (not partial pressure). It uses two wavelengths of light (red and infrared) and calculates the difference in absorption of light by oxyhaemoglobin and deoxyhaemoglobin. Oxygen saturation is then calculated from this data. Only the pulsation component of arterial blood is measured and the constant background (skin, fat, and venous blood) is subtracted. However, it has several drawbacks. It does not give a good indication of ventilation (better reflected by the partial pressure of CO_2). In the presence of carbon monoxide, pulse oximetry readings are unreliable. Carbon monoxide competes with oxygen binding to haemoglobin, forming carboxyhaemoglobin, which also appears bright red and gives falsely high saturation reading. Patients with poorly perfused peripheries, owing to hypotension or hypothermia, may also not give reliable saturation readings.

163. **B: It travels anterior to the vagus nerve**

The phrenic nerve arises from the anterior cervical rami of C3, 4, and 5, passing between scalanus medius and scalenus anterior, the latter of which it courses on in the neck. The right and left phrenic nerves travel anterior to the vagus nerve bilaterally.

The right phrenic nerve courses inferiorly, lateral to the superior vena cava, and onto the fibrous pericardium overlying the right atrium; it travels anterior to the root of the lung, then pierces the caval orifice of the diaphragm at T8.

The left phrenic nerve crosses anterior to the aortic arch (in contrast to the left vagus nerve, which crosses posteriorly) and courses inferiorly, anterior to the left pulmonary artery and fibrous pericardium of the left ventricle; after crossing the root of the left lung anteriorly, it passes through the central tendon of the diaphragm.

164. **A: Oesophageal atresia**

Oesophageal atresia is a congenital condition affecting 1 in 3000–4500 births. It is a developmental disorder of the oesophagus, which results in the oesophagus ending as a blind-ended pit. Only 10 per cent of those born with this congenital condition are born with this in isolation, with the remainder having some other form of congenital abnormality. Two-thirds of those born with this condition also have a tracheo-oesophageal fistula present. Other associated abnormalities include vertebral anomalies, anorectal anomalies, cardiac, renal, and limb malformations – the so-called VACTERL association. Diagnosis is confirmed by passing a nasogastric tube, which subsequently coils in the lower oesophagus and is visible on chest X-ray. It is considered a surgical emergency.

165. **D: Duodenal atresia**

The incidence of duodenal atresia is 1 in 5000 births in the UK. The 'double bubble' sign indicates gas in the stomach and proximal duodenum. If not treated it becomes fatal as a result of fluid shifts and electrolyte imbalances. Fullness in the epigastric region is a result of the stomach being full of gas. In oesophageal atresia the baby typically presents with choking rather than vomiting. In gastric outlet obstruction there is no bile in the vomit and, most importantly, it presents later at about 4 weeks whereas duodenal atresia presents at birth. In congenital intestinal obstruction a plain film will show more pathognomonic features of obstruction. There is an association of duodenal atresia with Down's syndrome.

166. **E: Meconium ileus**

Meconium ileus can cause neonatal intestinal obstruction and typically presents in patients with cystic fibrosis (CF) in 10 per cent of cases, where the deficiency of pancreatic enzymes causes the meconium to be thick and viscous. It presents within the first few hours of life with absolute constipation, bile-stained vomiting, and abdominal distension. Meconium is normally passed within the first 24 hours but this fails to occur. Abdominal X-ray (AXR) may display a mottled appearance from the lipid droplets within the meconium. It may be difficult to differentiate from Hirschsprung disease but this typically has multiple air fluid levels on erect AXR. Treatment is with gastrografin enema, provided that there is no evidence of perforation. Gastric outlet obstruction usually presents with non-bilious vomiting.

167. **C: Hirschsprung's disease**

Hirschsprung's disease is a congenital disease where the affected individuals lack mural ganglionic cells in the colon leading to constipation and abdominal distension. Rectal biopsy is the diagnostic investigation of choice to demonstrate the deficiency. Genes involved in the pathogenesis of Hirschsprung disease include RET (chromosome 10), EDNRB (chromosome 13), GDNF (chromosome 5), EDN3 (chromosome 20), SOX10 (chromosome 22), ECE1 (chromosome 1), NTN (chromosome 19), and SIP1 (chromosome 2).

168. **D: Rectus abdominis**

Direct inguinal hernias arise through Hesselbach's triangle, which is bordered by the inferior epigastric artery superiorly and laterally, the inguinal ligament inferiorly, and the lateral border of the rectus abdominis medially.

169. **C: Common hepatic duct, cystic duct, and inferior border of the liver**

There are many variations in biliary tree anatomy and therefore it is important to correctly identify the structures forming Calot's triangle before starting dissection in a cholecystectomy. The gallbladder is supplied by the cystic artery, a branch of the right hepatic artery, which requires ligation during the surgery. The cystic artery lies in Calot's triangle, which is bordered by the inferior border of the liver, the cystic duct, and the common hepatic duct.

170. **C: Long thoracic nerve**

The long thoracic nerve of Bell (C5, C6, C7) supplies the serratus anterior muscle and is responsible for lateral rotation and protraction of the scapula. Owing to its long, relatively superficial course it is susceptible to damage and can be damaged during breast surgery. Injuries can also result from direct trauma or stretching during sports. The winged scapula is most prominent when the patient pushes the outstretched arm against a wall.

171. **B: Ilioinguinal nerve**

     The ilioinguinal nerve innervates the muscles of the lower abdomen, specifically the skin overlying the inguinal region, upper part of the thigh, and anterior third of the scrotum or labia in women. This nerve is at risk in the muscle-splitting incision made for appendicectomy. Damage during appendicectomy would lead to the inability to pull the falx inguinalis over the thin area of weak fascia on the posterior wall of the inguinal canal, thereby predisposing the patient to develop a direct inguinal hernia.

172. **A: 70 mmHg**

     MAP is calculated using the formula: 1/3(pulse pressure) + diastolic pressure. In this case, MAP = 1/3(100 − 70) + 70 = 80 mmHg.

     CPP can be calculated using the MAP and ICP: CPP = MAP − ICP. In this case, CPP = 80 − 10 = 70 mmHg.

     Conservative management of raised ICP involves sedation, intubation keeping ICP at 10 mmHg and maintaining CPP at 60–70 mmHg. CPP is maintained by a phenomenon called autoregulation. Autoregulation is impaired in head injury patients and CPP <70 mmHg is associated with a poor outcome. Therefore, the priority is to maintain CPP as these patients are susceptible to brain injury caused by hypotension.

173. **B: *Pseudomonas aeruginosa***

     Of those organisms mentioned, Pseudomonas is the only Gram-negative bacillus and is typically seen in immunocompromised patients and hospital-acquired infections and is associated with respirators and drainage tubes. Listeria is a Gram-positive bacillus as is actinomyces. Moraxella is a Gram-negative coccus that is seen in atypical pneumonia. *Staphylococcus aureus* is a Gram-positive coccus.

174. **C: Ewing sarcoma**

     Ewing sarcoma is the second most common primary bone tumour in children. It typically affects the diaphysis of long tubular bones, particular the femur. Microscopic examination of the tumour reveals small, round blue cells of unknown origin. Patients typically present with pain and an enlarging mass. Osteosarcoma histology reveals malignant osteoblasts producing osteoid and are usually fairly aggressive tumours, with 20 per cent having pulmonary metastases on presentation. Myeloma is the most common primary bone tumour but typically affects patients over the age of 50. Malignant fibrous histiocytoma tumours on histology consist of spindle cells and giant cells.

175. **C: Parietal cells**

     The gastric parietal cells produce intrinsic factor which binds vitamin B_{12} in the stomach, thereby facilitating its absorption in the ileum. Post-gastrectomy patients require replacement because of the absence of the stomach. The G-cells are found in the antral mucosa and upper small bowel; they secrete gastrin, which stimulates secretion of acid by parietal cells. Goblet cells are found in the bowel, not stomach. Chief cells produce pepsinogen.

176. **E: Papillary**

Papillary thyroid carcinoma is the most common type of thyroid cancer, representing 70 per cent of these cancers in the UK. It typically affects young people and has good survival rates. Histology may demonstrate Orphan Annie nuclei and psammoma calcification, which, when seen, is diagnostic.

177. **C: Gastroduodenal artery**

The duodenum receives blood from the gastroduodenal artery, which is a branch of the common hepatic artery. The gastroduodenal artery lies just behind the superior part of the duodenum. It has two main branches: the right gastroepiploic and the superior pancreaticoduodenal, which is further divided into anterior and posterior parts. The left gastric vein is located in the lesser curvature of the stomach and the splenic vein joins the superior mesenteric vein to form the portal vein.

178. **B: 10**

The GCS offers a reliable, reproducible quantitative assessment of a patient's level of consciousness. It is measured on 3 scales, with the lowest possible score being 3 and highest 15.

Best Motor response:

- 6: Obeys command
- 5: Localises to pain
- 4: Withdraws from pain
- 3: Abnormal flexion
- 2: Extension
- 1: No response

Best Verbal response:

- 5: Orientated
- 4: Confused
- 3: Inappropriate words
- 2: Incomprehensible sounds
- 1: No speech

Best Eye-opening response:

- 4: Opens spontaneously
- 3: Opens to voice
- 2: Opens to pain
- 1: No response

This patient scores 4 on Motor response, 3 on Verbal response, and 3 on Eye response. Her score is therefore 10/15.

179. **E: Left gastroepiploic artery**

    The left and right gastroepiploic arteries supply the lower greater curvature and are the most likely source of bleeding. The fundus and upper left side of the greater curvature is supplied by the short gastric arteries. The lesser curvature is supplied from branches of the left and right gastric arteries.

180. **C: Iliacus**

    The lesser trochanter is on the medial aspect of the proximal femur and the psoas and ilacus muscles attach to this prominence. These muscles flex the hip. The femoral greater trochanter is on the lateral aspect of the hip joint and several muscles attach to this: piriformis, obturator internus and externus, gluteus medius and minimus, and the gemelli.

181. **D: 154 mM**

    The daily requirement of an adult's fluid intake equates to 3 L/day for an average adult. If an individual is placed nil by mouth (NBM) this requirement is easily achieved with three bags of intravenous fluids each run over 8 hours. One litre of normal saline contains 154 mM of Na+. The average adult requires 100 mM of Na+ per day, as well as 60 mM of potassium per day. Addition of 20 mM of potassium to each bag prescribed over the day will achieve this required amount of potassium.

182. **C: Equivocal**

    Triple assessment of any breast lump includes (1) history and examination; (2) mammography and ultrasound scan (USS); and (3) fine-needle aspiration (FNA) or core biopsy, either of which can be done clinically or stereotactically. FNA is performed using a green needle and syringe. The lump is aspirated, if possible, and the contents fixed to a slide before being sent to the laboratory. Once the sample is analysed, the results are graded as:

    - C1 = insufficient sample
    - C2 = benign
    - C3 = uncertain
    - C4 = suspected breast cancer
    - C5 = breast cancer

    A similar system is used for thyroid cytology (Thy 1-5 ratings).

183. **E: T2N1M0**

    TNM is a universally used cancer classification system (Tumour, Node, Metastases) and used in breast cancer. The staging system for breast cancer is:

    - T1 = <2 cm in diameter
    - T2 = 2–5 cm
    - T3 = >5 cm

- T4 = spread to chest wall or skin
- N0 = no palpable lymph nodes
- N1 = same side, mobile nodes
- N2 = same side, fixed nodes
- N3 = lymph nodes supra- or infra-clavicularly/arm lymphoedema
- M0 = no evidence of distant metastases
- M1 = presence of distant metastases

184. A: Benign paroxysmal positional vertigo (BPPV)

Benign paroxysmal positional vertigo (BPPV) occurs as a result of a degenerative condition of the inner ear where calcified particles are dislodged. The attacks of vertigo are short-lived (usually lasting a few seconds) and are provoked by turning of the head. BPPV can occur spontaneously, in cases of chronic otitis media, or secondary to head trauma. The Dix-Hallpike positional manoeuvre reproduces the symptoms achieved by rapidly turning the head when it is positioned and held below the horizontal plane of the body on an examination couch. Treatment is with the Epley manoeuvre. Ménière's disease is a triad of vertigo, deafness, and tinnitus. Acute labyrinthitis causes severe vertigo and loss of hearing.

185. A: Short gastric arteries

The splenic artery runs in the gastrosplenic ligament; this gives rise to the short gastric arteries which supply the fundus in addition to the superior part of the greater curvature. Branches of the left and right gastric arteries supply the lesser curvature of the stomach. The gastroduodenal artery gives rise to the right gastroepiploic artery and the splenic artery gives rise to the left gastro-epiploic artery. Both the right and left gastroepiploic arteries supply the inferior portion of the greater curvature of the stomach, as well as the greater omentum.

186. B: Parietal

The pterion is formed by the frontal, parietal, temporal, and greater wing of sphenoid bones, united by a H-shape formation of sutures. It is situated about 3 cm postero-superiorly to the level of the zygomatic process of the frontal bone. It is an important clinical landmark because it is the weakest part of the skull that is easily fractured by a blow to the side of the head. The anterior branch of the middle meningeal artery runs beneath the pterion and rupture of this vessel causes an extradural haemorrhage. An emergency burr hole may be required to decompress the brain in such situations.

187. D: Eosin

Lipofuscin is a brown pigment that accumulates in ageing cells. It is mainly formed from old cellular membranes that have become cross-linked as a result of free radical damage and which accumulate in residual bodies without being metabolised. It is also referred to as 'ageing pigment'.

188. **E: Telomerase**

    Histamine is stored in mast cells and causes vascular dilatation. Prostaglandins are derived from arachidonic acid and potentiate vascular permeability. Chemokines selectively attract various types of leucocytes to the site of inflammation. Mast cells have high concentration of 5-hydroxytryptamine, which causes vasoconstriction. The enzyme telomerase allows for replacement of short pieces of DNA known as telomeres, which are otherwise shortened when a cell divides via mitosis.

189. **D: *Clostridium perfringens***

    Gas gangrene is a form of spreading tissue necrosis that occurs when spores of *Clostridia perfringens* infect wounds with extensive soft tissue or muscle injury. Palpable crepitus and gas shadows on radiographs may be noted. Prompt diagnosis and definitive treatment with debridement of necrotic tissues, intravenous antibiotics, and supportive care such as hyperbaric oxygen therapy, are vital to prevent poor outcome.

190. **C: Morphogenetic**

    Apoptosis is a type of individual cell death associated with growth and morphogenesis. It can be triggered by factors outside the cell or can be an autonomous cell event ('programmed cell death').

    In embryological development there are 3 categories of autonomous apoptosis:

    - Morphogenetic
    - Histogenic
    - Phylogenetic

    Morphogenetic apoptosis occurs during embryological development involved in alteration of tissue form (e.g., interdigital cell death responsible for separating the fingers). Failure can lead to various pathologies such as syndactyly, cleft palate, spina bifida, and bladder diverticula/fistulae.

    Histogenic apoptosis occurs in the differentiation of tissues and organs, such as in the hormonally controlled differentiation of the accessory reproductive structures from the Mullerian and Wolffian ducts.

    Phylogenetic apoptosis is involved in removing vestigial structures from the embryo, such as the pronephros, a remnant from a much lower evolutionary level.

191. **A: Is a reversible transformation of one type of terminally differentiated cell into another fully differentiated cell type**

    Metaplasia occurs as a tissue response to environmental stress. This causes a reversible transformation of one type of terminally differentiated cell into another fully differentiated cell type, for example, glandular metaplasia of the lower oesophagus (Barrett's oesophagus) – a change from non-keratinising stratified squamous epithelium into columnar (glandular) epithelium.

192. **D: Peutz–Jeghers syndrome**

Peutz–Jeghers syndrome, also known as hereditary intestinal polyposis syndrome, is an autosomal dominant genetic disease characterised by the development of benign hamartomatous polyps in the gastrointestinal tract and hyperpigmented macules on the lips and oral mucosa.

193. **C: Osteosarcoma**

Papillary and follicular carcinomas of thyroid respond to growth-promoting effects of TSH. Oestrogens are associated with breast and endometrial carcinomas. Oestrogen receptor-modulating drug (tamoxifen) is used to blockade the oestrogen receptors in breast carcinoma. Prostatic epithelium and carcinomas are dependent upon androgenic stimulation for growth and survival.

194. **D: Calcitonin**

An innate immune system is formed by physical barriers, such as mucosal epithelium, and secretions with antibacterial activity, such as lactoferrin. Soluble mediators such as CRP and mannose-binding lectin help to enhance the activity of innate and specific responses to an antigen.

195. **D: Immunoglobulin G (IgG)**

B-lymphocytes initially produce IgM antibodies after encounter with an antigen as it is effective in complement fixation and opsonisation. IgM has a short half-life of approximately 5 days. Subsequently, the B-cell undergoes class-switching on T-cell recognition of an epitope on the same antigen. The B cell then produces IgA and IgE at around 1 week and IgG at around 3 weeks.

196. **D: Mucosal infections**

IgA is secreted onto mucosal surfaces. It prevents the initial adherence or mucosal penetration of bacterial and viral pathogens, thereby contributing to respiratory and gastrointestinal immunity. IgA deficiency along with absence of IgG is noted in primary antibody deficiency (PAD). Patients present with respiratory infections caused by encapsulated bacteria such as Haemophilus influenza, Streptococcus pneumonia, and mycoplasma. Gastrointestinal infections are caused by Giardia, Campylobacter, and Salmonella.

197. **C: Mycoplasma arthritis**

Primary antibody deficiency (PAD) syndromes are disorders of B-cell development or function with impaired or absent antibody production. A PAD presents with pneumonia, sinus, and gastrointestinal infections because of the absence of immunoglobulin G (IgG) and immunoglobulin A (IgA). PAD patients with low IgG levels are susceptible to Mycoplasma arthritis. It results in joint destruction and chronic pain. Treatment is with a combination of surgery and tetracycline.

198. **D: Natural killer cells**

Natural killer (NK) cells form part of the innate immune system. They make up about 10 per cent of the peripheral blood lymphocytes. They have no T-cell receptors; however, they have the ability to kill virally infected cells and tumour cells.

199. **B: Papillary thyroid carcinoma**

Psammoma bodies are concentric calcified structures that are a pathognomic feature of papillary carcinoma of thyroid. They are usually present in the cores of the papillae but may also be noted in draining lymph nodes and adjacent tissues. They may also be found in meningiomas and pituitary prolactinomas.

200. **B: Rhabdomyosarcoma**

Rhabdomyosarcoma is a malignant skeletal muscle neoplasm. It usually presents in children and adolescents and can occur in any skeletal muscle in the body. It has three variants: embryonal, alveolar, and pleomorphic. The rhabdomyoblast – the diagnostic cell in all types – contains eccentric eosinophilic granular cytoplasm rich in thick and thin filaments. The rhabdomyoblasts may be round or elongate; the latter are known as tadpole or strap cells and may contain cross-striations visible by light microscopy.

SECTION 2: SINGLE BEST ANSWER QUESTIONS

1. Analysis of arterial blood gases

   pH = 7.59, pCO_2 = 10 kPa,
   pCO_2 = 2.3 kPa, BE = −5.5

   Select the best answer from the options listed below:
   A Metabolic alkalosis
   B Metabolic alkalosis with compensation
   C Respiratory acidosis
   D Respiratory alkalosis
   E Respiratory alkalosis with compensation

2. A 35-year-old woman suffers from endometriosis and bleeds heavily every month. Her heart rate is 105 beats/min and all other parameters are normal. Select the degree of haemorrhagic shock.
   A Class I
   B Class II
   C Class III
   D Class IV
   E None of the above

3. A 45-year-old man is brought in from a road traffic accident. His pulse is 160 beats/min, BP is 75/50 mmHg, and he is unresponsive. Select the degree of haemorrhagic shock.
   A Class I
   B Class II
   C Class III
   D Class IV
   E None of the above

4. According to Wallace's rules, select the single best answer.
   A A man suffers full-thickness burns to his perineum. Degree of burns: 5 per cent
   B A man suffers full-thickness burns to the whole of his left arm. Degree of burns 9 per cent
   C A woman suffers full-thickness burns to her face and head. Degree of burns 18 per cent
   D A woman suffers full-thickness burns to the whole of her left leg. Degree of burns 27 per cent
   E A man suffers full-thickness burns to his back. Degree of burns 36 per cent

5. A 45-year-old woman presents to A&E with epigastric pain, jaundice, vomiting, and fever. Her bilirubin is 125 µmol/L, ALT 135 IU/L, alkaline phosphatase 700 IU/L, WBC 21 × 10⁹/L, and amylase 115 U/mL. On ultrasound the gallbladder wall measures 5 mm and gallstones are seen. The common bile duct measures 9 mm in diameter and the intrahepatic ducts are prominent. Select the likely diagnosis.
   A Carcinoma of head of pancreas
   B Cholangiocarcinoma
   C Pancreatitis
   D Gallstone ileus
   E Mirizzi syndrome

6. A 65-year-old woman presents to her GP with general malaise and grumbling abdominal pain. Her daughter thinks she is looking a little yellow. Her GP refers her for a specialist opinion and on examination there is a mass in the right upper quadrant. Select the likely diagnosis.
   A Carcinoma of head of pancreas
   B Prehepatic jaundice
   C Hepatocellular jaundice
   D Gallstone in common bile duct
   E Sclerosing cholangitis

7. A 45-year-old woman presents with epigastric tenderness and jaundice. She has deranged liver biochemistry and a long history of inflammatory bowel disease. Select the likely diagnosis.
   A Carcinoma of head of pancreas
   B Prehepatic jaundice
   C Hepatocellular jaundice
   D Gallstone in common bile duct
   E Sclerosing cholangitis

8. A 15-year-old boy of African origin presents with splenomegaly and jaundice. He is complaining of abdominal pain and his bilirubin is 100 μmol/L. Select the likely diagnosis.
   A Biliary colic
   B Prehepatic jaundice
   C Hepatocellular jaundice
   D Gallstone in common bile duct
   E Sclerosing cholangitis

9. An 8-month-old boy presents with vomiting and rectal bleeding. There is a sausage-shaped mass palpable in the left side of the abdomen. Select the appropriate diagnosis.
   A Volvulus
   B Intussusception

C Meconium ileus
D Hirschsprung's disease
E Meckel's diverticulum

10. A 3-day-old boy with Down's syndrome presents with vomiting and dehydration. A plain abdominal X-ray demonstrates two bubbles of gas in the upper abdomen. Select the appropriate diagnosis.
    A Gastro-oesophageal reflux disease
    B Pyloric stenosis
    C Duodenal atresia
    D Malrotation
    E Volvulus

11. A 7-week-old boy is brought into A&E. He presents with non-bilious vomiting and dehydration, and on examination there is an olive-sized mass in the right upper quadrant. Select the appropriate diagnosis.
    A Gastro-oesophageal reflux disease
    B Pyloric stenosis
    C Duodenal atresia
    D Malrotation
    E Volvulus

12. A 3-day-old girl with cystic fibrosis has a palpable mass in the right lower quadrant. A plain abdominal X-ray reveals dilated small bowel loops. Select the appropriate diagnosis.
    A Volvulus
    B Intussusception
    C Meconium ileus
    D Hirschsprung's disease
    E Meckel's diverticulum

13. A 35-year-old woman develops pain, swelling, and stiffness of her hands. On examination, 2 years after the onset of her

joint complaints, she is found to have swelling and tenderness in relation to the metacarpophalangeal joints. X-rays of the affected joints show diminution of joint space, osteoporosis, and marginal erosions of the articulating bones. Select the likely diagnosis.

A Osteoarthritis

B Gout

C Rheumatoid arthritis

D Tuberculosis arthritis

E Neuropathic joint disease

14. A 60-year-old woman complains of pain and swelling in both her knees of gradual onset over a duration of 2 years. On examination, there is evidence of excess synovial fluid and synovial thickening in both knee joints and local tenderness. Standing X-rays of her knees show diminution of joint space, sclerosis, and cysts in the adjacent bones. Osteophytes are also seen at the articular margins. Select the likely diagnosis.

A Osteoarthritis

B Gout

C Rheumatoid arthritis

D Tuberculosis arthritis

E Neuropathic joint disease

15. A 14-year-old boy has suffered with left knee pain, which has been gradually increasing in severity over the last month. It is constant in nature and keeps him awake at night. On examination, the overlying skin is warm and shiny. A radiograph of the knee joint demonstrates bone destruction in the metaphysis of the left femur with areas of new bone formation and periosteal elevation. Select the single most likely diagnosis.

A Osteosarcoma

B Osteomalacia

C Metastatic carcinoma

D Osteoblastoma

E Ewing's sarcoma

16. A 16-year-old boy presents with pain in his right upper arm. There is no history of trauma. On examination, he is well with a hot, hard swelling in the middle of his right arm. X-rays demonstrate an onion skin-shaped bone lesion in the medulla of the humerus. Select the single most likely diagnosis.

A Osteosarcoma

B Osteomalacia

C Metastatic carcinoma

D Osteoblastoma

E Ewing's sarcoma

17. A wholesale market producer has been experiencing pain in the lower back for 3 months. During the last 3 weeks he has noticed that the pain radiates down the back of his left leg and now he has difficulty walking. On examination, elevating his left lower limb aggravates the pain. There is diminished sensation on his left heel and along the lateral border of his left foot. The ankle jerk is absent on this side. Select the appropriate nerve.

A 4th lumbar nerve root

B 5th lumbar nerve root

C 1st sacral nerve root

D Sciatic nerve

E Tibial nerve

18. A construction worker presents with loss of sensation over the front and lateral side of his leg and foot. There is no foot drop, but he is unable to evert his foot. Select the appropriate nerve.
    A Sciatic nerve
    B Tibial nerve
    C Common peroneal nerve
    D Deep peroneal nerve
    E Superficial peroneal nerve

19. An 80-year-old retired builder presents with a chronic and slowly enlarging skin lesion over his left cheek. On examination, this lesion is pearly white with an associated telangiectasia. Select the appropriate diagnosis.
    A Basal cell carcinoma
    B Malignant melanoma
    C Squamous cell carcinoma
    D Solar keratosis
    E Keratocanthoma

20. An 82-year-old retired woman presents with a 2-month history of a facial skin lesion. The lesion has now disappeared. Select the appropriate diagnosis.
    A Basal cell carcinoma
    B Malignant melanoma
    C Squamous cell carcinoma
    D Solar keratosis
    E Keratocanthoma

21. A 34-year-old lawyer presents with an itchy brown pigmented lesion on her right lower limb. She states it occasionally bleeds. Select the appropriate diagnosis.
    A Basal cell carcinoma
    B Malignant melanoma
    C Squamous cell carcinoma
    D Solar keratosis
    E Keratocanthoma

22. A 39-year-old woman was a pedestrian hit by a car while crossing the road. She complains of chest and abdominal pains. On examination, her GCS score is 14/15 (E4, V4, M6). Her vital observations are as follows: BP 86/32 mmHg; pulse 145/min. She has bruising and tenderness over her lower left 9th and 10th ribs. She has rebound tenderness and guarding over the left upper quadrant of her abdomen. Her chest X-ray demonstrates left rib fractures affecting ribs 8–10. Select the likely diagnosis.
    A Tension pneumothorax
    B Cardiac tamponade
    C Flail segment
    D Ruptured spleen
    E Haemothorax

23. A 44-year-old man is involved in a road traffic accident. He was the driver of a delivery truck, travelling at 50 miles/h, and was hit from the side. On arrival at A&E he is unstable. His vital observations are as follows: BP 90/32 mmHg; pulse 160/min; respirator rate 45 breaths/min. On examination, his neck veins are engorged and distended. His trachea is central with quiet heart sounds. Select the likely diagnosis.
    A Tension pneumothorax
    B Cardiac tamponade
    C Flail segment
    D Ruptured spleen
    E Haemothorax

24. 24. A 72-year-old woman presents with an ulcer over the anteromedial aspect of the lower limb. It is

flat, with edges sloping towards the centre, and has seropurulent discharge. She does not recall any trauma. She has suffered 'for years' with an aching pain over the leg due to her varicose veins. Over the last 2 months she has noted that this area is now brown in colour. Select the likely diagnosis.

A Chronic obliterative arterial disease

B Venous ulcer

C Traumatic ulcer

D Rheumatoid arthritis

E Squamous cell carcinoma

25. An 80-year-old retired cook has noticed that the edge of an ulcer situated above the medial malleolus for 17 years has recently become 'heaped up' and bleeds easily on contact. Select the likely diagnosis.

A Chronic obliterative arterial disease

B Venous ulcer

C Traumatic ulcer

D Rheumatoid arthritis

E Squamous cell carcinoma

26. A 67-year-old man is admitted as an emergency with back pain. He is found to be shocked with a blood pressure of 90/40 mmHg. An epigastric mass is palpable and tender. Select the most appropriate investigation.

A Immediate ultrasound

B Insert intravenous lines, cross-match blood, and transfer to theatre

C Immediate CT head scan

D Immediate CT chest scan

E Immediate endovascular stenting

27. A 67-year-old man is admitted with a palpable expansive epigastric mass and thoracic back pain. His blood pressure is normal and there is gross widening of the mediastinum on chest X-ray. Select the most appropriate investigation.

A Immediate ultrasound

B Insert intravenous lines, cross-match blood, and transfer to theatre

C Immediate CT head scan

D Immediate CT chest scan

E Immediate endovascular stenting

28. A 26-year-old man is admitted following a sudden onset of severe headache coupled with photophobia and neck stiffness. Select the most appropriate investigation.

A Immediate ultrasound

B Insert intravenous lines, cross-match blood, and transfer to theatre

C Immediate CT head scan

D Immediate CT chest scan

E Immediate endovascular stenting

29. A 30-year-old woman with known pernicious anaemia suffers with dizzy spells, fatigue, and lethargy. Her investigations reveal a low blood pressure and high serum potassium concentration. Select the likely diagnosis.

A Cushing's syndrome

B Conn's syndrome

C Addison's disease

D Multiple endocrine neoplasia type 1 (Werner's syndrome)

E Multiple endocrine neoplasia type 2a

30. A 42-year-old woman presents with epigastric pain. Her past medical history includes: peptic

ulcers and hirsutism. She is under investigation for bilateral lower limb oedema. Her recent blood tests demonstrate hypercalcaemia and hypoglycaemia. Select the likely diagnosis.

A Cushing's syndrome
B Conn's syndrome
C Addison's disease
D Multiple endocrine neoplasia type 1 (Werner's syndrome)
E Multiple endocrine neoplasia type 2a

31. A 2-year-old boy is referred with a scrotal swelling during the day. At night, it resolves. On examination, there is a fluctuant transilluminable swelling in the right scrotum. It is not possible to get above the swelling. No bowel sounds are auscultated in the swelling. Select the likely diagnosis.

A Inguinal hernia
B Epispadias
C Hypospadias
D Non-communicating hydrocele
E Communicating hydrocele

32. A 55-year-old writer presents to A&E with abdominal pain and haematemesis. On examination, he is ethanolic with hepatomegaly. He is also noted to have spider naevi and palmar erythema. Select the appropriate diagnosis.

A Gastric volvulus
B Oesophageal varices
C Caecal carcinoma
D Strangulated hernia
E Achalasia

33. A 6-year-old boy presents with two episodes of vomiting, coupled with central abdominal pain. He

has a 2-day history of a sore throat and enlarged tonsils. On examination, he is apyrexial (but his mother reports a temperature of 38°C yesterday) with a pulse rate of 100/min. His mucosa membranes are dry with increased skin turgor. His tonsils are enlarged with obvious pus. His abdomen is soft, but tender to palpation.

A Hypertrophic pyloric stenosis
B Intussusception
C Gastro-oesophageal reflux
D Mesenteric adenitis
E Meckel's diverticulum

34. A 2-year-old boy presents with dark-red rectal bleeding and general pallor. There has been no vomiting and abdominal examination is unremarkable. Select the likely diagnosis.

A Hypertrophic pyloric stenosis
B Intussusception
C Gastro-oesophageal reflux
D Mesenteric adenitis
E Meckel's diverticulum

35. A 25-year-old woman is admitted to hospital with anorexia, abdominal pain, and diarrhoea over the previous 24 hours. She has vomited and has a low-grade pyrexia. She is tender in the lower abdomen and on rectal examination. Select the likely diagnosis.

A Non-bacterial food poisoning
B Carcinoma of the anus
C Typhoid fever
D Acute appendicitis
E Amoebic dysentery

36. A 70-year-old man recently returned from Bangladesh is admitted with a high temperature and persistent bloody diarrhoea

with a grossly abnormal rectal mucosa on sigmoidoscopy. Select the likely diagnosis.
A Non-bacterial food poisoning
B Carcinoma of the anus
C Typhoid fever
D Acute appendicitis
E Amoebic dysentery

37. A 64-year-old man is admitted with a 3-month history of inter-mittent diarrhoea, anorexia, and weight loss. He has a recent 1 week history of passing painless motions with dark-red blood mixed within the stool. Select the likely diagnosis.
A Non-bacterial food poisoning
B Carcinoma of the anus
C Typhoid fever
D Acute appendicitis
E Amoebic dysentery

38. A 75-year-old women pres-ents with a 4-month history of difficulty swallowing. She is now having difficulty swal-lowing fluids. Of note, she is a regular smoker. Select the likely diagnosis.
A Achalasia
B Oesophageal carcinoma
C Pharyngeal pouch
D Inflammatory stricture
E Plummer–Vinson syndrome

39. A 73-year-old homeless man has a history of recurrent sore throats for which he has completed a course of antibiotics, but there has been no improvement. He presents to A&E with a lump on the left side of his neck. Select the likely diagnosis.
A Achalasia
B Oesophageal carcinoma

C Pharyngeal pouch
D Inflammatory stricture
E Plummer–Vinson syndrome

40. A 25-year-old man discovers a hard lump on his left testicle. His GP has arranged a blood test (β-hCG) which is positive. Select the likely diagnosis.
A Seminoma
B Teratoma
C Torsion of testis
D Torsion of hydatid of Morgagni
E Inguinal hernia

41. An 18-year-old man, an avid football player, develops a sud-den onset of acute pain in his right testicle. There is no history of trauma. On examination, he is apyrexial and there is a small and very tender lump on the superior pole of the right testicle. The tes-ticle is located in a normal ana-tomical position. Select the likely diagnosis.
A Seminoma
B Teratoma
C Torsion of testis
D Torsion of hydatid of Morgagni
E Inguinal hernia

42. A 30-year-old man, with a 7-year history of ulcerative colitis, complains of fluctuating jaun-dice, right upper quadrant pain, and weight loss for the previous 6 months. Plasma alkaline phos-phatase is 20 U/L (normal range 30–130 U/L). Select the likely diagnosis.
A Primary biliary cirrhosis
B Ascending cholangitis
C Hepatic metastases
D Cholangiocarcinoma
E Primary sclerosing cholangitis

43. A 25-year-old man has noticed mild intermittent jaundice for the past 6 years. His blood tests demonstrate a moderate unconjugated hyperbilirubinemia with otherwise normal liver function tests and hepatic histology. Select the likely diagnosis.
    A Gilbert's syndrome
    B Common bile duct stone
    C Acute alcoholic hepatitis
    D Carcinoma of head of pancreas
    E Primary biliary cirrhosis

44. A 57-year-old woman presents with a 5-week history of jaundice, anorexia, and weight loss. She has a pyrexia of 37.8°C. She has a tender enlarged liver (12 cm), mild ascites, widespread spider naevi, and palmar erythema. Laboratory studies demonstrate a leucocytosis of 20×10^9/L, plasma alanine transaminase 280 U/L (normal range 2–50 U/L), plasma albumin 24 g/L (normal range 35–50 g/L), and prothrombin time (PT) of 20 seconds (control 13 s). Select the likely diagnosis.
    A Gilbert's syndrome
    B Common bile duct stone
    C Acute alcoholic hepatitis
    D Carcinoma of head of pancreas
    E Primary biliary cirrhosis

45. A 62-year-old man presents with a 3-month history of weight loss, increasing jaundice, and nocturnal epigastric pain. Five years ago he underwent an anterior resection of the rectum. On examination, there is a right upper quadrant mass that moves on respiration. Laboratory studies show plasma alkaline phosphatase of 752 U/L (normal range 30–130 U/L). Select the likely diagnosis.
    A Carcinoma of head of pancreas
    B Primary biliary cirrhosis
    C Ascending cholangitis
    D Hepatic metastases
    E Cholangiocarcinoma

46. A 45-year-old man presents with loin pain and haematuria. He has a palpable mass in his loin. Select the likely diagnosis.
    A Transitional cell carcinoma
    B Pelvi-ureteric junction obstruction
    C Renal cell carcinoma
    D Pyelonephritis
    E March haemoglobinuria

47. A 68-year-old man presents with acute painless frank haematuria. He had a similar episode several months ago. Moreover, he has noticed recent clots in his urine. On examination, his abdomen is soft and non-tender. Select the likely diagnosis.
    A Transitional cell carcinoma
    B Pelvi-ureteric junction obstruction
    C Renal cell carcinoma
    D Pyelonephritis
    E March haemoglobinuria

48. Select best pairing of wound classification with the description.
    A A 15-year-old man underwent an emergency appendicectomy for a perforated appendix. Classification of wound: Contaminated Class III
    B A 62-year-old man underwent an elective right-sided hemicolectomy for bowel cancer. Classification of wound: Dirty Class IV

C A 31-year-old man underwent an elective inguinal hernia repair. Classification of wound: Clean Contaminated Class III

D A 42-year-old woman underwent an open cholecystectomy. Classification of wound: Clean Contaminated Class II

E A 43-year-old man underwent an emergency repair for perforated small bowel following a stabbing. Classification of wound: Contaminated Class III

49. A 30-year-old man complains of polyuria and polydipsia. His fasting blood glucose is 4.7 mmol/L. Biochemical investigations reveal: Na 140 mmol/L; K 4.2 mmol/L; Ca 2.85 mmol/L; phosphate 0.4 mmol/L; PTH 4.2 pmol/L. Select the likely diagnosis.

(Normal ranges are: sodium 135–145 mmol/L; potassium 3.4–5.0 mmol/L; calcium 2.20–2.65 mmol/L; phosphate 0.8–1.4 mmol/L; PTH 1.1–6.8 pmol/L.)

A Addison's disease
B Cushing's syndrome
C Hypercalcaemia of malignancy
D Primary hyperparathyroidism
E Secondary hyperparathyroidism

50. A 50-year-old Asian woman complains of tingling in her hands and feet. On checking her blood pressure, her hands reveal carpal spasm. Her fasting blood glucose is 4.9 mmol/L. Biochemical investigations reveal: Na 141 mmol/L; K 4.1 mmol/L; Ca 1.85 mmol/L; phosphate 1.4 mmol/L; PTH 80 pmol/L. Select the likely diagnosis.

(Normal ranges are: sodium 135–145 mmol/L; potassium 3.4–5.0 mmol/L; calcium 2.20–2.65 mmol/L; phosphate 0.8–1.4 mmol/L; PTH 1.1–6.8 pmol/L.)

A Addison's disease
B Cushing's syndrome
C Hypercalcaemia of malignancy
D Primary hyperparathyroidism
E Secondary hyperparathyroidism

51. A 50-year-old Asian woman complains of nocturia and dizziness. Her fasting blood glucose is 3.9 mmol/L. Biochemical investigations reveal: Na 131 mmol/L; K 6.1 mmol/L; Ca 2.75 mmol/L; phosphate 1.0 mmol/L; PTH 1.3 pmol/L. Select the likely diagnosis.

(Normal ranges are: sodium 135–145 mmol/L; potassium 3.4–5.0 mmol/L; calcium 2.20–2.65 mmol/L; phosphate 0.8–1.4 mmol/L; PTH 1.1–6.8 pmol/L.)

A Addison's disease
B Cushing's syndrome
C Hypercalcaemia of malignancy
D Primary hyperparathyroidism
E Secondary hyperparathyroidism

52. A 60-year-old man complains of knee pain and examination reveals a moderate effusion. Withdrawal of fluid and microscopy reveals crystals, which on viewing under polarized light are positively birefringent. Select the likely diagnosis.

A Acute gout
B Ankylosing spondylitis
C Osteoarthritis
D Pseudogout
E Psoriatic arthropathy

53. A 21-year-old footballer presents to A&E with a stabbing pain above his right knee joint. He states the pain came on suddenly while he was sprinting. On examination he is unable to extend the leg and he walks with a limp. There is suprapatellar swelling and an absent knee jerk. What is the likely diagnosis?
    A Fracture of patella
    B Injury to posterior cruciate ligament
    C Tear of adductor magnus muscle
    D Tear of biceps femoris muscle
    E Tear of quadriceps tendon

54. During strenuous exercise, what else occurs besides tachycardia?
    A Rise in $PaCO_2$
    B Increased stroke volume
    C Rise in mixed venous blood O_2 saturation
    D No change to blood pressure
    E Increased renal blood flow

55. Which cells cannot regenerate?
    A Peripheral nerve cells
    B Schwann cells
    C Renal tubular cells
    D Mucosal cells
    E Liver cells

56. Which of the following is a feature of metastatic spread?
    A Commonly occurs transluminally
    B Basal cell carcinomas commonly spread via lymphatics
    C Osteosarcomas commonly spread via lymphatics
    D Prostatic carcinoma commonly spreads via the blood
    E Spread follows the pattern of venous drainage

57. In wound healing, which cells are responsible for wound contraction?
    A Fibroblasts
    B Macrophages
    C Reticulocytes
    D Giant cells
    E Lymphocytes

58. Which is a feature of an adenoma?
    A Typically encapsulated
    B Can arise in transitional epithelial cells
    C Typically invades the basement membrane
    D Typically annular lesions
    E Does not contain dysplastic cells

59. A singer complains of not being able to sing high notes following her thyroidectomy. What is the likely cause?
    A Damage to the recurrent laryngeal nerve
    B Damage to the external laryngeal nerve
    C Damage to the vagus nerve
    D Tracheal stenosis
    E Vocal cord hemiparalysis

60. When performing a left nephrectomy from a posterior approach, which of the following structures are encountered before reaching the kidney?
    A Peritoneum
    B Suprarenal gland
    C Subcostal nerve
    D Tail of pancreas
    E Right hemidiaphragm

61. When performing a right hemicolectomy, which of the following structures is encountered during dissection?
    A Caudate lobe of liver
    B Inferior vena cava

C Third part of duodenum

D Right ureter

E First part of duodenum

62. **What causes a reduction in pulmonary functional residual capacity?**

A Asthma

B Pulmonary fibrosis

C Emphysema

D Pneumonia

E Pulmonary oedema

63. **Which is a feature of the physiology of angiotensin II?**

A Stimulates renin release

B Inhibits aldosterone release

C Weak arteriolar vasoconstriction

D Converted from angiotensin I in the liver

E Released in hypovolaemia

64. **Which displaces the oxygen–haemoglobin curve to the left?**

A A decrease in pH

B Anaemia

C A rise in pCO_2

D A fall in pCO_2

E Pyrexia

65. **What factor decreases coronary perfusion?**

A Hypoxia

B Antidiuretic hormone (ADH)

C Alpha stimulation

D Beta stimulation

E Glyceryl trinitrate (GTN) spray

66. **Resection of the terminal ileum is associated with malabsorption of which of the following substances?**

A Calcium

B Folic acid

C Cholesterol

D Bile salts

E Potassium

67. **Which is a feature of the action of insulin?**

A Promotes protein synthesis

B Promotes gluconeogenesis

C Inhibits potassium entry into cells

D Promotes calcium release from bone

E Promotes phosphate release from bone

68. **Which causes prolonged vomiting due to pyloric stenosis?**

A A drop in serum urea

B A drop in bicarbonate

C A rise in serum potassium

D A rise in serum chloride

E A rise in arterial pCO_2

69. **A patient on the surgical ward has chronic renal impairment. The plasma creatinine is 225 µmol/L and the glomerular filtration rate (GFR) is 25 mL/min. Which statement is correct regarding the patient's renal function?**

A The GFR is the main factor determining the rate of urine production

B GFR can be measured by para-aminohippuric acid (PAH)

C The normal GFR is 50 mL/min

D Inulin clearance can be used to estimate GFR

E A normal plasma creatinine implies normal renal function

70. **Gastric acid secretion is stimulated by which of the following?**

A Somatostatin

B Gastrin

C Secretin

D The glossopharyngeal nerve

E Cholecystokinin

71. Carbon dioxide is principally transported in the blood in which form?
    A CO_2 physically dissolved in solution
    B Carboxyhaemoglobin
    C Bicarbonate
    D Carbaminohaemoglobin
    E Carbonic anhydrase

72. A patient with a 6 cm abdominal aortic aneurysm is scheduled for elective repair. As part of the preoperative workup, an echo-cardiogram is requested. The ejection fraction is defined as what?
    A The ratio of end-diastolic volume to stroke volume
    B The ratio of stroke volume to end-diastolic volume
    C End-diastolic volume minus end-systolic volume
    D End-systolic volume divided by stroke volume
    E The ratio of stroke volume to end-systolic volume

73. Bile salt reuptake principally occurs where?
    A In the duodenum
    B In the jejunum
    C In the ileum
    D In the colon
    E In the caecum

74. A 40-year-old patient is brought into the A&E unit with a head injury. The cardiovascular effects of raised intracranial pressure include (BP = blood pressure; HR = heart rate; CPP = cerebral perfusion pressure):
    A ↓ BP, ↓ HR, ↓ CPP
    B ↓ BP, ↑ HR, ↓ CPP
    C ↑ BP, ↑ HR, ↓ CPP
    D ↑ BP, ↓ HR, ↓ CPP
    E ↓ BP, ↑ HR, ↑ CPP

75. A patient is diagnosed with Conn's syndrome. Aldosterone is secreted from where?
    A Liver
    B Zona glomerulosa of the adrenal cortex
    C Juxtaglomerular apparatus
    D Adrenal medulla
    E Zona fasciculata of the adrenal cortex

76. Which of the following gastro-intestinal fluids is richest in potassium?
    A Salivary
    B Pancreatic
    C Gastric
    D Bile
    E Small bowel

77. Which of the following is a feature of the adaptive (acquired) immune response?
    A Acute inflammation
    B Secretion of tears
    C Natural killer cells
    D Surface epithelia
    E Self/non-self discrimination

78. With regard to the thyroid gland, which of the following is true?
    A Tri-iodothyronine is the principal hormone of the gland
    B Calcitonin is produced by follicu-lar cells
    C Organification involves the bind-ing of tetra-iodothyronine to amino acids
    D It is stimulated to produce thy-roxine (T4) by TRH
    E Thyroglobulin is stored in the colloid of follicles

79. Which one of the following is a depolarizing neuromuscular blocker?
    A Atracurium
    B Atropine
    C Guanethidine
    D Suxamethonium
    E Neostigmine

80. With regard to genital development:
    A The mesonephric (Wolffian) ducts differentiate into the female genitalia
    B Female development is hormonally regulated through the actions of anti-Mullerian hormone and testosterone
    C Gender is principally determined by the presence or absence of two X chromosomes
    D Anti-Mullerian hormone is secreted by Leydig cells
    E The testes and ovaries descend from their original position at the 10th thoracic level

81. With regard to visual field pathways:
    A The axons contained within the optic nerve are derived from photoreceptors
    B The optic tracts synapse in the medial geniculate nucleus of the thalamus
    C Decussation is complete at the optic chiasm
    D The macula region is grossly overrepresented in the visual cortex
    E Compression at the optic chiasm results in a homonymous hemianopia

82. With regard to neutrophils (polymorphonuclear leucocytes):
    A They are the predominant cell type in chronic inflammation
    B They have bilobed nuclei
    C They have a lifespan of only a few hours in inflamed tissue
    D They may fuse to form multinucleate giant cells
    E They carry out oxygen-dependent microbial killing by lysosomal enzymes

83. Which one of the following regarding myoglobin in skeletal muscle is correct?
    A It binds and stores oxygen for rapid release during falling P_{O_2}
    B It contains a magnesium cofactor
    C It releases oxygen at high P_{O_2}
    D It exhibits cooperative binding with O_2 (sigmoid dissociation curve)
    E It is devoid of iron

84. With regard to development of the limbs:
    A Occurs in the second trimester of pregnancy
    B Shaping of the hands and feet is brought about through apoptosis
    C Is independent of the apical ectodermal ridge
    D Thalidomide most commonly causes clinodactyly
    E Under some circumstances limb regeneration occurs to a small degree in adult humans following amputation

85. With regard to blood clotting:
    A The haemostatic response comprises two key events
    B Blood platelets have a small single-lobed nucleus
    C The conversion of fibrinogen to fibrin is catalysed by prothrombin
    D It is reversed by plasmin (fibrinolysin)
    E Liver failure results in a prothrombotic state

86. With regard to hepatitis B:
    A It is an RNA virus
    B Infection is more commonly cleared if acquired in childhood than later in life
    C It is the second most common human carcinogen worldwide
    D It is commonly acquired by the faeco-oral route
    E It is effectively treated by hepatitis B vaccination

87. A skydiver lands forcefully on his right lower limb and suffers a fracture of the acetabulum, with a dislocation of the femoral head into the pelvis. The acetabulum is formed by the ilium, ischium, and pubis. These three bones are completely fused by:
    A Birth
    B 6 years of age
    C Puberty
    D 16 years of age
    E 23 years of age

88. With regard to the microcirculation and formation of lymph:
    A At the arterial end of the capillary, the plasma colloid osmotic pressure exceeds the capillary hydrostatic pressure
    B At the venous end of the capillary, the capillary hydrostatic pressure exceeds the plasma colloid osmotic pressure
    C Oedema results from a rise in colloid osmotic pressure
    D Interstitial fluid hydrostatic pressure is normally negative
    E All the fluid that is filtered from the capillary flows into lymph vessels

89. Human immunodeficiency virus (HIV):
    A Is a DNA virus
    B Contains RNA polymerase

C Is transmitted by the faeco-oral route
D Establishes persistence through antigenic variation
E Principally targets CD8 T-cells

90. Typical physical and laboratory findings in hyperthyroidism include which of the following:
    A Bradycardia
    B Delayed reflexes
    C High serum cholesterol
    D Thick, rough skin
    E Tremor

91. With regard to cystic fibrosis:
    A Inheritance is sex-linked
    B It is caused by a genetic defect on chromosome 6
    C It is the most common inherited disease in Caucasians
    D Patients can expect a normal life expectancy
    E Gene therapy is a well-established treatment option

92. With regard to the cerebral circulation:
    A Cerebral blood flow is mainly governed by cardiovascular reflexes
    B Cerebral blood flow is very sensitive to changes in the pCO_2 of the perfusing blood
    C Cerebral blood flow increases steeply with increasing blood pressure
    D It comprises functional end-arteries
    E Raised intracranial pressure results in hypotension and tachycardia

93. With regard to influenza:
    A It is a DNA virus
    B It belongs to the Picornaviridae family of viruses

C Antigenic drift is responsible for pandemics

D Mutations in the haemagglutinin molecule are responsible for antigenic drift

E It can be prevented by administration of a live vaccine

94. **Risk factors for developing osteoporosis include:**

A Obesity

B Low calcium intake

C Late menopause

D Excessive rigorous physical exercise

E Abstinence from alcohol

95. **Haemophilia A:**

A Is more common in females than males

B Is due to an abnormal gene on the Y chromosome

C Is synonymous with Christmas disease

D Is due to a deficiency in factor IX

E Affects the intrinsic, rather than the extrinsic, pathway for blood coagulation

96. **With regard to the facial nerve:**

A It carries taste sensation from the posterior third of the tongue

B It innervates the levator palpebrae superioris muscle

C It is secreto-motor to the lacrimal gland

D It is associated with the 3rd branchial arch

E It supplies the principal muscles of mastication

97. **Which one of the following statements concerning lung volumes is true?**

A The functional residual capacity is the sum of the tidal volume and residual volume

B The vital capacity is the sum of the inspiratory reserve volume, the expiratory reserve volume, and the tidal volume

C The functional residual capacity can be measured directly by spirometry

D The residual volume is the volume of air left in the lungs after normal quiet expiration

E The normal tidal volume is approximately 2 L

98. **The pathogenicity of the tubercle bacillus is primarily due to which one of the following?**

A Ability to multiply within macrophages

B Delayed hypersensitivity reaction against the bacteria

C Direct toxic effect on host cells

D Effective antibody response

E Necrosis caused by expanding granulomas

99. **A 36-year-old man has a neck tumour. It has damaged his left cervical sympathetic chain ganglion. Which of the following physical signs would you expect?**

A Increased sweat secretion on the left side of the face

B Lateral deviation of the left eye

C Pale skin on the left side of his face

D Ptosis on the left

E Pupil dilatation of the left eye

100. **With regard to sickle cell anaemia:**

A The inheritance pattern is autosomal dominant

B It is caused by a mutation within the haemoglobin alpha chain

C Mutation is a valine–alanine substitution

D It is more common in regions of the world in which malaria is endemic

E It causes splenomegaly in adulthood

101. **With regard to the spinal cord and vertebral column:**
    A The spinal cord terminates at the level of L4
    B The intervertebral joints are secondary cartilaginous joints
    C It is supplied by two anterior spinal arteries and one posterior spinal artery
    D Batson's vertebral venous plexus contains valves
    E Intervertebral disc prolapse at L4/5 causes L4 root compression

102. **With regard to surfactant:**
    A It increases the surface tension of the film of liquid lining the alveoli
    B It reduces lung compliance
    C It is secreted by type I pneumocytes
    D The surface tension of fluid containing surfactant increases as the surface area of the fluid decreases
    E It helps to prevent the formation of pulmonary oedema

103. ***Mycobacterium tuberculosis*:**
    A Is a Gram-negative organism
    B Is an anaerobic microorganism
    C Typically affects the apical lung in post-primary TB
    D Is treated with penicillin
    E Is impossible to acquire following BCG vaccination

104. **What are the insensible losses of water (i.e., skin and lung) over 24 hours in a typical adult male at room temperature?**
    A 0 mL
    B 100–300 mL

C 500–1000 mL
D 2500–3500 mL
E 4000–5000 mL

105. **With regard to disorders of haemoglobin:**
    A Sickle cell disease is due to the decreased production of normal globin
    B Haemoglobin binds more avidly to oxygen than carbon monoxide
    C Defective haem synthesis results in porphyria
    D Thalassaemia is due to the production of abnormal globin
    E Cyanide kills by blocking the interaction between oxygen and haemoglobin

106. **With regard to pulmonary blood flow:**
    A Dilatation of pulmonary blood vessels occurs in response to hypoxia
    B The pulse pressure in the pulmonary artery is about the same as that in the aorta
    C During exercise, blood flow to the upper portion of the lung increases
    D The ventilation/perfusion ratio is the same in all parts of the lung in a standing man
    E Pulmonary vascular resistance is six times greater than that of the systemic circulation

107. **With regard to tetanus:**
    A It is caused by a Gram-negative bacillus
    B It is caused by an aerobic organism
    C It results from the secretion of exotoxin
    D It is caused by *Clostridium perfringens*
    E It is caused by bacterial invasion of the nervous system

108. Nitric oxide (NO) results in induction of vascular smooth muscle relaxation in response to acetylcholine. The production of NO requires which amino acid?
     A Lysine
     B Glutamine
     C Cysteine
     D Aspargine
     E Arginine

109. In a certain trial, the mean ± standard error is 0.5 ± 0.2, with a *p*-value under 0.005. This implies that:
     A Ninety-five per cent of the values lie between 0.1 and 0.9
     B This difference would have arisen by chance alone less than one time in 200
     C This difference would have arisen by chance alone less than one time in 20,000
     D One can be 95 per cent confident that the true population mean lies somewhere within the interval 0.3–0.7
     E There is a 2.5 per cent chance that the true population mean lies outside the range 0.1–0.9

110. With regard to the inguinal canal:
     A The superficial inguinal ring is a hole in transversalis fascia
     B The canal runs from the anterior superior iliac spine to the pubic tubercle
     C The conjoint tendon is formed by fusion of external and internal oblique muscles
     D The posterior wall of the canal is bounded by transversalis fascia and the conjoint tendon medially

E A direct inguinal hernia passes through both the deep and superficial inguinal rings

111. With regard to the juxtaglomerular apparatus:
     A The macula densa is a specialized region of the afferent arteriole
     B Renin is secreted at the macula densa
     C Renin is secreted in response to a raised sodium at the macula densa
     D A fall in pressure in the afferent arteriole promotes renin secretion
     E The juxtaglomerular (granular) cells are located in the wall of the distal convoluted tubule

112. Which of the following malignant neoplasms rarely metastasizes to distant sites:
     A Bronchial carcinoma
     B Breast carcinoma
     C Astrocytomas
     D Renal-cell carcinoma
     E Melanoma

113. A 56-year-old man presents with a productive cough and weight loss. Chest X-ray demonstrates a large hilar mass. Sputum cytology shows oval cells with hyperchromatism, paucity of cytoplasm, and inconspicuous nuclei. These malignant cells are most likely associated with:
     A Clara cells
     B Metaplastic bronchial epithelial cells
     C Neuroendocrine cells
     D Type I alveolar pneumocytes
     E Type 2 alveolar pneumocytes

114. The following table shows the results for a screening test for pancreatic cancer in 100 people:

	Disease positive	Disease negative
Test positive	4	5
Test negative	1	90

Which of the following is true?
A The positive predictive value is 0.95
B The sensitivity is 0.95
C The specificity is 0.8
D The negative predictive value is 0.99
E The sensitivity and specificity depends on the disease prevalence

115. With regard to the epiploic foramen (of Winslow), which of the following is true?
A The posterior wall is formed from the lesser omentum
B The portal vein lies in its posterior wall
C Superiorly lies the quadrate lobe of the liver
D The common bile duct sits in the free edge of the greater omentum anteriorly
E It forms the entrance to the lesser sac

116. With regard to ADH (arginine vasopressin):
A It increases in response to a loss of circulating volume of at least 10 per cent
B It is secreted by the pars distalis (adenohypophysis)
C Increased secretion occurs in response to hypo-osmolar blood

D It causes water reabsorption from the loop of Henle
E Insufficiency results in diabetes mellitus

117. One sensitive indicator of heavy alcohol dependence is:
A Decreased mean cell volume (MCV)
B Decreased serum alkaline phosphatase
C Elevated serum creatinine
D Elevated serum gamma-glutamyl transpeptidase
E Elevated serum indirect bilirubin

118. Which of the following are features of small bowel?
A Valvulae conniventes
B Haustra
C Sacculations
D Appendices epiploicae
E Taeniae coli

119. With regard to acid–base balance:
A The normal pH of arterial blood is 7.85–7.95
B The pH of the blood fluctuates widely
C The kidneys respond most rapidly to a change in pH
D The kidney is able to generate new bicarbonate from glutamine
E The renal tubule reabsorbs hydrogen ions and actively excretes bicarbonate

120. Which is true of tumour kinetics?
A The smallest clinically detectable tumour is 1000 cells
B Tumour growth obeys Gompertzian kinetics
C In most tumours, the growth fraction is greater than 90 per cent

D Tumour growth is characterized by contact inhibition

E The clinical phase of tumour growth is long in comparison to the preclinical phase

121. With regard to the gallbladder:
A Epithelium is stratified squamous
B It has a normal capacity of around 10 mL
C It is supplied by the cystic artery, a branch of the left hepatic artery
D It is stimulated to contract by cholecystokinin
E It is essential for life

122. With regard to renal blood flow:
A The kidneys receive 5 per cent of the cardiac output
B Angiotensin II vasoconstricts the afferent more than the efferent arteriole
C It can be accurately measured by the use of inulin
D The low blood flow in the vasa recta assists in the formation of concentrated urine
E A fall in arterial blood pressure decreases GFR

123. With regard to angiogenesis:
A It is the process of programmed cell death
B It is highly dependent on vascular endothelial growth factor (VEGF)
C It is impaired when tumours grow larger than 1 mm^3
D It is always pathological
E Granulation tissue is rich in cytokines that inhibit angiogenesis

124. With regard to gallbladder disease:
A Courvoisier's law states that in the presence of obstructive jaundice an impalpable gallbladder is always due to gallstones
B It may refer pain to the right shoulder tip
C The surface marking of the gallbladder is the right sixth intercostal space, mid-clavicular line
D Gallstones are usually composed of calcium carbonate
E Gallstones always cause symptoms

125. With regard to glomerular filtration:
A The GFR is the main factor determining the rate of urine production
B GFR can be measured by PAH
C The normal GFR is 50 mL/min
D The glomerular filtration barrier comprises three layers
E A normal plasma creatinine implies normal renal function

126. An increased frequency of tumours caused by occupational carcinogen exposure has been proven in the following groups, *except*:
A Transitional cell carcinoma bladder in dye workers
B Scrotal carcinoma in chimney sweeps
C Mesothelioma with asbestos exposure
D Hepatocellular carcinoma with polyvinyl chloride exposure
E Malignant melanoma with sunlight exposure

127. Which of the following decreases insulin resistance:
A Cortisol
B Exercise
C Obesity
D Pregnancy
E Growth hormone

128. With regard to the liver:
   A It is completely surrounded by the peritoneum
   B The ligamentum venosum is a remnant of the umbilical vein
   C It receives oxygen from the hepatic artery only
   D It is surrounded by Gerota's fascia
   E The right subhepatic space or hepatorenal pouch (of Rutherford–Morison) is the most dependent part of the peritoneal cavity

129. With regard to tubular function:
   A Fifty per cent of the filtered sodium is reabsorbed in the distal convoluted tubule
   B Most glucose is reabsorbed in the loop of Henle
   C The ascending limb of the loop of Henle is permeable to water
   D Drinking seawater is better than drinking nothing at all if lost at sea
   E The maximum concentrating ability of the human kidney is 1200 mOsm/L

130. For which one of the following tumours is there an association with Epstein–Barr virus (EBV) infection?
   A Bronchial carcinoma
   B Cervical carcinoma
   C Burkitt's lymphoma
   D Hepatocellular carcinoma
   E Kaposi's sarcoma

131. Which of the following is the most common thyroid neoplasm in the UK?
   A Medullary thyroid cancer
   B Lymphoma
   C Papillary thyroid cancer
   D Follicular cancer
   E Metastases

132. With regard to portosystemic anastomoses:
   A They occur at sites at which arterial blood meets venous blood
   B They feature at the lower end of the oesophagus
   C They become highly significant in renal failure
   D They are most clinically significant at the lower end of the anal canal
   E They feature at the splenic hilum

133. With regard to oncogenes:
   A They behave in a dominant fashion
   B They encode proteins that negatively regulate growth
   C BRCA1 is an oncogene implicated in breast carcinoma
   D Transcription of oncogenes is dysregulated in normal cells
   E Oncogenes are present only in tumour cells

134. The neurotransmitter released from the cerebellar Pukinke cells is:
   A Glutamate
   B GABA
   C Acetylcholine
   D Glycine
   E Serotonin

135. With regard to the spleen:
   A It lies under cover of ribs 9–11 on the right
   B It is the major site of erythropoietin secretion
   C It is normally the site of haematopoiesis in adults
   D Accessory spleens are rare
   E Splenectomized patients are at high risk of post-splenectomy sepsis

136. Which of the following cells secretes intrinsic factor?
   A Goblet cells
   B Kupffer cells
   C Peptic cells
   D Chief cells
   E Parietal cells

137. With regard to acute inflammation:
   A The predominant cell type involved is the macrophage
   B Inflammation is usually initiated by cell-mediated immunity
   C Inflammation may last for many months
   D Inflammation is intimately connected with the clotting system
   E Inflammation is always due to infection

138. A man is bleeding from the carotid artery. In order to temporarily control the bleeding, the surgeon should compress the artery against the anterior tubercle of which of the following?
   A 2nd cervical vertebra
   B 3rd cervical vertebra
   C 4th cervical vertebra
   D 5th cervical vertebra
   E 6th cervical vertebra

139. With regard to the spermatic cord:
   A It contains within it the ilioinguinal nerve
   B It contains the femoral branch of the genitofemoral nerve
   C It is surrounded by two fascial coverings
   D It contains the pampiniform plexus
   E It has dartos muscle contained in its wall

140. With regard to intestinal absorption:
   A A greater volume of water is absorbed from the colon than from the small intestine
   B Gastric acid assists in the absorption of iron
   C Glucose is absorbed by a potassium-cotransport mechanism
   D Vitamin B_{12} is absorbed from the duodenum
   E Sodium is absorbed at a rate proportional to body needs

141. The following are possible outcomes of acute inflammation, *except*:
   A Resolution
   B Chronic inflammation
   C Abscess formation
   D Amyloidosis
   E Death

142. With regard to the testis:
   A It is supplied by the testicular artery which arises from the internal iliac artery
   B It drains via the pampiniform plexus to the inferior vena cava
   C Lymph drainage is to the inguinal group of lymph nodes
   D It is supplied by T10 sympathetic nerves
   E A fluid collection around the testis is known as a varicocele

143. In the setting of starvation:
   A Glycogen stores last for 2 weeks
   B Glucose is the only metabolic fuel that can be used by neurones
   C The brain uses free amino acids when glucose levels begin to fall
   D Protein is spared until relatively late
   E Death occurs at around 21 days

144. With regard to chronic inflammation:
    A It is always preceded by an acute inflammatory phase
    B It usually heals by organization and repair
    C It is characterized by less tissue destruction than acute inflammation
    D It usually results in resolution
    E Neutrophils are the predominant cell type

145. Under normal conditions, virtually 100 per cent of the filtered load of glucose is reabsorbed by the kidney tubules. Which part of the nephron is expected to have the highest reabsorption of glucose?
    A Proximal convoluted tubule
    B Thin descending loop of Henle
    C Thick ascending limb of loop of Henle
    D Distal convoluted tubule
    E Collecting duct

146. With regard to the ovary:
    A It is retroperitoneal
    B It lies medial to the obturator nerve and anterior to the ureter
    C It drains lymph to the internal iliac nodes
    D It receives a parasympathetic supply from the pudendal nerve
    E It gives rise to referred pain in the suprapubic region

147. Which one of the following hormones is secreted by the anterior pituitary?
    A Testosterone
    B Oxytocin
    C Thyroid-stimulating hormone (TSH)
    D Corticotropin-releasing hormone (CRH)
    E ADH

148. Which of the following inflammatory processes often involves granulomas?
    A Lobar pneumonia
    B Bronchopneumonia
    C Tuberculosis
    D Granulation tissue
    E Ulcerative colitis

149. An intravenous drug user presents with pyrexia and haematuria. Clinical examination demonstrates splenomegaly and splinter haemorrhages. Of which of the following heart valves would vegetations be expected?
    A Aortic
    B Pulmonary
    C Mitral
    D Tricuspid
    E Bicuspid

150. With regard to the rectum:
    A It is drained by tributaries of both the inferior mesenteric and internal iliac veins
    B It is suspended by a mesentery
    C It receives its blood supply from the external iliac artery
    D It is lined by transitional epithelium
    E It is supplied by parasympathetic nerve fibres from the vagus

151. Which one of these statements regarding type 2 diabetes mellitus is true?
    A It usually presents with weight loss
    B Ketones are found
    C It is associated with HLA DR3/4

D Identical twins show 90 per cent concordance

E It usually presents in the teen years

152. With regard to wound healing:
A Granulation tissue actively contracts
B Granulation tissue is defined by the presence or absence of granulomas
C Repair implies the complete restitution of normal tissue architecture and function
D In first-intention healing, the wound is unapposed
E Scar formation is absent in second-intention healing

153. A 62-year-old industrial chemist presents with painless haematuria, urinary frequency, and urgency. He is diagnosed with bladder cancer. Which is the most likely type?
A Adenocarcinoma
B Sarcoma
C Papilloma
D Squamous cell carcinoma
E Transitional cell carcinoma

154. With regard to the uterus:
A It usually lies in a retroverted, anteflexed position
B The broad ligament is a remnant of the gubernaculum
C The pouch of Douglas lies between the bladder anteriorly and uterus posteriorly
D The ovarian artery is intimately related to the ureter
E The ureter is closely related to the lateral fornix of the cervix

155. A 7-year-old girl presents with bleeding in joints. She has a prolonged activated partial thromboplastin time (APTT) and bleeding time, normal PT time, and a normal platelet count. Which one of the following factors is deficient?
A Factor IX
B Factor VIII
C Factor X
D von Willebrand factor
E Protein C

156. In amyloidosis, β-pleated sheets will be seen using which of the following?
A X-ray crystallography
B Transmission electron microscopy
C Scanning electron microscopy
D Western blot
E Congo red stain

157. Which of the following enzymes helps protein digestion in the stomach?
A Trypsin
B Chymotrypsin
C Pepsin
D Carboxypeptidase
E Proelastase

158. Which of the following is the site of red blood cell formation in adults?
A Liver
B Spleen
C Kidneys
D Long bones
E Membranous bones

159. Which one of the following electrolytes is not found in Hartmann's solution?
A Potassium
B Lactate
C Magnesium
D Sodium
E Chloride

160. Which one of the following is not involved in the intrinsic pathway of clotting?
    A Factor XII
    B Factor XI
    C Factor IX
    D Factor VII
    E Calcium

161. Which one of the following causes the sigmoid shape of the oxygen–haemoglobin dissociation curve?
    A The Bohr effect
    B The binding of one oxygen molecule increases the affinity of binding of other oxygen molecules
    C The binding of one oxygen molecule decreases the affinity of binding of other oxygen molecules
    D Adenosine diphosphate (ADP) in the cells
    E Surfactant

162. Which one of the following molecules is used for cell signalling?
    A CO_2
    B O_2
    C NO
    D N_2
    E HCO_3^-

163. Carbon dioxide is primarily transported in the arterial blood as which one of the following?
    A Dissolved CO_2
    B Carbonic acid
    C Carbaminohaemoglobin
    D Bicarbonate
    E Calcium carbonate

164. You are concerned about myocardial ischaemia in a postoperative patient who is complaining of chest pain. The electrocardiogram (ECG) shows tachycardia and isolated ST-segment depression in leads V1 and V2. Which coronary artery is most likely to be responsible?
    A Circumflex coronary artery
    B Left anterior descending coronary artery
    C Posterior descending coronary artery
    D Left main stem coronary artery
    E Right coronary artery

165. A 56-year-old man awoke with paraplegia following a thoraco-abdominal aneurysm repair. What is the most likely cause?
    A Cord compression
    B Cord infarction
    C Brain infarction
    D Myocardial infarction
    E Cord haemorrhage

166. Which one of the following is the terminal group of lymph nodes involved in colonic lymphatic drainage?
    A Pre-aortic
    B Intermediate
    C Paracolic
    D Epicolic
    E Subpectoral

167. Which of the following characteristics are helpful in differentiating between cervical and lumbar vertebra?
    A Foramen transverserium
    B Transverse process
    C Shape of spinous process
    D Heavy vertebral body
    E Facets for articulation

168. Meralgia paraesthetica results from the involvement of which one of the following?
    A The sural nerve
    B The femoral nerve
    C The common peroneal nerve
    D The medial cutaneous nerve of the thigh
    E The lateral cutaneous nerve of the thigh

169. Common peroneal nerve injury is related to fracture of which one of the following?
    A Shaft of the tibia
    B Neck of the fibula
    C Lower tibio-fibular joint
    D Shaft of the fibula
    E Shaft of the femur

170. Which one of the following is not contained in the carpal tunnel?
    A Median nerve
    B Flexor pollicis longus
    C Flexor digitorum profundus
    D Flexor digitorum superficialis
    E Palmaris longus

171. Fascia around nerve bundle of brachial plexus is derived from which one of the following?
    A Prevertebral fascia
    B Clavipectoral fascia
    C Deep cervical fascia
    D Pectoral fascia
    E Fascia lata

172. A 70-year-old woman falls and sustains a humeral fracture on the left side affecting the area of the spiral groove. Which nerve is most likely to be affected by this injury?
    A Ulnar nerve
    B Radial nerve
    C Axillary nerve

D Median nerve
E Posterior interosseous nerve

173. In a subcostal flank approach to the kidney, which of the following may be incised to increase upward mobility of the 12th rib?
    A The latissimus dorsi muscle
    B The lumbodorsal fascia
    C The quadratus lumborum muscle
    D The costovertebral ligament
    E The intercostal muscles between ribs 11 and 12

174. A young man sustains a skull-base fracture at the middle cranial fossa that injures his right abducens (VI) nerve. Which of the following signs is most likely to be present on clinical examination?
    A There is ptosis on the right side
    B The pupil on the right side is constricted and fails to respond to light
    C The right eyelid is numb
    D The patient is unable to deviate his right eye medially
    E The patient is unable to deviate his right eye laterally

175. The blade of a retractor has rested on the psoas muscle during a lengthy operative procedure. This has resulted in femoral nerve palsy. In the postoperative period the patient will experience which one of the following?
    A Inability to flex the knee only
    B Inability to flex the knee and numbness over the thigh
    C Numbness over the anterior thigh only

D Inability to extend the knee and numbness over the anterior thigh

E Inability to flex the hip and numbness over the anterior thigh

176. Which one of the following is a function of the psoas major muscle?
   A Flexes the thigh at the hip joint
   B Extends the thigh at the hip joint
   C Adducts the thigh at the hip joint
   D Abducts the thigh at the hip joint
   E Assists in the full contraction of the diaphragm

177. Which one of the following is the narrowest part of the male urethra?
   A The navicular fossa
   B Site of seminal colliculus
   C Membranous urethra
   D External urethral orifice
   E Bulbous urethra

178. A 35-year-old woman attends clinic complaining of pins and needles affecting the radial (lateral) three digits of her hand. The symptoms are worse at night and after driving long distances. Which of the following motor signs would confirm the likely diagnosis?
   A Inability to flex the radial three digits
   B Inability to adduct all the fingers of her hand
   C Inability to abduct all the fingers of her hand
   D Weakness of opposition of the thumb
   E There will be no motor deficit

179. A patient develops common peroneal nerve palsy following treatment with a below-knee cast for 6 weeks for an undisplaced ankle fracture. Which one of the following statements is true?
   A The patient is unable to stand on tiptoe
   B There would be complete sensory loss below the knee
   C There would be no dorsiflexion of the foot
   D The patient would complain of complete sensory loss on the sole of the foot
   E Sensation would be normal on the dorsum of the foot

180. A 40-year-old man presents with pins and needles on the lateral and anterior aspect of his left thigh. On examination, there is no motor deficit. There is no history of trauma. Which of the following is likely to be causing the problem?
   A Lateral cutaneous nerve of the thigh lesion
   B L2 root lesion
   C L3 root lesion
   D Femoral nerve lesion
   E Saphenous nerve lesion

181. A 20-year-old motor cyclist is involved in a road traffic accident. He is found to have weakness of right shoulder abduction and forearm flexion, as well as some sensory loss over the lateral aspect of his upper arm. The right biceps and brachioradialis reflexes are absent. Which of the following is the likely level of maximal plexus injury?
   A C4/C5 root
   B C5/C6 root
   C C6/7 root
   D C7/C8 root
   E C8/T1 root

182. A 50-year-old woman presents with varicosities around the lateral malleolus and further varicosities on the posterolateral aspect of the leg up to the level of the knee joint. Which one of the following statements is the single best answer?
    A The patient has varicosities of the long saphenous vein
    B There is incompetence at the saphenofemoral junction
    C The incompetent valve is unlikely to be in the popliteal fossa
    D Both short and long saphenous veins are affected
    E The patient has varicosities of the short saphenous system

183. A patient undergoes a radical parotidectomy for a malignant parotid tumour, at which time it is found necessary to perform a total division of the left facial (VII) nerve. Postoperatively, which is the most likely sequela?
    A Loss of left-sided frown in all cases
    B Numbness over the cheek on the left side
    C Ptosis of the upper eyelid on the left side
    D Tendency for food and fluids to collect in the buccal sulcus after meals
    E Loss of taste sensation over the anterior two-thirds of the tongue on the left side

184. Which of the following is a boundary of the omental foramen (epiploic foramen or foramen of Winslow)?
    A Anteriorly the hepatic artery
    B Posteriorly the hepatic vein

C Superiorly the quadrate lobe of the liver
    D Inferiorly the hepatic vein
    E Inferiorly the 2nd part of the duodenum

185. Which of the following structures is located in the anterior mediastinum as seen on computed tomography (CT)?
    A Thymus
    B Oesophagus
    C Aorta
    D Heart
    E Trachea

186. From lateral to medial, which of the following describes the structures in the femoral triangle?
    A Femoral vein, femoral artery, femoral nerve
    B Femoral nerve, femoral vein, femoral artery
    C Femoral nerve, femoral artery, femoral vein, long saphenous vein
    D Long saphenous vein, femoral vein, femoral artery, femoral nerve
    E Short saphenous vein, femoral vein, femoral artery, femoral nerve

187. 79-year-old woman suffers a displaced transverse fracture of her left olecranon. The fracture is treated conservatively in a cast. Which of the following functions is she most likely to have difficulty with?
    A Brushing her hair
    B Fastening buttons
    C Pouring a kettle
    D Pushing to standing from an armchair
    E Reaching into a high cupboard

188. A dental surgeon carries out a block of the inferior alveolar nerve by infiltrating local anaesthetic at the mandibular foramen. Which clinical feature may result from this procedure?
    A Ineffective block for the incisor teeth
    B Numbness of the lower lip on the injected side
    C Numbness of the side of the tongue
    D Inability of the patient to clench his jaws
    E Transient weakness of the facial muscles on the injected side

189. Following open reduction internal fixation of both the distal tibia and the distal fibula, a patient complains of numbness along the lateral side of the foot. Which nerve is likely to have been injured?
    A Deep peroneal nerve
    B Saphenous nerve
    C Superficial peroneal nerve
    D Tibial nerve
    E Sural nerve

190. A 3-year-old boy is about to undergo bronchoscopy for a suspected inhaled peanut. Which of the following is the most likely site for the inhaled peanut?
    A Right middle lobe bronchus
    B Left lower lobe bronchus
    C Right superior lobe bronchus
    D Left superior lobe bronchus
    E Right lower lobe bronchus

191. Action potentials cause changes in membrane potential by which one of the following mechanisms?
    A Chloride ions outwards
    B Potassium ions inwards
    C Potassium ions outwards
    D Sodium ions inwards
    E Sodium ions outwards

192. The serum of a patient needing a transfusion reacts (agglutinates) with blood from Group B and the blood cells of this patient react (agglutinate) with the antisera anti-A and anti-D. Which of the following is the blood group of this patient?
    A A-Positive
    B A-Negative
    C B-Positive
    D B-Negative
    E O-Negative

193. With regards to the anticoagulation effect of warfarin:
    A Patients on warfarin have a decreased PT
    B Warfarin is monitored using the APTT
    C Upon initiation of treatment with warfarin patients are temporarily at increased risk of thrombosis
    D Warfarin is safe for use during pregnancy as it does not cross the placenta
    E Warfarin is the treatment of choice following myocardial infarction

194. A patient under general anaesthesia rapidly develops muscle rigidity, tachypnoea, and a temperature of 40°C. Malignant hyperthermia is suspected and the patient is treated with dantrolene. Which of the following is the likely cause of malignant hyperthermia?
    A Decreased convectional heat loss from skin caused by drapes
    B Increased blood levels of interleukin-1

C Increased heat production in skeletal muscle

D A change in hypothalamic temperature set point

E Increased immune system activity against gut and lung commensals

195. How do skeletal muscles differ from both cardiac and smooth muscle?

A Voluntary control

B Involuntary control

C Striated

D Fusiform

E Branching cellular chains

196. What is the function of the ductus arteriosus?

A Bypass brain in the fetus

B Bypass lungs in the fetus

C Bypass liver in the fetus

D Supply brain in the fetus

E Supply lungs in fetus

197. A 23-year-old man has acute appendicitis, which is exacerbated by external rotation and extension of the leg. Which muscle is being irritated?

A Rectus femoris

B Adductor longus

C Hamstrings

D Psoas major

E Adductor magnus

198. Foot drop can occur from a fracture of what structure?

A Tibial plateau

B Fibular neck

C Patella

D Femoral neck

E Talar dome

199. A patient injured his left index finger and now cannot bend his fingertip at the distal interphalangeal joint. What is the most likely cause?

A Injury to the median nerve

B Avulsion of extensor digitorum

C Avulsion of flexor digitorum superficialis

D Avulsion of flexor digitorum profundus

E Avulsion of flexor pollicis longus

200. Which muscle divides the posterior triangle of the neck into the supraclavicular and occipital triangles?

A Superior belly of omohyoid

B Inferior belly of omohyoid

C Sternocleidomastoid

D Posterior scalene

E Trapezius

SECTION 2: SBA ANSWERS AND EXPLANATIONS

1. **E: Respiratory alkalosis with compensation**

   The pH is high = alkalosis; the pCO_2 is low = respiratory cause; the base excess is negative = metabolic compensation.

2. **A: Class I**

   Class I shock = 0–15 per cent of circulatory volume blood loss. There is only tachycardia.

3. **D: Class IV**

   Class IV shock = >40 per cent of circulatory volume blood loss. There is extreme tachycardia, tachypnoea, often undetectable, anuria, unconscious.

4. **B: A man suffers full-thickness burns to the whole of his left arm. Degree of burns 9 per cent**

   Apply Wallace's rules of 9s:

   - 1 per cent for perineum
   - 9 per cent for each arm
   - 9 per cent for face and head
   - 18 per cent for each leg
   - 18 per cent for the back of trunk

   Burns can cause the release of myoglobin secondary to rhabdomyolysis. This may block the renal tubules, resulting in acute renal failure and consequently hyperkalaemia.

5. **E: Mirizzi syndrome**

   Mirizzi syndrome occurs when a gallstone in the gallbladder causes compression on the common bile duct resulting in obstructive jaundice. There is gallstone cholecystitis here as well.

6. **A: Carcinoma of head of pancreas**

   This obeys Courvoisier's law which states that a palpable gallbladder in the presence of jaundice is more likely to be malignancy than gallstones.

7. E: Sclerosing cholangitis

This woman has ulcerative colitis which is associated with sclerosing cholangitis.

8. A: Biliary colic

This boy is in sickle cell crisis with haemolytic jaundice. Sickle cell anaemia almost exclusively occurs in black Americans and black Africans.

9. B: Intussusception

This is the classic story of intussusception, which occurs in young children and is most often idiopathic. There is redcurrant jelly stool due to bleeding. Intussusception is an invagination of one segment of bowel into another segment of bowel. Peristalsis lengthens the invaginated portion and each peristaltic wave results in a bout of colic. A viral illness is thought to enlarge Peyer's patches, resulting in an intussusception. In the adult population, this may also be associated with intestinal polyps or tumours. Early symptoms are nausea, vomiting, and abdominal pain. Later, rectal bleeding ('redcurrant stool') and a sausage-shaped mass may be palpable in the abdominal examination. An ileocaecal intussusception is the most common type. The investigations of choice are an ultrasound and barium enema. A barium enema can be diagnostic and therapeutic (inflation of air). Further treatment includes an urgent laparotomy for reduction with or without bowel resection.

10. C: Duodenal atresia

This is the double-bubble sign seen on plain X-ray and represents dilated proximal duodenum and stomach due to duodenal atresia. It is associated with Down's syndrome.

11. B: Pyloric stenosis

This is the classic story of pyloric stenosis and most commonly affects males in the first few months of life. They usually present with non-bilious projectile vomiting. Hypertrophic pyloric stenosis is an obstruction of the pyloric lumen due to pyloric muscular hypertrophy. It affects 1 in 250 infants, is more common in firstborn males, and occurs at age 2–6 weeks. The typical infant presents with non-bilious projectile vomiting and dehydration. On examination, gastric peristaltic waves may be present and a discrete 2–3 cm firm movable 'olive-like' mass may be palpable. The classic laboratory finding is a hypochloraemic, hypokalaemic metabolic alkalosis. Repeated vomiting results in a loss of HCl, causing the hypochloraemic metabolic alkalosis. The patient is likely to be dehydrated from repeated gastrointestinal loss and poor oral intake. The diagnosis is confirmed by abdominal ultrasound. Initial treatment is correction of the dehydration and electrolyte abnormality. Definitive treatment is a longitudinal pyloromyotomy.

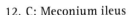

12. **C: Meconium ileus**

Most patients with meconium ileus have cystic fibrosis. Meconium is foetal stool and in this case is impacted in the ileum and can be felt as a mass. The obstructing meconium leads to dilatation of small bowel loops more proximally.

13. **C: Rheumatoid arthritis**

The patient has rheumatoid arthritis. In this chronic inflammatory disorder, patients present with bilateral and symmetrical polyarthropathy affecting the small joints of the hand with sparing of the distal interphalangeal (DIP) joints and involvement of the metacarpophalangeal (MCP) and proximal interphalangeal (PIP) joints. X-ray findings include narrowing of joint space, periarticular osteopenia, juxta-articular bony erosions (non-cartilage protected bone), subluxation with gross deformity, and periarticular soft tissue swelling.

14. **A: Osteoarthritis**

The patient has osteoarthritis (OA). In degenerative joint disease, patients present with joint pain, tenderness, and stiffness due to the process of progressive deterioration of articular cartilage and formation of new bone (osteophytes) at the joint surface. While OA can affect any joint in the body, the disorder commonly affects the hands, hips, knees, neck, and lumbar spine. In the hands, OA typically targets the proximal interphalangeal joints, distal interphalangeal joints, and the first carpometacarpal joints. X-ray shows that the affected joint spaces are narrowed with reactive subchondral sclerosis (eburnation). Bony erosions are centrally located (in contrast to the marginal erosions in rheumatoid arthritis). Other classic radiographic findings include osteophytes and subchondral cysts. Heberden's nodes at the DIP joints and Bouchard's nodes at the PIP joints of the hands are areas of osteophyte formation. Moreover, periarticular soft tissue swelling, intra-articular loose bodies, and osseous fusion can also be seen.

15. **A: Osteosarcoma**

The patient has osteosarcoma of the left femur. These highly malignant lesions appear in two age groups: between 10 and 20 years, and those aged over 50 (secondary to Paget's disease). Osteosarcoma usually occurs at the metaphysis of long bones and presents with pain, associated with a history of trauma. X-ray findings include periosteal new bone formation, which produces a speckled triangle (Codman's triangle) with a 'sun-ray speculation'. Resectable tumours are now treated with cytotoxic therapy, followed by surgical resection. The 5-year survival rate is 50 per cent.

16. **E: Ewing's sarcoma**

Ewing's sarcoma is a rare malignant bone tumour. The common areas in which it occurs are the pelvis, ribs, humerus, and femur (in the long bone medullary cavity).

It is more common in males and usually presents in childhood or early adulthood, with a peak between 10 and 20 years of age. Patients usually present with bone pain. Radiological findings are a permeative lytic lesion with periosteal reaction. The classic description of lamellated or 'onion skin' type periosteal reaction is often associated with this lesion.

17. **C: First sacral nerve root**

Compression of the first sacral nerve root results in pain in the posterior leg and ankle, reduced plantar flexion, reduced sensation in the lateral aspect of the foot, and loss of the ankle reflex (Table 4).

Table 4 Lumbar radiculopathy secondary to lumbar disc protrusions

	L4/L5	L4/L5	L5/S1
Disc	5%	45%	50%
Root	L4	L5	S1
Reflex	Knee	–	Ankle
Motor	Knee extension	Extensor hallucis longus	Plantar flexion
		Tibialis anterior	
Sensory	Medial calf	Lateral calf	Lateral foot
Pain	Anterior thigh	Posterior leg	Posterior leg
			Ankle

18. **E: Superficial peroneal nerve**

The superficial peroneal nerve supplies the peroneal muscles, hence the loss of ankle eversion. It should be differentiated from the common peroneal nerve injury, which involves loss of function in both superficial and deep peroneal nerves. The deep peroneal nerve supplies the anterior compartment of the leg; injury causes inability to dorsiflex the foot.

19. **A: Basal cell carcinoma**

Basal cell carcinoma is the most common type of skin cancer. It is considered malignant because it can cause significant local destruction by invading into the surrounding tissues. Most lesions are located on the patient's head and neck (80 per cent). It occurs more often in men than in women. Most basal cell carcinomas are seen in patients over the age of 40 years. Patients present with a shiny and pearly white nodule on sun-exposed areas.

20. **E: Keratocanthoma**

Keratocanthoma is a benign lesion that originates in the pilosebaceous glands and closely resembles squamous cell carcinoma. In most cases, a keratocanthoma is characterized by rapid growth over a few weeks to months, followed by spontaneous resolution over 4–6 months. It usually appears as a volcano-like bump on the sun-exposed skin of middle-aged and elderly individuals. Most lesions cause minimal skin destruction, but a few behave more aggressively and can spread to regional lymph nodes.

21. **B: Malignant melanoma**

Malignant melanoma is a tumour of melanocytes. The cells are found in the skin, bowel, and eye. There are 5 types of malignant melanoma of the skin:

- *Superficial spreading (most common)*: Usually palpable with an irregular edge
- *Lentigo maligna (least common)*: Least malignant, usually located on the face of the elderly (Hutchinson's freckle)
- *Nodular*: Most malignant, affects the young and may ulcerate and bleed
- *Acral*: Affects palms and soles (includes subungual tumours) and has poor overall prognosis
- *Amelanotic*: Pink in colour but usually pigmented at base; poor prognosis

Patients present with changes to the shape or colour of existing moles or appearance of new skin lesions. They cause pruritus, ulceration, or bleeding. Urgent excisional biopsy is recommended.

Resection on a malignant melanoma is based on Breslow staging (Table 5).

Table 5 Breslow staging of melanoma

Depth of lesion (mm)	Recommended width of excision (mm)
<0.75	2
0.76–1.5	20
1.6–3.0	50
>3.0	50

22. **D: Ruptured spleen**

This patient is presenting with a ruptured spleen (left lower rib fractures with associated hypotension) secondary to trauma. Patients present with abdominal pain, left shoulder tip pain (Kehr's sign), hypotension, and tachycardia. Bruising

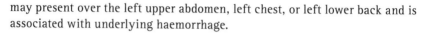

may present over the left upper abdomen, left chest, or left lower back and is associated with underlying haemorrhage.

23. **B: Cardiac tamponade**

The patient has a cardiac (pericardial) tamponade. The clinical syndrome is caused by accumulation of fluid in the pericardial space, which results in reduced ventricular filling and subsequent haemodynamic compromise. Cardiac tamponade presents with Beck's triad: quiet and muffled heart sounds, hypotension, and distended neck vein (jugular venous distention). An emergency pericardiocentesis is the life-saving treatment of choice.

24. **B: Venous ulcer**

Venous ulcers are commonly secondary to venous stasis from varicose veins and/or deep vein thrombosis. They invariably begin after the skin of the leg has been injured. However, the patient may not recall the initial insult. Chronic venous insufficiency may occur secondary to longstanding high pressure in the veins. This high venous pressure results in reflux (reverse flow) in the veins. Characteristic changes occur at the medial gaiter area of the leg. The classical changes include ulceration, haemosiderin deposition, thrombophlebitis, venous eczema and scars, lipodermatosclerosis, 'inverted champagne bottle leg', pitting oedema, healed ulceration (atrophie blanche), ankle flare (corona phlebectatica), and loss of hair.

25. **E: Squamous cell carcinoma**

A chronic venous ulcer may rarely undergo metaplasia to form an ulcerating squamous cell carcinoma, which is called a Marjolin's ulcer. In 1828, Dr Jean Nicolas Marjolin first described the occurrence of ulcerating lesions within scar tissue. Marjolin's ulcer is the term given to these aggressive epidermoid tumours that arise from areas of chronic injury (burn injuries, osteomyelitis, post-radiotherapy).

26. **B: Insert intravenous lines, cross-match blood, and transfer to theatre**

An aneurysm is an abnormal, permanent dilation of a blood vessel to 1.5–2 times its normal diameter. Patients who present with back pain and shock should be managed as a high index of suspicion as having a leaking abdominal aortic aneurysm (AAA). They need immediate resuscitation and reconstruction surgery, as 50 per cent of patients die before reaching hospital, and of those who arrive, 50 per cent die either of shock before theatre and renal failure after surgery. An elective operation has under 6 per cent mortality rate. Thus, asymptomatic aneurysms are regularly followed up with ultrasound or CT scan. This is because an AAA with a diameter of more than 6 cm has a high chance of rupture within 1 year. The immediate management of this patient is to insert intravenous lines, cross-match, and transfer to theatre.

27. **D: Immediate CT chest scan**

A patient with a widened mediastinum on chest X-ray needs to have the diagnosis of a thoracic aortic aneurysm excluded. The gold standard investigation to detect this abnormality is an angiogram. However, a CT scan is easier, time-efficient, and non-invasive. Both investigations will demonstrate whether the aneurysm is secondary to an aortic dissection. As this patient is cardiovascularly stable, there is time to undergo formal investigations.

28. **C: Immediate CT head scan**

The patient's history is suggestive of a subarachnoid haemorrhage secondary to an aneurysmal bleed. In general, patients present with a sudden onset of a severe headache coupled with neck pain, vomiting, and photophobia. The diagnosis of a subarachnoid haemorrhage is confirmed with a CT head scan. The Fisher grade classifies the appearance of the subarachnoid haemorrhage on a CT head scan (Table 6).

Table 6 **Fisher grading for subarachnoid haemorrhage**

Grade	Appearance
1	None evident
2	Less than 1 mm thick
3	More than 1 mm thick
4	Any thickness with intraventricular haemorrhage or parenchymal extension

The World Federation of Neurosurgeons (WFNS) classification uses the Glasgow Coma Scale (GCS) score and focal neurological deficit to classify the severity of symptoms (Table 7). A cerebral angiogram will identify the underlying aneurysm.

Table 7 **World Federation of Neurosurgeons classification**

Grade	GCS score	Focal neurological deficit
1	15	Absent
2	13–14	Absent
3	13–14	Present
4	7–12	Present or absent
5	<7	Present or absent

29. **C: Addison's disease**

In 60 per cent of cases, Addison's disease, an adrenocortical insufficiency, is caused by an autoimmune disorder. There is an association with other autoimmune conditions (i.e., chronic thyroiditis, Graves' disease, hypoparathyroidism, hypopituitarism, myasthenia gravis, or pernicious anaemia). Other causes include tuberculosis, metastases (lung cancer), amyloidosis, and bleeding. Patients present with muscle weakness, fatigue, loss of appetite, weight loss, dizzy spells (low blood pressure), nausea, diarrhoea, vomiting, irritability, and depression. Routine investigations may reveal hypercalcaemia, hypoglycaemia, hyponatraemia, hyperkalaemia, eosinophilia, lymphocytosis, and metabolic acidosis.

30. **E: Multiple endocrine neoplasia type 2a**

Multiple endocrine neoplasia is due to neoplasia of amine precursor uptake and decarboxylation (APUD) cells. Inheritance may be sporadic or autosomal dominant. They are classified into 3 types:

- *MEN 1*: Parathyroid gland, pancreatic islet cells, and pituitary gland (common), thyroid and adrenal cortex (rare)
- *MEN 2a*: Parathyroid hyperplasia, medullary thyroid carcinoma, and phaeochromocytoma
- *MEN 2b*: MEN 2a and neurofibromatosis

This patient is suffering from MEN1. Her signs and symptoms can be classified by organ system.

- *Parathyroid*: Hyperparathyroidism is present in 90 per cent or more of patients
- *Pancreas*: Pancreatic islet cell tumours occur in 60–70 per cent of patients. Approximately 40 per cent of islet tumours originate from beta-cells, secrete insulin (insulinoma), and cause hypoglycaemia. Most islet tumour cells secrete pancreatic polypeptides. Gastrin is secreted by many non-B-cell tumours (increased gastrin secretion is linked to the duodenum). Increased gastrin secretion increases gastric acid production, which may inactivate pancreatic lipase leading to diarrhoea and steatorrhoea. Increased gastrin secretion also leads to peptic ulcer formation in more than 50 per cent of MEN 1 patients
- *Pituitary*: Pituitary tumours can occur In MEN 1. The majority are prolactinomas, followed by tumours that secrete growth hormone and prolactin, and ACTH. Excess hormones may lead to other clinical syndromes (i.e., excess prolactin: galactorrhoea; excess growth hormone: acromegaly; excess ACTH: Cushing's disease)

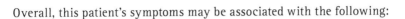

Overall, this patient's symptoms may be associated with the following:

- Hypercalcaemia from hyperparathyroidism
- Excess steroid production from Cushing's disease
- Zollinger–Ellison syndrome

31. E: Communicating hydrocele

The testis descends from the posterior wall of the abdomen into the scrotum via the inguinal canal. It carries a pouch of peritoneum called the processus vaginalis. In a child's first year, the processus vaginalis becomes obliterated, leaving the tunica vaginalis surrounding the testis. If this does not occur, the scrotal sac fills with peritoneal fluid via a communicating hydrocele. Owing to the continuity with the peritoneal cavity, the swelling will increase in size during standing and resolve when lying down. If the sac fills with bowel contents, an inguinal hernia will be present. A non-communicating hydrocele occurs when the processus vaginalis has closed, but the reabsorption of fluid from the tunica vaginalis is incomplete. This condition is present at birth and does not change in size.

32. B: Oesophageal varices

This patient has haematemesis (vomiting blood) secondary to oesophageal varices. Oesophageal varices are dilated submucosal veins in the lower oesophagus. They are often a consequence of portal hypertension. Cirrhosis is a common cause of portal hypertension. The patient's history of alcohol use, hepatomegaly, and peripheral stigmata of liver disease (spider naevi and palmar erythema) is in keeping with this underlying diagnosis. His portal hypertension is a result of enlarged collateral channels between the portal and systematic circulation (at points of portal systemic anastomosis: Table 8).

Table 8 Sites of portosystemic anastomosis

Site	Portal circulation	Systemic circulation
Oesophagus	Left gastric vein	Azygous vein
Paraumbilical	Paraumbilical vein	Superior epigastric vein
Retroperitoneal	Right, left, and middle colic veins	Renal, suprarenal, paravertebral, and gonadal veins
Patent ductus venosus	Left branch of portal vein	Inferior vena cava
Rectal	Superior rectal vein	Middle and inferior rectal veins

33. D: Mesenteric adenitis

This child is presenting with mesenteric adenitis. This condition is a self-limiting inflammatory process that affects the mesenteric lymph nodes in the right lower quadrant of the abdomen. It is frequently caused by a viral pathogen. The patient has a history of fever, enlarged lymph nodes, and generalized abdominal pain. The abdominal pain and tenderness are often centred in the right lower quadrant, but they may be more diffuse than appendicitis. The site of tenderness may shift when the position of the patient changes. The clinical presentation of mesenteric adenitis may mimic appendicitis. With appendicitis, children often present with pyrexia, facial flushing, and localized abdominal pain.

34. E: Meckel's diverticulum

Meckel's diverticulum is the most common congenital abnormality of the small intestine. It is caused by an incomplete obliteration of the vitelline duct. It is present in approximately 2 per cent of the population, with a male predominance. The rule of 2's may be applied:

- 2 per cent of the population
- 2 types of ectopic tissue (gastric and pancreatic)
- 2 years of age at time of presentation
- 2 times more common in males to be affected

The most common presenting symptom is painless rectal bleeding followed by intestinal obstruction, volvulus, and intussusception.

35. D: Acute appendicitis

Appendicitis is a result of acute inflammation of the appendix. The main symptom is abdominal pain. The pain is generalized and then localizes to the right lower quadrant (McBurney's point). On clinical examination, rebound tenderness is noted. Rectal examination may also illicit tenderness. Patients also present with loss of appetite, which can progress to nausea and vomiting. Other symptoms include constipation or diarrhoea, low-grade fever, and abdominal swelling. The diagnosis is based on patient history and physical examination supported by an elevated neutrophilic white cell count.

36. E: Amoebic dysentery

Amoebic dysentery is transmitted through contaminated food and water sources and is caused by the amoeba *Entamoeba histolytica*. Patients can present with frequent, loose, and bloodstained stools; weight loss; dehydration; indigestion; colic abdominal pain; and rectal bleeding. The most frequent sites of infection are the caecum, ascending colon, and sigmoid

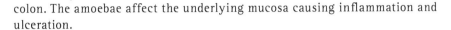

colon. The amoebae affect the underlying mucosa causing inflammation and ulceration.

37. **B: Carcinoma of the anus**

Anal carcinoma, typically a squamous cell carcinoma, arises near the squamo-columnar junction. The adult population is most commonly affected (average age of presentation is 60 years). Right-sided colon cancer commonly presents with anaemia and weight loss, whereas transverse and left-sided colon cancer presents with change in bowel habit, blood mixed with stool, and weight loss. Risk factors for this condition include human papillomavirus, smoking, immunosuppression, benign anal lesions (inflammatory bowel disease, haemorrhoids, fistulae), and sexual activity (multiple sexual partners and anal intercourse).

38. **B: Oesophageal carcinoma**

Oesophageal cancer can be divided into various subtypes based on anatomical location. In general, a cancer in the upper two-thirds is a squamous cell carcinoma and one in the lower third is an adenocarcinoma. In cases of squamous cell carcinoma, which are similar to head and neck cancers, there is an association with tobacco and alcohol excess. Cases of adenocarcinoma are often associated with gastro-oesophageal reflux disease and Barrett's oesophagus. Patients present with dysphasia, odynophagia, and weight loss. Initially, patients have difficulty with swallowing hard and bulky substances but will progress to having difficulty with soft foods and liquids.

39. **C: Pharyngeal pouch**

Pharyngeal pouches occur most commonly in patients aged over 70 years. Typical symptoms include dysphagia, regurgitation, chronic cough, aspiration, and weight loss. The aetiology remains unknown, but many theories centre upon a structural or physiological abnormality of the oesophageal muscles. The pharyngeal pouch is thought to be due to a mucosal out-pouching between the two parts of the inferior constrictor: thyropharyngeus above and cricopharyngeus below. The potential gap is called Killian's dehiscence. Food is propelled from the pharynx to the oesophagus by a series of sequential contractions of the superior, middle, and thyropharyngeus constrictors. Then the cricopharyngeus, which acts as a sphincter, relaxes to allow food to enter the oesophagus. If it fails to relax, the pressure above will produce a posterior out-pouching through the weak Killian's dehiscence. It cannot expand posteriorly because of the adjacent vertebrae, so it descends down the back of the oesophagus to present as a lump in the posterior triangle of the neck. This is usually on the left as the oesophagus lies on the left side of the vertebral bodies. The diagnosis is confirmed on barium studies.

40. **B: Teratoma**

    Teratomas are germ cell tumours commonly composed of multiple cell types derived from one or more of three germ layers. They belong to a class known as non-seminomatous germ cell tumours (NSGCTs). All of this class are the result of abnormal development of pluripotent cells: germ cells and embryonic cells. Histologically, teratomas have contained hair, teeth, and bone. The age of onset is 20–30 years. Formal investigations include blood tests (α-fetoprotein and β-hCG) and radiological imaging (ultrasound and CT scan of abdomen and pelvis). Surgical treatment is the mainstay, but teratomas are also chemosensitive.

41. **D: Torsion of hydatid of Morgagni**

    A cyst of the hydatid of Morgagni is also known as an 'appendix testis'. It is a remnant of the Mullerian duct and located at the top of the testis. It is comparable to the fimbriated end of the fallopian tube in females. It may become twisted upon itself, causing a painful lump, which remains in a similar anatomical position. In cases of testicular torsion, the testicle will reside in a higher position and may be rotated.

42. **E: Primary sclerosing cholangitis**

    Primary sclerosing cholangitis (PSC) is a chronic liver disease caused by progressive inflammation and scarring of the bile ducts of the liver. The inflammation impedes the flow of bile to the gut, which can ultimately lead to liver cirrhosis, liver failure, and liver cancer. The underlying cause of the inflammation is believed to be autoimmunity. Patients present with fatigue, lethargy, jaundice, malabsorption, steatorrhoea, cirrhosis, and dark urine. There is an association of PSC with ulcerative colitis: as many as 5 per cent of patients with ulcerative colitis may progress to develop PSC, and about 70 per cent of people with PSC have ulcerative colitis. The following blood studies may suggest the diagnosis of PSC:

    - Elevated alkaline phosphatase or γ-glutamyltransferase (GGT)
    - Elevated serum transaminase level (but may be normal)
    - Elevated serum bilirubin level (in advanced stages)
    - Serum albumin and prothrombin time abnormal (with advanced disease)
    - Immunoglobulin IgG and IgM levels elevated in 48 and 80 per cent of cases, respectively
    - The presence of perinuclear antineutrophil cytoplasmic autoantibodies (p-ANCAs) in 60–82 per cent of patients

    Radiological imaging can aid diagnosis: endoscopic retrograde cholangiopancreatography (ERCP) and magnetic resonance cholangiopancreatography (MRCP).

43. **A: Gilbert's syndrome**

Gilberts' syndrome is a common hereditary cause of increased unconjugated bilirubin in the bloodstream. Mild jaundice may appear with exertion, stress, fasting, and infections (but there may be no symptoms). It has an autosomal dominant pattern of inheritance.

44. **C: Acute alcoholic hepatitis**

Acute alcoholic hepatitis is an acute inflammation of the liver secondary to alcohol excess. Symptoms include jaundice, hepatomegaly, ascites, fatigue, and hepatic encephalopathy. Peripheral stigmata of cirrhosis also include spider naevi, scleral icterus, palmar erythema, gynaecomastia, and asterixis. The diagnosis is made by taking a full medical history, physical examination, ultrasound, and bloods tests (abnormal liver and clotting function tests: aspartate aminotransferase [AST], alanine aminotransferase [ALT], and prothrombin time [PT]).

45. **D: Hepatic metastases**

Hepatic metastases is a malignant neoplasm that has spread to the liver from a primary site. Colon cancer can spread to other organs in the body including the lungs and liver (stage III disease). Between 20 and 25 per cent of patients with colorectal cancer have liver metastases at the time of their diagnosis. Patients present with jaundice, anorexia, nausea, fevers, pain in the upper right part of the abdomen, and weight loss. Blood tests demonstrate elevated plasma alkaline phosphatase and carcinoembryonic antigen. An ultrasound and CT scan of the abdomen will confirm the diagnosis.

46. **C: Renal cell carcinoma**

Renal cell carcinoma is also known as hypernephroma, Grawitz tumour, or clear cell carcinoma. The classical triad of presentation occurs in 10–15 per cent of patients: haematuria, flank pain, and a loin mass. Patients can also present with malaise, weight loss, anorexia, polycythaemia (secondary to excess erythropoietin production), anaemia (secondary to depression of erythropoietin), varicocele (secondary to obstruction of the testicular vein), hypertension (secondary to renin secretion by the tumour), hypercalcaemia (secondary to ectopic parathormone production by the tumour), cannonball metastases (which may disappear after nephrectomy), pyrexia of unknown origin, and nephritic syndrome.

47. **A: Transitional cell carcinoma**

Transitional cell carcinoma of the bladder is the most common cause of painless haematuria. Transitional epithelium lines the entire urinary tract, so these tumours may arise from the renal pelvis to the end of the urethra in females and to the end of the prostatic urethra in males. Patients commonly present with haematuria, dysuria, polyuria, and nocturia. If left untreated, local invasion of the bladder neck may lead to incontinence. Obstructive hydronephrosis and clot retention are also recognized complications. There are recognized *risk factors:*

- *Cigarette smoking*: Smoking increases the risk of developing bladder cancer nearly five-fold. As many as 50 per cent of all bladder cancers in men and 30 per cent in women are linked to cigarette smoke

- *Chemical exposure at work*: About one in four cases of bladder cancer are caused by exposure to carcinogens. Dye workers, rubber workers, aluminium workers, leather workers, truck drivers, and pesticide applicators are at the highest risk. Arylamines are the chemicals most responsible

- *Radiation and chemotherapy*: Women who received radiation therapy for the treatment of cervical cancer have an increased risk of developing transitional cell bladder cancer. Some patients who have received chemotherapy with cyclophosphamide (Cytoxan) are also at an increased risk

- *Parasite infection*: In developing countries, infection with schistosomiasis has been linked to bladder cancer

48. **D: A 42-year-old woman underwent an open cholecystectomy. Classification of wound: Clean Contaminated Class II**

- Patient A has a dirty wound. Examples are wounds made in the presence of pus, a perforated viscus, or traumatic wounds. The infection rate is 40 per cent

- Patient B has a contaminated wound. Examples are incisions contaminated by opening the colon, open fractures, or animal bites. The infection rate is 20 per cent

- Patient C has a clean wound. Examples are incisions through uninfected skin that do not breach any hollow viscus (inguinal hernia repair). The infection rate is 2 per cent

- Patient D has a clean contaminated wound. Examples are incisions that breach a hollow viscus other than the colon (open cholecystectomy). The infection rate is below 10 per cent

- Patient E has a dirty wound following a perforated viscera. The infection rate is 40 per cent

49. D: Primary hyperparathyroidism

The diagnosis is primary hyperparathyroidism. This patient has symptomatic hypercalcaemia with polyuria and polydipsia. The high calcium fails to suppress PTH secretion, making a parathyroid adenoma most likely. This is an important point – a normal PTH in this instance is *abnormal,* since in normal individuals a high calcium would suppress PTH secretion and one should expect in such instances a *low* PTH. The low phosphate fits with primary hyperparathyroidism since PTH has a phosphaturic effect at the level of the renal tubules. Other symptoms of hypercalcaemia may be remembered by 'bones, stones, abdominal moans, and psychotic groans' (i.e., bony pains, renal stones, constipation, abdominal pains, and psychiatric disturbances). Management consists of control of calcium with fluids, furosemide, and bisphosphonates. An ultrasound and/or Sestamibi scan may be used to localize the parathyroid adenoma. Definitive treatment is surgical: neck exploration and parathyroidectomy.

50. E: Secondary hyperparathyroidism

The diagnosis is secondary hyperparathyroidism. This patient demonstrates symptomatic hypocalcaemia with acroparasthesia (pins and needles in the peripheries) and an elevated PTH. Chvostek's sign (gentle tapping over the facial nerve causing twitching of the facial muscles) and Trousseau's sign (carpopedal spasm) would be expected to be positive.

Secondary hyperparathyroidism is physiological compensatory hypertrophy of all parathyroid glands because of hypocalcaemia, such as occurs in renal failure or vitamin D deficiency. PTH levels are raised due to loss of the inhibitory feedback effect of calcium on the parathyroid glands. PTH levels fall to normal on correction of the cause of hypocalcaemia where this is possible.

51. A: Addison's disease

This patient has Addison's disease (primary hypoadrenalism), as manifested by hypotension, hypoglycaemia, hyponatraemia, and hyperkalaemia, as a result of mineralocorticoid and glucocorticoid deficiency. Diagnosis is confirmed by a short synACTHen (synthetic ACTH) test, whereby the endocrine response of the adrenal gland (cortisol production) is measured in response to a given bolus of synthetic ACTH. An absent or impaired cortisol response is seen in Addison's disease.

52. D: Pseudogout

Crystal-related arthropathy defines a syndrome of synovitis in response to crystal deposition/formation in the joint. There are two main forms: gout and pseudogout. Gout is the more common entity. The main distinguishing features are given in Table 9.

Table 9 Gout and pseudogout

Gout	Pseudogout
Affects smaller joints	Affects large joints
Pain intense	Pain moderate
Joint inflamed	Joint swollen
Hyperuricaemia	Chondrocalcinosis
Uric acid (monosodium urate) crystals: • Needle-like • 5–20 μm long • Exhibit strongly negative birefringence under plane polarized light • Often associated with increased polymorphs	Calcium pyrophosphate crystals: • Rhomboid • Slightly smaller than urate crystals (<10 μm) • Show positive birefringence under plane polarized light
Treatment is analgesia and prophylaxis	Treatment is analgesia; no prophylaxis available

53. E: Tear of quadriceps tendon

A 21-year-old male has sustained an injury of sudden onset, associated with swelling and an inability to extend at the knee joint and an absent knee reflex. This is consistent with an injury to the quadriceps group of muscles that lie in the anterior compartment of the thigh and act as the principal extensors of the knee joint. The mechanism of injury is inconsistent with a fractured patella.

54. B: Increased stroke volume

During strenuous exercise there is an increase in heart rate, stroke volume, and cardiac output. Remember cardiac output is a function of heart rate and stroke volume. During exercise, there is an increase in respiratory rate (hyperventilation) which will lead to a reduction in PCO_2. During exercise the oxygen demand of skeletal muscle rises, therefore leading to a reduction in mixed venous blood oxygen concentration. Renal blood flow is autoregulated, so renal blood flow is preserved and will tend to remain the same. Mean arterial blood pressure (MABP) is a function of cardiac output and total peripheral resistance and will increase with exercise, mainly as a result of the increase in cardiac output that occurs.

55. C: Renal tubular cells

Peripheral nerve cells, unlike nerve cells of the central nervous system, do regenerate following injury. It is a slow process that occurs at about 1 mm/day and may be followed with nerve conduction studies. Schwann cells are responsible for myelination of nerve fibres which increases the axonal speed of conduction. Following injury (Wallerian degeneration), they are able to regenerate. Mucosal cells are epithelial cells which behave like stem cells and can therefore continuously renew themselves. Liver cells (hepatocytes) under certain circumstances can be stimulated to divide. Renal tubular cells lack the ability to regenerate following injury. This is why renal blood flow is so carefully autoregulated. It is also why acute tubular necrosis is taken so seriously, because damage to renal tubular cells is irreversible and will lead to end-stage renal failure, requiring renal replacement therapy in the form of dialysis or transplantation.

56. D: Prostatic carcinoma commonly spreads via the blood

Metastasis may be defined as the survival and growth of cells that have migrated or have otherwise been transferred from a malignant tumour to a site or sites distant from the primary. Tumours commonly spread via the lymphatic and haematogenous routes, so spread generally follows the pattern of these two routes. Other routes are less common (transcoelomic, perineural spread, through cerebrospinal fluid, iatrogenic). Although there are some exceptions, as a general rule, adenocarcinomas spread via the lymphatic route and sarcomas typically spread haematogenously (through the bloodstream). Therefore, osteosarcomas typically spread via the bloodstream. Basal cell carcinomas rarely metastasize (thereby excluding answer B) and tend to cause destruction through local invasion. Adenocarcinoma of the prostate tends to metastasize haematogenously through the basivertebral vertebral venous plexus to bone.

57. A: Fibroblasts

The stages of wound healing include:

- Haemostasis/coagulation
- Acute inflammation
- Formation of granulation tissue (endothelial cells, fibroblasts, macrophages)
- Angiogenesis
- Epithelialization, fibroplasia, wound contraction (myofibroblasts)
- Remodelling

During the wound contraction phase (which is responsible for forming a mature scar), fibroblasts change phenotypes and take on contractile properties (forming myofibroblasts). They are primarily responsible for drawing the two wound edges together. Macrophages are responsible for engulfing foreign and particulate matter through phagocytosis and also release cytokines that assist in the inflammatory and healing phases of the injury response. Reticulocytes are immature red blood cells (erythrocytes) and play no significant role in wound contraction. Giant cells are formed from a coalescence of macrophages and are seen in granulomatous conditions but again play no significant role in wound contraction.

58. **A: Typically encapsulated**

An adenoma is defined as a benign tumour of epithelial cells. Table 10 distinguishes the main features of benign and malignant tumours.

Table 10 Features of benign and malignant tumours

Benign	Malignant
Non-invasive	Invasive
No metastasis	Capable of metastasis
Resembles tissue of origin (well-differentiated)	Variable resemblance to tissue of origin
Slowly growing	Rapidly growing
Normal nuclear morphology	Abnormal nuclear morphology
Well circumscribed	Irregular border
Rare necrosis/ulceration	Common necrosis/ulceration

Benign tumours do *not* spread beyond the basement membrane, nor metastasize to distant sites. They are typically encapsulated and have a pseudocapsule caused by compression of the normal surrounding tissues as a result of their slow growth.

Some cells may be dysplastic within a benign tumour (dysplasia means 'precancerous', or disordered, cells but importantly without the ability to invade through the basement membrane and metastasize to distant sites, so technically by definition are still benign). Dysplasia represents an important step in the progression to a malignant tumour and severe dysplasia is synonymous with carcinoma-*in situ*. Examples of adenomas that may contain dysplastic cells include some types of bowel polyps (e.g., tubular, villous, and tubulovillous polyps/adenomas).

Most adenomas are solid nodules, rather than being annular or circumferential lesions. Rectal carcinomas (that are malignant) can form annular or circumferential lesions.

59. B: Damage to the external laryngeal nerve

Two important nerves are at risk in a thyroidectomy.

- The recurrent laryngeal nerve supplies all the intrinsic muscles of the larynx with the exception of the cricothyroid muscle. Damage on either side leads to vocal fold paralysis and resulting hoarseness. Bilateral injury leads to stridor which may necessitate a tracheostomy to maintain a reasonable airway (Semon's law)
- The external branch of the superior laryngeal nerve supplies the cricothyroid which is responsible for lengthening and shortening of the vocal cords, thereby controlling voice pitch

60. C: Subcostal nerve

When the kidney is approached surgically through a posterior approach, the subcostal nerve is usually superficial and encountered before reaching the kidney. The kidney lies extraperitoneally (retroperitoneal) and therefore A is incorrect. B and D are incorrect because the question is asking which structure is encountered before reaching the kidney. E is incorrect because the left kidney is being operated on and therefore the right hemidiaphragm should not be encountered. Always remember to read the question carefully!

61. D: Right ureter

There are 3 important structures at risk in a right hemicolectomy that also form important relations to the right hemicolon:

- Right ureter
- Right gonadal vessels
- Second part of the duodenum

Vigilance and careful identification of these structures are needed to prevent inadvertent injury to them at the time of surgery.

62. B: Pulmonary fibrosis

Pulmonary functional residual capacity (FRC) is the volume of air present in the lungs at the end of passive expiration. Obstructive diseases (e.g., emphysema, chronic bronchitis, asthma) lead to an increase in FRC due to an increase in lung compliance and air trapping. Restrictive diseases (e.g., pulmonary fibrosis) result in stiffer, less compliant lungs, and a reduction in FRC.

63. E: Released in hypovolaemia

Angiotensin II is one of the most potent vasoconstrictors in the human body. It is released as part of the renin–angiotensin system and is derived from angiotensin I (Figure 5). Angiotensinogen is converted to angiotensin I by renin. Angiotensin I is converted to angiotensin II by angiotensin-converting enzyme

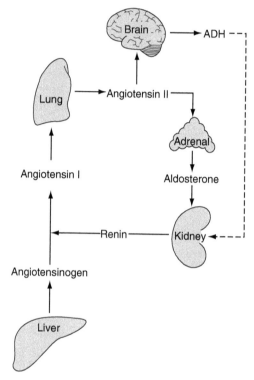

Figure 5 The renin–angiotensin–aldosterone system. Angiotensin I is a decapeptide and angiotensin II is an octapeptide. Renin is a proteolytic enzyme; angiotensin II is a converting enzyme. ADH, antidiuretic hormone.

(ACE) in the lungs. Angiotensin II stimulates secretion of aldosterone from the adrenal cortex (zona glomerulosa layer).

Hypovolaemia results in a decrease in intrarenal blood pressure which is sensed by the juxtaglomerular apparatus of the kidney, resulting in renin secretion and a rise in the levels of angiotensin II.

64. **D: A fall in pCO$_2$**

The oxygen–haemoglobin dissociation curve is shifted to the right by a fall in pH (increased hydrogen ion concentration, or acidosis), a rise in temperature, an increase in 2,3-DPG (2,3-diphosphoglycerate), a rise in pCO$_2$, exercise, and HbS (sickle-cell haemoglobin). The dissociation curve is shifted to the left by a rise in pH, a fall in temperature, a decrease in 2,3-DPG, a fall in pCO$_2$, fetal haemoglobin, high carbon monoxide levels (carboxyhaemoglobin), and methaemoglobinaemia (Figure 6).

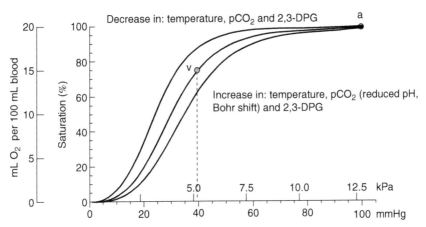

Figure 6 The carriage of oxygen by blood. v, venous; a, arterial.

Anaemia has no effect on the dissociation curve as the graph represents the degree of oxygen saturation of the existing haemoglobin, rather than the amount, or concentration, of haemoglobin in the blood.

65. **A: Hypoxia**

The dominant control process of coronary perfusion is metabolic hyperaemia. GTN spray is used in angina and increases coronary blood flow through the vasodilatatory action of nitric oxide (NO). Alpha-adrenoceptor stimulation increases systemic blood pressure and thereby increases coronary artery perfusion. All beta-adrenoceptor agonists dilate the coronary vessels thereby increasing coronary perfusion. ADH, or vasopressin, causes a strong vasoconstriction in most tissues, but the cerebral and coronary vessels, by contrast, respond to vasopressin with an EDRF-mediated dilatation (thereby increasing coronary flow). Vasopressin thus produces a redistribution of cardiac output in favour of brain and heart, which seems appropriate in hypovolaemia. Hypoxia reduces myocardial contractility and thereby decreases coronary perfusion.

66. **D: Bile salts**

Resection of the terminal ileum interferes with the enterohepatic circulation, which is the route by which bile salts are recirculated in the body. Resection of the terminal ileum (e.g., in Crohn's disease) may therefore lead to a deficiency in bile salts. The clinical consequences of this are an increased risk of cholesterol gallstones. Vitamin B_{12} is also reabsorbed in the terminal ileum, so resection may also lead to deficiencies in vitamin B_{12} levels through malabsorption.

67. **A: Promotes protein synthesis**

Insulin is produced by the beta-cells of the islets of Langerhans in the pancreas and has various actions, including promoting uptake of glucose into cells, glycogen synthesis (glycogenesis), protein synthesis, and stimulation of lipogenesis (formation of fat). Insulin functions to drive potassium into cells and is used to treat hyperkalaemia. Parathyroid hormone and activated vitamin D are the principal hormones involved in calcium/phosphate metabolism, rather than insulin.

68. E: A rise in arterial pCO_2

Prolonged vomiting will lead to a hypochloraemic metabolic alkalosis (a rise in pH; raised bicarbonate), in addition to causing a hypokalaemia as gastric juices are rich in potassium. A hypovolaemic state will ensue with a raised urea concentration. pH compensation occurs through the respiratory system, resulting in hypoventilation which will tend to increase arterial pCO_2 levels.

69. D: Inulin clearance can be used to estimate GFR

In the normal adult human, the GFR (or normal renal clearance) averages 125 mL/min, or 180 L/day. The entire plasma volume (about 3 L) can therefore be filtered and processed by the kidney approximately 60 times each day. The rate of urine production in humans is dominated by tubular function and not by GFR. The GFR remains relatively constant through autoregulation.

After 35 years of age, GFR falls at about 1 mL/min/year. By the age of 80, GFR has fallen to about 50 per cent of its youthful level. GFR can decrease by as much as 50 per cent before plasma creatinine rises beyond the normal range. Consequently, a normal creatinine does not necessarily imply normal renal function, although a raised creatinine does usually indicate impaired renal function.

A substance used to measure the GFR must be freely filtered at the glomerulus, not be secreted by the tubules, not be reabsorbed, not be metabolized or synthesized in the body, not alter the renal function/GFR, and be non-toxic and soluble in plasma. Such a substance is the polyfructose molecule, inulin. However, it is too cumbersome to use in routine clinical practice. Instead, GFR is more commonly quantified by measuring the 24-hour urinary creatinine excretion. Para-aminohippuric acid is used to measure renal blood flow and not GFR.

70. B: Gastrin

Gastric acid is *stimulated* by 3 factors:

- Acetylcholine, from parasympathetic neurones of the vagus nerve that innervate parietal cells directly
- Gastrin, produced by pyloric G-cells
- Histamine, produced by mast cells. This stimulates the parietal cells directly and also potentiates parietal cell stimulation by gastrin and neuronal stimulation. H_2 blockers such as ranitidine are therefore an effective way of reducing acid secretion

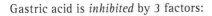

Gastric acid is *inhibited* by 3 factors:

- Somatostatin
- Secretin
- Cholecystokinin

There are *3 classic phases of gastric acid secretion*:

- *Cephalic* (preparatory) phase [significant]: Results in the production of gastric acid before food actually enters the stomach – triggered by the sight, smell, thought, and taste of food acting via the vagus nerve
- *Gastric* phase [most significant]: Initiated by the presence of food in the stomach, particularly protein-rich food
- *Intestinal* phase [least significant]: The presence of amino acids and food in the duodenum stimulate acid production

71. **C: Bicarbonate**

Carbon dioxide is transported in the blood in various forms:

- Bicarbonate accounts for about 80–90 per cent of the total CO_2 in the blood
- Carbamino compounds account for 5–10 per cent
- Only 5 per cent is physically dissolved in solution

Carbon dioxide is carried on the haemoglobin molecule as carbamino-haemoglobin; carboxyhaemoglobin is the combination of haemoglobin with carbon monoxide.

Erythrocytes contain the enzyme carbonic anhydrase that catalyses the reaction $CO_2 + H_2O = H^+ + HCO_3^-$ and requires zinc as a cofactor. This plays an important role in carbon dioxide transport and in the buffering of pH.

72. **B: The ratio of stroke volume to end-diastolic volume**

During diastole, filling of the ventricles normally increases the volume of each ventricle to about 120 mL. This volume is known as the end-diastolic volume. Then, as the ventricles empty in systole, the volume decreases about 70 mL, which is known as the stroke volume. The remaining volume in each ventricle, about 50 mL, is known as the end-systolic volume and acts as a reserve which can be utilized to increase stroke volume in exercise.

The fraction of end-diastolic volume that is ejected is called the 'ejection fraction' – usually equal to about 60 per cent. The ejection fraction is often used clinically as an indirect index of contractility. It is particularly useful in assessing the state of the myocardium prior to aortic aneurysm repair where cross-clamping of the aorta places particular stress on the myocardium.

73. **C: In the ileum**

Between 90 and 95 per cent of the bile salts are absorbed from the small intestine and then excreted again from the liver; most are absorbed from the terminal ileum. This is known as the enterohepatic circulation. The entire pool recycles twice per meal and approximately 6–8 times per day.

Disruption of the enterohepatic circulation, either by terminal ileal resection or through a diseased terminal ileum (e.g., Crohn's disease), results in decreased fat absorption and cholesterol gallstone formation. The latter is believed to result because bile salts normally make cholesterol more water-soluble through the formation of cholesterol micelles. Loss of reuptake also results in the presence of bile salts in colonic contents, which alters colonic bacterial growth and stool consistency.

74. **D: ↑BP, ↓HR, ↓CPP**

The important relationship between cerebral perfusion pressure (CPP), MABP, and intracranial pressure (ICP) is as follows: CPP = MABP − ICP. It stems from the fact that the adult brain is enclosed in a rigid, incompressible box, with the result that the volume inside it must remain constant (Monro–Kelly Doctrine). A rise in ICP therefore decreases CPP (and hence cerebral blood flow).

In raised ICP, as the brainstem becomes compressed, local neuronal activity causes a rise in sympathetic vasomotor drive and thus a rise in blood pressure. This is known as the Cushing's reflex. This elevated blood pressure evokes a bradycardia via the baroreceptor reflex. The Cushing's reflex helps to maintain cerebral blood flow and protect the vital centres of the brain from loss of nutrition if the ICP rises high enough to compress the cerebral arteries.

75. **B: Zona glomerulosa of the adrenal cortex**

The adrenal gland comprises an outer cortex and an inner medulla, which represent two developmentally and functionally independent endocrine glands within the same anatomical structure. The adrenal medulla secretes adrenaline (70 per cent) and noradrenaline (30 per cent). The adrenal cortex consists of three layers, or zones. The layers from the surface inwards may be remembered by the mnemonic GFR:

G = zona Glomerulosa (secretes aldosterone)

F = zona Fasciculata (secretes cortisol and sex steroids)

R = zona Reticularis (secretes cortisol and sex steroids)

Aldosterone is a steroid hormone that facilitates the reabsorption of sodium and water and the excretion of potassium and hydrogen ions from the distal convoluted tubule and collecting ducts. Conn's syndrome is characterized by increased aldosterone secretion from the adrenal glands.

76. **A: Salivary**

In humans, about 1–1.5 L of saliva are secreted each day. Secretion is an active process. The two-stage hypothesis of salivation states that a primary secretion is first formed by secretory end pieces (that resembles an ultrafiltrate of plasma), which is then modified as it flows along the duct system. Na^+ and Cl^- are absorbed and K^+ and HCO_3^- are secreted as saliva flows along the ductal system. In addition, the ducts have a low water permeability.

The final saliva is hypotonic with respect to plasma and contains a higher potassium concentration than any other gastrointestinal secretion of the body. Any abnormal state in which saliva is lost to the exterior of the body for long periods can lead to a serious depletion of potassium, leading in occasional circumstances to serious hypokalaemia and paralysis.

77. **E: Self/non-self-discrimination**

Innate (natural) immunity comprises:

- Physical barriers (skin, mucosal membranes)
- Physiological factors (pH, temperature, oxygen tension; e.g., low pH of stomach inhibits microbial growth, commensal flora)
- Protein secretions (e.g., lysozyme in saliva and tears, complement, cytokines, acute phase proteins)
- Phagocytic cells (neutrophils, macrophages, natural killer cells)
- Acute inflammation (including mast cells, histamine etc.)

The two key features of adaptive (acquired) immunity are its specificity and memory.

The adaptive (acquired) arm of the immune response operates through both humoral and cell-mediated mechanisms and has a number of key features. Immunological tolerance is the exposure to self-components in foetal life that leads to a state of specific immunological unresponsiveness (anergy). In adulthood the adaptive immune system is therefore able to discriminate self from non-self, which is essential in preventing one's own immune system mounting a response against tissues. It may become defective resulting in autoimmune disease.

Immunological memory is a feature of the adaptive immune response and is essential for the rapid response to subsequent exposure of antigens. This concept is central to understanding how vaccines work.

78. **E: Thyroglobulin is stored in the colloid of follicles**

The thyroid gland produces 3 hormones: tetra-iodothyronine (T4), which is the principal hormone; tri-iodothyronine (T3), which has shorter duration but is more potent than T4; and calcitonin, which is produced by parafollicular C-cells and is involved in calcium balance. The steps in the production of T4 and T3 can be summarized as follows:

An active pump concentrates iodine into the thyroid follicular cells.

- Iodine is oxidized into its active form (by peroxidase)
- Iodine binds with tyrosine, to form tyrosyl units (organification)
- Tyrosyl units bind to a protein core, to form thyroglobulin
- Tyrosyl units combine while bound to the protein core, to form either T3 or T4
- Thyroglobulin molecules are stored as colloid in follicles
- TRH (from the hypothalamus) stimulates the anterior pituitary gland to produce TSH
- TSH (thyroid-stimulating hormone) stimulates the release of T3 and T4 into the blood

79. D: Suxamethonium

Neuromuscular blockers are commonly used drugs in anaesthetics. By specific blockade of the neuromuscular junction (NMJ) they relax skeletal muscles and induce paralysis. This enables light levels of anaesthesia to be employed with adequate relaxation of the muscles of the abdomen and diaphragm, thereby facilitating surgery. They also relax the vocal cords and allow the easy passage of a tracheal tube at anaesthetic induction, a procedure known as endotracheal intubation. They can be used *only* when mechanical ventilation is available because such drugs also paralyse the main muscles of respiration. Neuromuscular blockers can be divided into 2 main types: depolarizing and non-depolarizing.

Non-depolarising blockers (e.g., atracurium), also known as competitive muscle relaxants, compete with acetylcholine for receptor sites at the NMJ and their action can be reversed with anticholinesterases, such as neostigmine. Atropine is a muscarinic antagonist and is often given with neostigmine in order to prevent the muscarinic (parasympathomimetic) side effects of anticholinesterases (such as bradycardia, excessive salivation, etc.).

Depolarizing blockers (e.g., suxamethonium, also known as succinylcholine) act by mimicking the action of acetylcholine at the NMJ but hydrolysis is much slower than for acetylcholine because it is resistant to degradation by cholinesterase. Depolarization is therefore prolonged, resulting in sodium-channel inactivation and neuromuscular blockade. Unlike non-depolarizing agents, its action cannot be reversed and recovery is spontaneous. Indeed, anticholinesterases such as neostigmine potentiate the neuromuscular block. Anticholinesterases are also used in myasthenia gravis to enhance neuromuscular transmission by prolonging the action of acetylcholine.

Suxamethonium has a half-life of only a few minutes and is rapidly hydrolysed by pseudocholinesterase. In patients with deficient or atypical pseudocholin-esterase enzyme (an autosomal recessive condition), the metabolism is reduced and the half-life and duration of action of suxamethonium are prolonged, resulting in 'scoline apnoea', or prolonged paralysis. Assisted ventilation should be continued until muscle function is restored. In addition, suxamethonium may be responsible for triggering malignant hyperthermia (MH) in susceptible individuals – an autosomal dominant disorder that results in intense muscular spasm and hyperpyrexia and is associated with a high mortality.

Guanethidine inhibits the release of noradrenaline from postganglionic sympa-thetic nerve terminals. It has largely fallen out of use but is extremely effective in lowering blood pressure and may be useful in cases of resistant hypertension.

80. **E: The testes and ovaries descend from their original position at the 10th thoracic level**

Genital development is principally determined by the presence or absence of a Y chromosome. Thus, XO individuals (Turner's syndrome) are female and XXY individuals (Klinefelter's syndrome) are male. Presence of the sex-determining region of the Y chromosome (SRY) results in male development, absence of SRY leads to female development.

If the embryo is male, the SRY gene is transcribed and this initiates a cascade of events. The sex cord forms the seminiferous tubules, some of the support cells become Sertoli cells and produce a hormone known as anti-Mullerian hormone (AMH), while other support cells become Leydig cells and secrete testosterone. This has the consequence that the paramesonephric (Mullerian) ducts regress due to AMH and the external genitalia become male (conversion of testosterone to dihydrotestosterone in the genital fold results in the formation of the penis and scrotum). The mesonephric (Wolffian) ducts grow to form the vas deferens and associated ducts. In females, where there is no SRY gene, the support cells do not form Sertoli cells. This has the consequence that no AMH is produced and no testosterone-secreting cells develop. The paramesonephric (Mullerian) ducts remain and form the uterus and fallopian tubes, the mesonephric (Wolffian) ducts regress, and female external genitalia develop (labia majora and minora, clitoris). Aberrations of this process may lead to ambiguous genitalia and problems with gender assignment.

During embryonic and foetal life, the testes and the ovaries both descend from their original position at the 10th thoracic level. This explains the long course taken by the gonadal arteries and the site of referred pain from the gonads to the umbilicus (T10 dermatome). Descent is genetically, hormonally, and anatomi-cally regulated and depends on a ligamentous cord known as the gubernaculum. Furthermore, descent of the testis through the inguinal canal into the scrotum depends on an evagination of peritoneum known as the processus vaginalis. This normally obliterates at birth. Gonadal descent is a complicated process and therefore there are many ways in which it can go wrong. Most commonly, an undescended or maldescended testis may occur (cryptorchidism). A patent processus vaginalis may lead to the formation of a congenital hydrocele, or inguinal hernia.

81. **D: The macula region is grossly over-represented in the visual cortex**

The visual pathway may be summarized as follows:

- Photoreceptors (rods, cones) within the retina convert light energy into electrical impulses (phototransduction)
- This is transmitted to ganglion cells, directly via bipolar cells, or indirectly via horizontal and amacrine cells
- Ganglion cells are the output cells of the retina. Axons from ganglion cells converge at the optic disc (blind spot) and travel in the optic nerve
- Incomplete decussation occurs at the optic chiasm; those from the nasal half of each retina (corresponding to the temporal halves of the visual field) cross over (decussate), while those from the temporal halves of each retina stay on the same side
- The optic tracts synapse in the various layers of the lateral geniculate nucleus of the thalamus before being relayed to the primary visual cortex in the occipital lobe via the optic radiation

The macula is a region of the retina that subserves highest visual acuity. It is grossly over-represented in the visual cortex in a phenomenon known as 'cortical magnification'. This may partly explain why lesions located within the visual cortex may result in macula sparing.

The effects of lesions to the visual pathway may be easily predicted utilizing the earlier information:

- Lesions anterior to the optic chiasm (i.e., a transected optic nerve) result in a unilaterally blind eye
- Lesions of the optic chiasm (commonly from a pituitary tumour) result in a bitemporal hemianopia
- Lesions posterior to the optic chiasm (commonly due to ischaemic events) result in a homonymous hemianopia, with or without macula sparing

82. **C: They have a lifespan of only a few hours in inflamed tissue**

Neutrophils are the most common type of leukocyte in the blood. They are present in large numbers in acute inflammation, but in chronic inflammation macrophages predominate. They have multilobed rather than bilobed nuclei, with 4–5 lobes but rising to 6–7 lobes in patients with vitamin B_{12} or folate deficiency. The ability to form multinucleate giant cells is a characteristic of macrophages rather than neutrophils and is classically seen in granulomatous conditions such as tuberculosis.

The phagocytic ability of neutrophils plays a vital role in the host defence against infection. Microbial killing results from both oxygen-dependent and oxygen-independent mechanisms. The former is more important and depends on the 'respiratory burst'. The respiratory burst follows activation of cell membrane NADPH oxidase by phagocytosis and results in the formation of powerful bacteriocidal agents (H_2O_2, superoxide anion and singlet oxygen). Oxygen-independent microbial killing is carried out by lysosomal enzymes, such as lysozyme. The importance of oxygen-dependent bacterial mechanisms is illustrated by the congenital disorder, chronic granulomatous disease. It results from inherited defects in the genes encoding several components of NADPH oxidase, rendering the patient susceptible to recurrent bacterial infections.

Neutrophils have a lifespan of only a few hours in an inflammatory lesion, sometimes less. A severe local infection quickly becomes a graveyard of thousands of neutrophils. Their content, especially enzymes, spill out and may cause additional damage to host tissues. This is known as immune pathology and is the price to be paid for having a sophisticated immune system.

83. **A: It binds and stores oxygen for rapid release during falling P_{O_2}**

Myoglobin is a single-chain globular protein containing a haem group (iron-containing porphyrin) with eight alpha helices and a hydrophobic core. Being monomeric, it has instant binding with oxygen rather than the cooperative binding seen in haemoglobin. It has a hyperbolic dissociation curve. Its function is to store oxygen in muscle tissues for rapid release during times of need, as in exercise.

84. **B: Shaping of the hands and feet is brought about through apoptosis**

The limb is the organ whose development is probably best understood and to understand abnormalities it is necessary to understand how the limb develops. Limb development takes places over a 4-week period, and by the end of the eighth week all the components of the upper and lower limbs are distinct. During this critical period, limb development is susceptible to the harmful effects of environmental teratogens, resulting in limb anomalies.

The limbs develop from small protrusions (the limb buds) that arise from the body wall of the embryo. Positioning and patterning the limb involves cellular interactions between the ectoderm surrounding the limb bud (apical ectodermal ridge) and the mesenchymal cells that form the core of the limb bud.

As the limb grows out the cells acquire a positional value that relates to their position in the bud with respect to all three axes: proximodistal, anteroposterior, and dorsoventral. These positional values largely determine how the cells will develop. The positional value of the cells is acquired in the progress zone at the tip of the growing bud. Thalidomide, a drug commonly used in the late 1950s and early 1960s for morning sickness, was later found to interfere with the normal processes of limb development resulting in major limb defects such as phocomelia (short, ill-formed limbs resembling the flippers of a seal) and amelia (absent limbs).

Separation of the digits occurs by apoptosis (or programmed cell death). This is a good example of a situation in which apoptosis is physiological, rather than pathological.

Adult human limbs never regenerate following amputation, under any circumstances. Adult human limb loss is permanent and irreversible. Some amphibians, however, are unique among vertebrates in being able to regenerate entire limbs. This relates to their ability to revert to an embryonic state (dedifferentiate) in order to recapitulate embryogenesis. Elucidation of the mechanisms involved in amphibians and their possible relationship to limb development in higher organisms may one day enable us to regenerate a lost limb following an amputation.

85. **D: It is reversed by plasmin (fibrinolysin)**

One of the drawbacks of having a high-pressure circulation is that even slight damage to blood vessels, especially on the arterial side, can lead to a rapid loss of circulatory blood volume. To prevent bleeding, we have developed quite complicated responses to vessel damage designed to stop bleeding. Three key physiological events occur upon the onset of bleeding:

- Vasoconstriction
- Platelet aggregation to form the primary haemostatic plug
- Activation of the clotting cascade to form a fibrin plug (secondary or stable haemostatic plug)

The balance of all components – vessel wall, platelets, adhesive and coagulation proteins, and regulatory mechanisms – determines the effectiveness of the haemostatic plug in maintaining the structural and functional integrity of the circulatory system.

Blood platelets are formed from megakaryocytes in the bone marrow. They are anucleate, but the cytoplasm contains electron-dense granules, lysosomes, and mitochondria. Each megakaryocyte is responsible for the production of around 4000 platelets. The half-life of platelets in the blood is about 8–12 days.

The clotting cascade involves a series of several highly specific serine proteases which activate each other in a stepwise manner. In this way a rapid response is achieved because at each step the signal is amplified. Clotting factors are produced in the liver so that liver failure results in a tendency to bleed (anticoagulant state). The final stage of the clotting cascade involves the conversion of fibrinogen to fibrin; this is catalysed by thrombin, not prothrombin, which is the inactive precursor of thrombin.

Plasmin acts as a regulatory mechanism to keep the clotting cascade in check and to prevent the over-clotting of blood which could have disastrous consequences (such as the occlusion of blood vessels). It degrades both fibrin and fibrinogen to products that can inhibit thrombin. Fibrinolytic agents are widely used in clinical practice, a good example being the use of thrombolytics in acute myocardial infarction.

86. **C: It is the second most common human carcinogen worldwide**

A third of the world's population are currently infected with the hepatitis B virus. Hepatitis B is a double-stranded DNA virus, usually transmitted haematogenously, by sexual intercourse, or vertically from mother to baby. Hepatitis A (not hepatitis B) is acquired by the faeco-oral route. Infection during childhood leads to a high rate of chronic carriage of the virus, with only 10 per cent of children clearing the virus. This chronic carrier state is associated with long-term complications in later life. Ninety per cent of adults, on the other hand, clear the virus, with only 10 per cent of adults becoming chronic carriers of the virus.

Hepatic complications of hepatitis B infections include:

- Acute viral hepatitis
- Fulminant hepatic failure
- Chronic active and chronic persistent viral hepatitis
- Cirrhosis
- Hepatocellular carcinoma

Chronic carriage of the virus is facilitated by the ability of the hepatitis B virus to integrate into the DNA and to infect hepatocytes which normally express low levels of MHC class I on their cell surface. Both these strategies help the virus to evade the host's defence mechanisms. Damage to the liver usually results from the host's immune response in an attempt to clear the virus (so-called immune pathology).

It is now well recognized that hepatitis B is a risk factor for the development of primary liver cancer (hepatocellular carcinoma). Indeed, after tobacco smoking, hepatitis B is the second most common human carcinogen worldwide.

Hepatitis B is effectively prevented (not treated) by hepatitis B vaccination. Vaccination is mandatory for all healthcare professionals who regularly come into contact with blood products. Hepatitis B is treated with serum immunoglobulin and antiviral agents (α-interferon, lamivudine).

87. **E: 23 years of age**

Fusion of the ilium, ischium, and pubis at the acetabulum is usually complete by the age of 23. From birth to the early twenties, the three bones are held together by Y-shaped cartilage.

88. D: Interstitial fluid hydrostatic pressure is normally negative

Four primary forces determine the movement of fluid across the capillary membrane (Starling's forces):

- *Capillary hydrostatic pressure*: 'Forces fluid out'
- *Plasma colloid osmotic pressure*: 'Pulls fluid in'
- *Interstitial fluid hydrostatic pressure*: 'Pushes fluid in'
- *Interstitial fluid colloid osmotic pressure*: 'Pulls fluid out'

At the arterial end of the capillary, the capillary hydrostatic pressure exceeds the plasma colloid osmotic pressure and fluid is drawn out of the capillary into the interstitium. By this means, transport of nutrients to the tissues occurs. However, as one moves along the capillary the capillary hydrostatic pressure falls such that, at the venous end of the capillary, the plasma colloid osmotic pressure exceeds the capillary hydrostatic pressure and fluid moves back into the capillary, removing cellular excreta. In this way, about 90 per cent of the fluid that has filtered out of the arterial ends of capillaries is reabsorbed at the venous ends. Only the remainder flows into the lymph vessels.

Interstitial fluid hydrostatic pressure is normally subatmospheric (negative). This results from the suction effect of the lymphatics returning fluid to the circulation. This maintains the structural integrity of the tissues, keeps the interstitial spaces small, and reduces distances for diffusion.

Movement of lymph in one direction along the lymphatics depends on:

- Filtration pressure from capillaries
- Action of local muscles
- Action of local arterial pulsation
- Respiratory movement (thoraco-abdominal pump) with intermittent negative pressures in the brachiocephalic veins
- Smooth muscle in the walls of larger lymphatics (sympathetically controlled)
- Valves within

Oedema (excess fluid accumulation in the extracellular spaces) results from:

- Elevated capillary pressure
- Decreased plasma colloid osmotic pressure
- Increased interstitial fluid protein
- Increased capillary permeability
- Blockage of lymph return (lymphoedema)

Diffusion distances are greatly increased as a result of oedema and this can interfere with cell nutrition.

89. D: Establishes persistence through antigenic variation

HIV is an enveloped RNA retrovirus containing two copies of genomic RNA and three viral enzymes (reverse transcriptase, protease, and integrase). HIV RNA is transcribed by viral reverse transcriptase into DNA that integrates into the host-cell genome. HIV is transmitted by three routes: sexual contact, blood-borne transmission (transfusions or contaminated needles), or vertically from mother to baby (transplacental or via breast milk).

The CD4 antigen on helper T-cells is the receptor for the gp120 viral envelope protein, allowing HIV to infect CD4 T-cells (helper T-cells). The destruction of CD4 cells is central to the pathogenesis of HIV infection. CD4 cells play a pivotal role in the orchestration of both humoral and cell-mediated immune responses. Therefore, by directly infecting and eliminating CD4 cells, the HIV virus leads to a slow and progressive decline in immune function. The end result is AIDS (acquired immunodeficiency syndrome) where the body opens up a whole range of opportunistic infections, the consequences of which are often fatal.

There are several ways in which the HIV evades the host immune system and establishes persistence. For example:

- By directly infecting cells of the immune system, thereby enabling the virus to 'hide' from the immune system
- By infecting macrophages and dendritic cells in addition to CD4 cells, thereby establishing an important reservoir of infection in lymphoid tissues and forming a site for continued viral replication
- By directly integrating into the host cell DNA
- By constantly mutating in a process known as antigenic variation

The generation of new antigenic variants is primarily a function of the high intrinsic error rate present in the reverse transcriptase enzyme (1 in 1000 base-pair error rate). The huge number of variants of HIV in a single infected patient during the course of infection eventually swamps the immune system, leading to its collapse.

90. E: Tremor

Hyperthyroidism is associated with tremor, tachycardia, low serum cholesterol, and hyperreflexia. All the other options are classical findings of hypothyroidism.

91. C: It is the most common inherited disease in Caucasians

Cystic fibrosis (also known as mucoviscidosis) is an autosomal recessive condition, caused by a genetic mutation in the cystic fibrosis transmembrane regulator (CFTR) on chromosome 7. It is the most common inherited disease in Caucasians, affecting 1 in 2500 children. Cystic fibrosis carriers are believed to offer a selective advantage to the population by being relatively more resistant to cholera. This may explain the fact that, on the basis of the frequency of affected homozygotes in the white population, 2–4 per cent must be heterozygote carriers (using the Hardy–Weinberg equation).

Clinical manifestations relate mainly to the lungs (chronic lung infections, especially caused by *Pseudomonas aeruginosa,* bronchiectasis) and the digestive system (meconium ileus, pancreatic insufficiency, failure to thrive). There is no cure for cystic fibrosis. Treatment is mainly supportive, through a multidisciplinary approach, consisting of vigorous chest physiotherapy, mucolytics, antibiotics to treat chest infections, pancreatic enzyme replacement (Creon), and in some cases heart–lung transplantation may be an option in the final stages of the disease. Life expectancy is markedly reduced with a median survival of around 35 years. End-stage lung disease is the principal cause of death.

Gene therapy is not a well-established treatment option and is still best confined to clinical trials. The main problems that have been encountered in the application of gene therapy to clinical practice concern the targeting of vectors to specific sites and integration into the genome.

92. **B: Cerebral blood flow is very sensitive to changes in the pCO_2 of the perfusing blood**

The cerebral circulation does not consist of functional end-arteries. Rather, a rich vascular anastomosis known as the circle of Willis surrounds the base of the brain, into which all the main arteries to the brain connect so that if one artery should block, the brain can still be supplied by the other arteries in this anastomotic arrangement.

Cerebral blood flow is little affected by cardiovascular reflexes (i.e., the autonomic nervous system). Carbon dioxide is the most important determinant of cerebral blood flow, via its local vasodilator action (in underperfused areas carbon dioxide accumulates and this leads to vasodilatation and restoration of normal cerebral perfusion). Hyperventilation leads to washout of carbon dioxide from the blood and constriction of cerebral blood vessels. This may result in syncope following a panic attack. In addition, it explains why hyperventilating prior to diving into water can result in syncope underwater and drowning. The local effect of carbon dioxide on the cerebral vasculature is deliberately utilized in the management of head injury where hyperventilation is used to reduce raised ICP.

The rate of cerebral blood flow remains essentially stable, up to a point, with changing blood pressure owing to local autoregulation of flow. Autoregulation is very well developed in the brain; a fall in blood pressure causes the resistance vessels to dilate and thereby maintain flow. Cerebral autoregulation seems to involve both myogenic and metabolic mechanisms.

The important relationship between the cerebral perfusion, mean arterial blood pressure, and ICP is as follows:

$$CPP = MABP - ICP$$

It stems from the fact that the adult brain is enclosed in a rigid, incompressible box, with the result that the volume inside it must remain constant (Monro–Kelly Doctrine). A rise in ICP therefore decreases CPP (and hence cerebral blood flow). In raised ICP, as the brainstem becomes compressed, local neuronal activity causes a rise in sympathetic vasomotor drive and thus a rise in blood pressure. This is known as the Cushing's reflex. This elevated blood pressure evokes a bradycardia via the baroreceptor reflex. The Cushing's reflex helps to maintain cerebral blood flow and protect the vital centres of the brain from loss of nutrition if the ICP rises high enough to compress the cerebral arteries.

93. **D: Mutations in the haemagglutinin molecule are responsible for antigenic drift**

Viruses can be classified according to:

- Particle structure (i.e., virus family)
- Genomic type – RNA or DNA, single-stranded or double-stranded
- In addition, single-stranded RNA viruses can be divided into positive-stranded (coding) and negative-stranded (non-coding) RNA

Influenza is a member of the Orthomyxoviridae family of viruses and has a negative single-stranded RNA genome. The spherical surface of the virus is a lipid bilayer (envelope) containing the viral haemagglutinin (HA) and neuramidase (NA) which determine the subtype of the virus. The HA molecule mediates the entry of the virus into host cells. The NA molecule may be important in the release of viruses from host cells.

Epidemics of influenza occur through mutations, resulting in amino acid substitutions of the HA and NA that allow the virus to escape most host antibodies (antigenic drift). Pandemics, which tend to be longer and more widespread then epidemics, may occur when both the HA and NA are replaced through recombination of RNA segments with those of animal viruses, making all individuals susceptible to the new influenza virus (antigenic shift). The most notable influenza pandemics occurred in 1918, 1957, and 1968, resulting in millions of deaths worldwide. The virus that caused the last pandemic (H3N2) has been drifting ever since and we have no idea when the next pandemic will occur.

Transmission of influenza occurs by droplet inhalation. The initial symptoms of influenza are due to direct viral damage and associated inflammatory responses. Life-threatening influenza is often due to secondary bacterial infection as a result of the destruction of the respiratory epithelium by the influenza virus.

Influenza may be prevented by a vaccine that consists of inactivated preparations of the virus. It provides protection in up to 70 per cent of individuals for about one year. It is recommended for those only at high risk of acquiring the virus. The vaccines in use contain the HA and NA components in relation to the prevalent strain or strains of influenza circulating the previous year. Each year the World Health Organization recommends which strains should be included.

94. **B: Low calcium intake**

High dietary intake of calcium promotes calcium absorption, suppresses PTH release and bone dissolution, and thus protects against osteoporosis. Excess alcohol intake, sedentary lifestyle, early menopause, and a thin body habitus all promote bone loss.

95. **E: Affects the intrinsic, rather than the extrinsic, pathway for blood coagulation**

Haemophilia A is a sex-linked (X-linked recessive) disorder that results in a reduction in the amount or activity of the clotting factor, factor VIII, a member of the intrinsic pathway. Since the inheritance pattern is X-linked the disorder primarily affects males, since female individuals who carry the affected gene usually do not have bleeding manifestations. Clinically there is a tendency toward easy bruising and haemorrhage after trauma or operative procedures. In addition, spontaneous haemorrhages are frequently encountered in regions of the body normally subject to trauma, particularly the joints (haemarthroses).

Factor IX deficiency is known as haemophilia B (or Christmas disease) and is clinically indistinguishable from haemophilia A. Treatment of haemophilia A includes clotting factor replacement with recombinant factor VIII. The continued presence of this devastating disease throughout history may be explained by the protective effect against ischaemic heart disease in haemophilia carriers (by reducing the 'stickiness' of the blood; a similar effect to aspirin).

96. **C: It is secreto-motor to the lacrimal gland**

The facial, or 7th cranial, nerve has a variety of different functions and is important clinically. Its functions may be summarized as follows:

- Is associated developmentally with the 2nd branchial arch
- Supplies the muscles of facial expression
- Gives special taste sensation to the anterior two-thirds of the tongue via the chorda tympani nerve
- Carries secreto-motor fibres to the lacrimal gland through the greater petrosal nerve
- Is secreto-motor to the submandibular and sublingual glands
- Gives somatic sensation to the external auditory meatus

Special taste from the posterior third of the tongue is carried by the glossopharyngeal nerve. The levator palpebrae superioris muscle, responsible for elevating the eyelid, is not a muscle of facial expression – it is innervated by the occulomotor nerve and sympathetics. The orbicularis oculi muscle, responsible for blinking and for screwing the eye tight, is regarded as a muscle of facial expression and is supplied by the facial nerve.

The four principal muscles of mastication (temporalis, medial, and lateral pterygoids, masseter) are all supplied by the mandibular division of the trigeminal nerve. Note buccinator is not a muscle of mastication and is innervated by the facial nerve.

Understanding the earlier helps to explain what happens when things go wrong. A facial nerve (Bell's) palsy results in weakness of the muscles of facial expression down one side of the face, leading to a droop. Note that this is a lower motor neurone palsy and that all the muscles down the side of the face are affected including the forehead muscles. This is in sharp contrast to a cerebrovascular accident, or upper motor neurone facial palsy, where the upper (forehead) muscles are spared since they are bilaterally innervated from both cerebral cortices.

Beside a droopy face, however, a Bell's palsy also results in loss of sensation to the anterior two-thirds of the tongue and hyperacusis (sensitivity to sounds) as a result of denervation of the stapedius muscle, which normally serves to dampen down sounds in the middle ear. Dry eyes occur as a result of the loss of the secreto-motor supply to the lacrimal gland (and hence the need to protect the eye to prevent keratitis and corneal ulceration in a facial nerve palsy). This is exacerbated by the denervation of the orbicularis oculi muscle which normally functions to spread the tear film over the surface of the cornea with the blinking reflex.

Although it may not seem very important, the small somatic sensory branch of the facial nerve (that supplies the external auditory meatus) may explain why in Ramsey–Hunt syndrome (herpes zoster infection of the geniculate ganglion) herpes vesicles are found around the external auditory meatus.

This question illustrates nicely how a good understanding of anatomy may help the student in future clinical practice.

97. **B: The vital capacity is the sum of the inspiratory reserve volume, the expiratory reserve volume, and the tidal volume**

Spirometry traces are easy to understand if you remember the following 2 rules:

- There are 4 lung volumes and 5 capacities that you need to remember
- A capacity is made up of 2 or more lung volumes

The *4 lung volumes* are:

- *Tidal volume* = volume of air inspired or expired with each normal breath in quiet breathing, approximately 500 mL
- *Residual volume* = the volume of air that remains in the lung after forced expiration
- *Inspiratory reserve volume* = extra volume of air that can be inspired over and above the normal tidal volume
- *Expiratory reserve volume* = extra volume of air that can be expired by forceful expiration after the end of a normal tidal expiration

The *5 lung capacities* are:

- *Functional residual capacity* = the volume of air that remains in the lung at the end of quiet expiration – equal to the sum of the residual volume and the expiratory reserve volume
- *Inspiratory capacity* = inspiratory reserve volume + tidal volume
- *Expiratory capacity* = expiratory reserve volume + tidal volume
- *Vital capacity* = inspiratory reserve volume + tidal volume + expiratory reserve volume (or total lung capacity minus residual volume)
- *Total lung capacity* = vital capacity + residual volume

The residual volume (and therefore FRC and total lung capacity) cannot be measured directly by spirometry. They are measured by either whole-body plethysmography, or by using the helium dilution or nitrogen washout techniques.

98. **B: Delayed hypersensitivity reaction against the bacteria**

Mycobacteria stimulate a specific T-cell response of cell-mediated immunity resulting in granuloma formation. While this is effective in reducing the infection, the delayed hypersensitivity (type IV) reaction also damages the host tissues. Damage therefore primarily results from the host's immune response in an attempt to clear the body of infection – so-called immune pathology. The formation of granulomas is the host's attempt to wall off the mycobacteria from the rest of the body, thereby preventing dissemination. When an individual is immunosuppressed (in HIV for example), dissemination therefore occurs more readily with disastrous consequences.

The tubercle bacilli can survive within macrophages and this may account for latent infections and reactivation of tuberculosis in later life. There is no significant humoral response to mycobacteria. Necrosis does occur in tuberculosis, but it is usually within the granuloma (caseous necrosis). *M. tuberculosis* causes little or no direct or toxin-mediated damage.

99. **D: Ptosis of the left eye**

This patient has Horner's syndrome. Unilateral loss of sympathetic innervation of the face results in ptosis, pupil constriction (miosis), anhidrosis, facial flushing, and enophthalmos. Lateral deviation of the eye would suggest damage to the 3rd cranial nerve.

100. **D: It is more common in regions of the world in which malaria is endemic**

Sickle cell anaemia is an autosomal recessive condition, caused by a single base change in the DNA coding for the amino acid in the 6th position of the beta-haemoglobin chain (adenine is replaced by thymine). This leads to an amino acid change from glutamic acid to valine. The resultant haemoglobin, HbS, has abnormal physiochemical properties that leads to sickling of red bloods cells and sickle cell disease. Homozygosity at the sickle cell locus is known as sickle cell anaemia, while heterozygosity at the same locus is known as the sickle cell trait. Where malaria is endemic, as many as 30 per cent of black Africans are heterozygous. This frequency may be related in part to the slight protection against *Plasmodium falciparum* afforded by HbS.

Clinical manifestations do not occur until around 3–6 months after birth when the main switch from foetal to adult haemoglobin occurs (foetal haemoglobin does not contain β-haemoglobin chains). Clinical manifestations relate to the sickling of red blood cells as a result of the production of a structurally abnormal haemoglobin. This includes haemolysis (the average red cell survival is shortened from the normal 120 days to approximately 20 days) and occlusion of small blood vessels resulting in ischaemic tissue damage (so-called painful vaso-occlusive crises). The latter crises are precipitated by factors such as infection, acidosis, dehydration, or hypoxia. Homozygotes sickle at Po_2 levels of 5–6 kPa (i.e., normal venous blood) and thus sickling takes place all the time. Heterozygotes sickle at Po_2 levels of 2.5–4 kPa and therefore only sickle at extremely low oxygen tensions.

The spleen is enlarged in infancy and childhood, as a result of extramedullary haematopoiesis, but later is often reduced in size (autosplenectomy) as a result of erythrostasis within the spleen leading to thrombosis, autoinfarction, or at least marked tissue hypoxia. Therefore, one should not expect to find a palpable spleen on examining an adult with sickle cell anaemia.

101. **B: The intervertebral joints are secondary cartilaginous joints**

The spinal cord terminates at the level of L1/L2. Below this, only nerve roots exist within the vertebral canal (cauda equina). It is therefore safe to perform a lumbar puncture at the level of L3/4 or L4/5. Fortunately for the purpose of a lumbar puncture, the dural sac containing the cerebrospinal fluid does not terminate until the level of S2.

The intervertebral joints are secondary cartilaginous joints. Between each vertebral body lies an intervertebral disc which is predominantly created from an annulus fibrosus of fibrocartilage with an internal nucleus pulposus, a bubble of semiliquid gelatinous substance derived from the embryonic notochord. With age the fibrocartilaginous annulus does deteriorate and may weaken, often in the lower lumbar region, giving rise to a slipped, or prolapsed, disc. In such cases, the nucleus pulposus is typically extruded posterolaterally.

The relationship of the nerve roots to intervertebral discs is of great importance. At the level of the L4/5 disc, the 4th lumbar nerve roots within their dural sheath have already emerged from the intervertebral foramen and so are not lying low enough to come into contact with the disc. The roots that lie behind the posterolateral part of this disc are those of the 5th lumbar nerve and these are the ones likely to be irritated by the prolapse. Thus, the general rule throughout the vertebral column is that when a disc herniates (usually posterolaterally, rather than in the midline) it may irritate the nerve roots numbered one below the disc.

The spinal cord is supplied by the single, anterior spinal artery and two (right and left) posterior spinal arteries. Since there is only one anterior spinal artery, the spinal cord is vulnerable to anterior ischaemia (the anterior spinal artery syndrome). The posterior columns (mediating light touch and proprioception) remain intact, but most of the rest of the cord below the level of the lesion is affected, leading to weakness (corticospinal tract involvement) and loss of pain/ temperature sensation (anterolateral, or spinothalamic, tract involvement).

The richly supplied red marrow of the vertebral body drains through its posterior surface by large basivertebral veins into Batson's internal vertebral venous plexus, which lies inside the vertebral canal, but outside the dura (in the extradural space). It drains into the external vertebral venous plexus and thence into regional segmental veins. These veins are valveless and often act as a subsidiary route for blood flow when the inferior vena cava cannot cope with a sudden flush of blood resulting from a sudden increase of intra-abdominal pressure (e.g., straining, coughing, sneezing). A rise in pressure on the abdominal and pelvic veins would tend to force the blood backward out of the abdominal and pelvic cavities into the valveless veins within the vertebral canal. The existence of this venous plexus may explain how carcinoma of the prostate, kidney, breast, bronchus, and thyroid may metastasize to the vertebral column.

102. **E: It helps to prevent the formation of pulmonary oedema**

Surfactant is formed in and secreted by type II pneumocytes. The active ingredient is dipalmitoyl phosphatidylcholine. It helps prevent alveolar collapse by lowering the surface tension between water molecules in the surface layer. In this way it helps to reduce the work of breathing (makes the lungs more compliant) and permits the lung to be more easily inflated.

Since the surfactant remains at the water-air interface, the space between surfactant molecules decreases as the surface area is reduced; this is equivalent to raising its concentration, which lowers surface tension. This prevents alveolar collapse. Likewise, the decreasing effect of surfactant as the lungs inflate helps to prevent overinflation. This unique property of surfactant helps to stabilize different sizes of alveoli (otherwise the smaller alveoli would empty into the larger alveoli by LaPlace's law).

Surfactant is not produced in any significant quantity until the 32nd week of gestation and it then builds up to a high concentration by the 35th week (the normal gestation period is 39 weeks). Premature delivery may therefore result in inadequate surfactant production and respiratory distress syndrome of the newborn (hyaline membrane disease).

Surfactant also plays an important role in keeping the alveoli dry. Just as the surface tension forces tend to collapse alveoli, they also tend to suck fluid into the alveolar spaces from the capillaries. By reducing these surface forces, surfactant prevents the transudation of fluid. In this way surfactant acts as an important safety mechanism against the formation of pulmonary oedema.

103. **C: Typically affects the apical lung in post-primary TB**

One-third of the world's population are infected with *Mycobacterium tuberculosis*. It is a major cause of death worldwide and is rapidly increasing in prevalence, in part because of the sharp increase in the number of individuals infected with HIV and because of the recent emergence of multi-drug resistant TB. Mycobacteria are obligate aerobic, rod-shaped, non-spore forming, non-motile bacilli with a waxy coat that causes them to retain certain stains after being treated with acid and alcohol; they are therefore known as acid–alcohol-fast bacilli (AAFB). Mycobacteria do not readily take up the Gram stain but they would be Gram-positive if the Gram stain could penetrate their waxy walls. The Ziehl–Neelsen stain is used instead to visualize the organisms, which stain pinkish red.

The pattern of host response depends on whether the infection represents a primary first exposure to the organism (primary TB) or secondary reactivation or reinfection (post-primary or secondary TB). Primary TB is most often subpleural, most often in the periphery of one lung, in the mid-zone. The residuum of the primary infection is a calcified scar in the lung parenchyma (Ghon focus) along with hilar lymph node enlargement, together referred to as the Ghon complex. Secondary TB most often occurs at the lung apex (Assman lesion) of one or both lungs which may cavitate and heal by dense fibrosis. The apex of the lung is more highly oxygen-ated, allowing the aerobic mycobacteria to multiply more rapidly. Involvement of extrapulmonary sites (kidney, meninges, bone, etc.) is not uncommon.

M. tuberculosis is resistant to penicillin and requires multimodal antibiotic ther-apy (which may be remembered by RIPE) to prevent the emergence of resistance:

- Rifampicin (main side effect, liver toxicity)
- Isoniazid (main side effect, peripheral neuropathy)
- Pyrazinamide (main side effect, liver toxicity)
- Ethambutol (main side effect, optic neuropathy with visual disturbances)

Several months of combination treatment are required to treat *M. tuberculosis*. Pyridoxine (vitamin B$_6$) should be given with isoniazid to prevent isoniazid neuropathy.

M. tuberculosis can be prevented by immunization with BCG, a vaccine made from non-virulent tubercle bacilli. However, the protective efficacy of the vaccine is variable, ranging from 0 to 80 per cent depending on the part of the world in which it is administered.

104. **C: 500–1000 mL**

Fluid balance is maintained by water intake that is equal to losses in urine, stool, sweat, and insensible losses (through skin and lungs).

105. **C: Defective haem synthesis results in porphyria**

- Sickle cell disease is due to the production of abnormal globin
- Thalassaemia is due to the decreased production of normal globin

Both sickle cell and thalassaemia seemingly developed as a form of carrier resistance against malaria, and as such are widespread in areas profoundly affected by malaria, predominantly Africa, South East Asia, the Mediterranean, and the Middle East.

The porphyrias are a group of genetic diseases resulting from errors in the pathway of haem biosynthesis, resulting in the toxic accumulation of porphyrin precursors. Interestingly, porphyria has been suggested as an explanation for the origin of vampire and werewolf legends and is believed to have accounted for the insanity exhibited by King George III that may have cost Britain the American War of Independence.

Carbon monoxide binds 250 times more avidly to haemoglobin than oxygen, resulting in the formation of carboxyhaemoglobin. The result is a decrease in the oxygen-carrying capacity of the blood. Carbon monoxide is a colourless, odourless, and tasteless gas, so poisoning often occurs unnoticed. Levels of carboxyhaemoglobin >50–60 per cent result in death. The treatment is 100 per cent oxygen which competitively displaces carbon monoxide from the haemoglobin, thereby decreasing the half-life of carboxyhaemoglobin from around 4 hours to 30 minutes.

Cyanide binds more strongly than oxygen to the iron atom present in the enzyme, cytochrome oxidase. This deactivates the enzyme and the final transport of electrons from cytochrome oxidase to oxygen cannot be completed. As a result, oxidative phosphorylation is disrupted, meaning that the cell can no longer produce ATP for energy. Tissues that mainly depend on aerobic respiration, such as the central nervous system and heart, are particularly affected, rapidly resulting in death.

106. C: During exercise, blood flow to the upper portion of the lung increases

Systolic and diastolic pressures in the pulmonary artery are about one-sixth those in the aorta and so is the pulse pressure. This is because the pulmonary vascular resistance is about one-sixth of the systemic vascular resistance. The blood flow is the same in both circulations, otherwise blood would accumulate in one or the other bed.

In a standing subject, blood flow is less in the upper parts of the lung than the lower regions, but this is not matched by the differences in ventilation, so that the ventilation/perfusion ratio is not the same in all parts of the lung. A standing subject has a higher ventilation/perfusion ratio at the apex than the base.

During exercise, recruitment of the apical vessels occurs to accommodate the increase in cardiac output and pulmonary blood flow that occurs with exercise. This has the effect of increasing the area of capillaries available for gas exchange.

The pulmonary vasculature exhibits a peculiar property found nowhere else in the circulation, known as hypoxic pulmonary vasoconstriction. It consists of contraction of smooth muscle in the walls of the small arterioles in response to hypoxia – the opposite effect to that normally observed in the systemic circulation. The mechanism remains obscure. It has the effect of directing blood flow away from hypoxic regions of the lung (e.g., poorly ventilated areas of the diseased lung in adults) and in this way helps to optimize the local ventilation/perfusion ratios.

107. C: It results from the secretion of exotoxin

All members of the *Clostridia* group of organisms have the following properties:

- Gram-positive bacilli
- Obligate anaerobes
- Spore-forming
- Saprophytic (e.g., live in the soil)
- Motile (but non-invasive)
- Exotoxin-producing

Clostridia are responsible for causing several diseases in man: *C. tetani* (tetanus); *C. botulinum* (botulism); *C. perfringens,* formerly known as *C. welchii* (gas gangrene and food poisoning); and *C. difficile* (pseudomembranous colitis).

Tetanus is typically a disease of soldiers, farmers, or gardeners. It is caused by deep penetrating wounds caused by objects contaminated with soil, which introduces spores into the tissue. As soon as the wound becomes anaerobic, the tetanus spores germinate to produce vegetative cells, which then multiply and release a potent neurotoxin called tetanospasmin. Only the tiniest quantities of exotoxin are required for the disease to develop. The bacteria producing the exotoxin are entirely non-invasive and lack all other virulence factors apart from the capacity to produce toxin. The exotoxin binds to local nerve endings, travels up the axon to the spinal cord, traverses a synaptic junction, and finally gains entry to the cytoplasm of inhibitory neurones. Within these cells the toxin exerts a highly specific proteolytic activity on one of the proteins (synaptobrevin) present in the vesicles that is responsible for the normal trafficking of inhibitory neurotransmitter to the synaptic junction. As a result, the inhibitory neurone cannot transmit its impulse and there is unopposed stimulation of skeletal muscles by motor neurones. Death is normally due to muscular spasm (spastic paralysis) extending to involve the muscles of the chest so that the patient is unable to breathe.

As in other diseases caused entirely by an exotoxin, tetanus can be treated by passive immunization with antitoxin, and prevented by vaccination with toxoid. However, antitoxin cannot neutralize any toxin that has already entered neurones. Antibiotics are of limited value against anaerobic bacteria like *Clostridia* because they cannot penetrate the necrotic infected area in sufficient concentrations to be effective; surgical debridement of wounds is far superior.

108. **E: Arginine**

Nitric oxide (NO) is generated from arginine in a reaction catalysed by NO synthase. The other product of the reaction is citrulline.

109. **B: This difference would have arisen by chance alone less than one time in 200**

Do not confuse the terms standard error and standard deviation. The standard deviation gives a measure of the spread of the distribution. The smaller the standard deviation (or variance), the more tightly grouped the values are. If the values are normally distributed, approximately 95 per cent of values lie within two standard deviations of the mean (not standard errors!).

The standard error is a measure of how precisely the sample mean reflects the population mean. The standard error can be used to construct confidence intervals. Typically, a 95 per cent confidence interval is quoted, which means that we are 95 per cent certain that the true population mean lies within the interval given by mean $\pm$ 1.96 standard errors. In this case the 95 per cent confidence interval is approximately 0.5 $\pm$ 0.4, or 0.1–0.9. There is therefore a 5 per cent chance that the true population mean lies outside the range 0.1–0.9.

The p-value is a probability that derives from statistical significance tests. It takes a value between 0 and 1. Values close to zero suggest that the null hypothesis is unlikely to be true. The smaller the p-value, the more significant the result. A significant result is normally taken as a p-value <0.05 (or 5 per cent), meaning that the difference would have arisen by chance alone in less than 1 time in 20. A *p*-value <0.005 (or 0.5 per cent) is highly significant, meaning that the difference would have arisen by chance alone less than 1 time in 200.

110. **D: The posterior wall of the canal is bounded by transversalis fascia and the conjoint tendon medially**

Many students are troubled by the anatomy and significance of the inguinal canal. Its boundaries are:

- *Anterior wall*: Skin, superficial fascia, external oblique (for whole length), internal oblique for lateral one-third
- *Posterior wall*: Transversalis fascia (for whole length), conjoint tendon, and pectineal (Cooper's) ligament medially
- *Floor*: Inguinal ligament (Poupart's ligament)
- *Roof*: Arching fibres of internal oblique and transversus abdominus which fuse to form the conjoint tendon on the posteromedial aspect of the canal

The inguinal canal is an oblique passage that runs from the deep to the superficial inguinal rings and serves to transmit the testis (in the developing male) and spermatic cord in adulthood. It therefore functions to exteriorize the testis so that an optimal temperature can be obtained in order for spermatogenesis to proceed. In the female the inguinal canal transmits the round ligament of the uterus and by this means helps to maintain and support the uterus in its typical anteverted, anteflexed position.

The deep inguinal ring is a hole in the transversalis fascia and lies a finger-breadth above the mid-point of the inguinal ligament (i.e., halfway between the anterior superior iliac spine and pubic tubercle). The superficial inguinal ring is a hole in the external oblique aponeurosis. The key to understanding the inguinal canal is to concentrate on the internal oblique layer which laterally forms the anterior wall of the inguinal canal. The internal oblique then arches over the top of the canal forming its roof and then blends with the transversus abdominus layer posteriorly and medially to form the conjoint tendon.

A hernia is simply a protrusion of a viscus, or part of a viscus, outwith its normal position. A femoral hernia can be distinguished from an inguinal hernia by its position. An inguinal hernia lies above and medial to the pubic tubercle, while a femoral hernia lies below and lateral to the pubic tubercle. The pubic tubercle is thus an important landmark in differentiating a femoral from an inguinal hernia. In addition, an inguinal hernia may be either direct or indirect. A direct hernia passes straight through a weakness in the anterior abdominal wall and passes through the superficial ring only. An indirect hernia, in contrast, passes through both the deep and superficial inguinal rings and thereby passes along the entire length of the inguinal canal.

111. **D: A fall in pressure in the afferent arteriole promotes renin secretion**

The juxtaglomerular apparatus is a specialization of the glomerular afferent arteriole and the distal convoluted tubule of the corresponding nephron and is involved in the regulation of extracellular volume and blood pressure via the renin–angiotensin system.

The juxtaglomerular apparatus has 3 components:

- Macula densa – Specialized epithelial cells lining the distal convoluted tubule
- Juxtaglomerular cells (also known as granular cells) of the afferent arterioles – Modified smooth muscle cells that are renin-secreting
- Extraglomerular mesangial cells (also known as Lacis cells or Goormaghtigh cells) – Their function remains obscure

The extraglomerular mesangial cells contain contractile proteins that are instrumental in the fine tuning of glomerular filtration. They have phagocytic properties and may act as antigen-presenting cells. They may also be the site of secretion of the hormone erythropoietin.

The renin–angiotensin system is triggered to release renin under 3 circumstances:

- Fall in the renal perfusion pressure detected by baroreceptors in the afferent arterioles
- Activation of the sympathetic nervous system – this occurs when there is a fall in arterial blood pressure
- Reduced sodium delivery to the macula densa (as detected by osmoreceptors) – this occurs when there is also a fall in renal perfusion pressure

An unknown paracrine factor is believed to act between the macula densa and juxtaglomerular cells to stimulate renin release (a prostaglandin or NO has been postulated).

The renin–angiotensin system is strongly implicated in the pathogenesis of hypertension secondary to renal artery stenosis. The juxtaglomerular apparatus of the affected kidney responds to decreased perfusion pressure by increasing renin secretion (Goldblatt hypertension).

112. **C: Astrocytomas**

It is estimated that 50 per cent of bronchial carcinomas have metastasized by the time of clinical presentation. Breast carcinoma metastasizes readily to sites such as the lung, bone, and brain. Melanoma is an aggressive tumour that can metastasize to virtually any site within the body. It therefore carries an extremely poor prognosis. Renal cell carcinomas characteristically invade the renal veins and extend into the inferior vena cava (sometimes reaching as far up as the right atrium), so that blood-borne metastases are common, especially to the lungs, liver, and bone.

Astrocytomas (and even the poorly differentiated form, glioblastoma multiforme), rarely metastasize to sites outside of the central nervous system since they are contained by the blood–brain barrier. They usually metastasize outside the central nervous system *only* if there is a breach in the blood–brain barrier, or if there is an artificial connection (such as a ventriculoperitoneal shunt) connecting the central nervous system with another part of the body.

113. C: Neuroendocrine cells

Small-cell undifferentiated pulmonary carcinoma (oat-cell carcinoma) is closely linked to smoking. This malignancy is thought to arise from neuroendocrine cells of the bronchial mucosa. Clara cells may give rise to certain pulmonary adenocarcinomas, and metaplastic bronchial epithelium is a likely source of squamous cell carcinomas. Alveolar pneumocytes rarely undergo malignant transformation.

114. D: The negative predictive value is 0.99

The *sensitivity* indicates how sensitive the test is at picking up those people who have the disease. It is equal to the number of people who are both disease-positive and test-positive divided by the number who are disease-positive. In this example, it is 4/5. The *specificity* indicates how good the test is at picking up those people who do not have the disease. It is equal to the number of people who are both disease-negative and test-negative divided by the number of people who are disease-negative. In this example it is 90/95.

The *positive predictive value* estimates the probability that a subject, who has a positive test, truly has the disease. In this example, it is 4/9. The *negative predictive value* estimates the probability that a subject who has a negative test truly does not have the disease. Here it is 90/91. The sensitivity and specificity are independent of disease prevalence.

115. E: It forms the entrance to the lesser sac

The greater and lesser sacs of the peritoneal cavity communicate with each other by way of the epiploic foramen (of Winslow). This is therefore a key landmark within the abdomen both anatomically and clinically. The boundaries of the epiploic foramen are as follows:

- *Anteriorly*: The lesser omentum with the common bile duct, portal vein, and common hepatic artery in its free edge
- *Posteriorly*: Inferior vena cava
- *Superiorly*: The caudate (not quadrate) lobe of the liver
- *Inferiorly*: First part of duodenum
- *Medially*: Lesser sac (posterior to stomach)
- *Laterally*: Greater sac

From a clinical standpoint, the epiploic foramen is important for two reasons. First, it may be the site of internal herniation of bowel. Second, compression of the common hepatic artery in the free edge of the lesser omentum by a carefully placed hand in the epiploic foramen may be a life-saving manoeuvre at laparotomy to control bleeding from the liver (Pringle's manoeuvre).

116. **A: It increases in response to a loss of circulating volume of at least 10 per cent**

ADH synthesis occurs in the cell bodies of the magnocellular neurones in the supraoptic (5/6) and paraventricular nuclei (1/6) of the hypothalamus. From there, ADH is transported down the axons of these neurones to their endings in the posterior pituitary (neurohypophysis or pars nervosa) where they are stored as secretory granules prior to release. Release is controlled directly by nerve impulses passing down the axons from the hypothalamus; this process is known as neurosecretion.

Increased secretion of ADH occurs in response to two main stimuli: an increase in plasma osmolality and a decrease in effective circulating volume. Significant changes in secretion occur when osmolality is changed as little as 1 per cent. Such a change is detected by osmoreceptors that lie outside the blood–brain barrier and appear to be located in the circumventricular organs, particularly the organum vasculosum of the lamina terminalis. In this way, the osmoreceptors rapidly respond to changes in plasma osmolality and in normal individuals plasma osmolality is maintained very close to 285 mOsm/L. ADH secretion is considerably more sensitive to small changes in osmolality than to similar changes in blood volume. Plasma ADH levels do not increase appreciably until blood volume is reduced by about 10 per cent, when ADH plays a significant role in the response to haemorrhage.

ADH has two main actions: it increases free-water absorption from the collecting ducts of the kidney (thereby conserving water), and it is a potent vasoconstrictor. The mechanism by which ADH exerts its antidiuretic effect is through the action on V2 receptors and insertion of protein water channels (aquaporins) in the luminal membranes of collecting-duct cells. Aquaporins are stored in endosomes inside cells and ADH causes their translocation to the cell membrane via a cyclic AMP pathway. In this way, the urine becomes concentrated and its volume decreases in response to an increase in plasma osmolality and a rise in ADH; this osmoregulatory action of ADH is a good example of a homeostatic mechanism. Vasoconstriction is mediated via V1 receptors (and the phosphoinositol pathway). The latter effect has an important role in maintaining arterial blood pressure in haemorrhagic shock.

Hypersecretion of ADH occurs in the syndrome of inappropriate ADH release (SIADH). Diabetes insipidus is the syndrome that results when there is ADH deficiency (cranial form), or when the kidney fails to respond to the hormone (nephrogenic form). It should not be confused with diabetes mellitus; the term 'diabetes' is derived from the Greek meaning 'siphon', and simply reflects the excessive passing of urine in both conditions.

117. **D: Elevated serum gamma-glutamyl transpeptidase**

Elevated serum gamma-glutamyl transpeptidase (GGT) may be the only laboratory abnormality in patients who are dependent on alcohol. Heavy drinkers may also have an increased MCV.

118. **A: Valvulae conniventes**

The following distinguish the large bowel from small bowel in the cadaver, at laparotomy, and on imaging. Large bowel has the following 3 characteristic features:

- Haustra (synonymous with sacculations)
- Appendices epiploicae
- *Taeniae coli*

Valvulae conniventes (synonymous with plica circulares) are a feature of small bowel rather than large bowel.

119. **D: The kidney is able to generate new bicarbonate from glutamine**

The precision with which hydrogen ion concentration is regulated emphasizes its importance to the various cell functions. The normal pH of the blood is held remarkably constant in the range 7.35–7.45. It is essential that the pH be kept within these stringent limits to prevent the denaturing of body proteins and enzymes. This is yet another example of homeostasis, whereby the constancy of the 'internal milieu' is essential to life.

There are 3 primary systems that regulate the pH in the body:

- The chemical buffer systems of the body fluids
- The respiratory system (which regulates the removal of CO_2 and therefore carbonic acid from the blood)
- The kidneys

The bone and liver also play a small role in the regulation of pH. When there is a change in pH, the buffer systems work fastest (within a fraction of a second) to minimize the change in pH. Of these, the bicarbonate buffer system is the most important extracellular buffer. The second line of defence is the respiratory system which acts within a few minutes. These first two lines of defence keep the pH constant until the more slowly responding third line of defence, the kidneys, can eliminate the excess acid or base from the body. Although the kidneys are relatively slow to respond compared with the other defences (taking hours to days), they are the most powerful of the acid–base regulatory systems.

The renal tubule actively secretes hydrogen ions and reabsorbs bicarbonate ions. Acute renal failure therefore results in an inability to excrete acid and metabolic acidosis. There are 3 main methods by which the kidney absorbs bicarbonate:

- Replacement of filtered bicarbonate with bicarbonate that is generated in tubular cells
- Generation of new bicarbonate by the phosphate buffer system which carries excess hydrogen ions into the urine
- Generation of new bicarbonate from glutamine molecules that are absorbed by the tubular cell (the ammonia buffer system)

120. B: Tumour growth obeys Gompertzian kinetics

Consider the growth of a tumour. A cell divides to form two cells, these divide to form four cells, and so on. Assuming no cell losses, the tumour will double in cell numbers every few days (a typical cell cycle in a mammalian cell is about 24 hours). Cells continue to multiply because there is loss of the normal regulatory mechanisms that restrict tissue growth (such as contact inhibition). It is unusual for a tumour to become clinically obvious until there are about 10^9 cells (30 divisions), or 1 gram of tumour cells (corresponding to a tumour diameter of approximately 1 cm).

However, as the tumour continues to grow it begins to outstrip its own blood supply so that an increasing number of cells are lost by apoptosis. Also, as the tumour expands, more and more cells are shed through exfoliation, hypoxia, non-viability, metastasis, and host defences. The result of this is two-fold. First, the rate of tumour growth begins to slow down from the initial exponential pattern. The tumour growth curve therefore tends to assume a sigmoidal shape (Gompertzian kinetics).

Second, it means the growth fraction (the proportion of cells within the tumour population that are in the proliferative pool) of smaller tumours is greater than that of larger tumours. As tumours continue to grow, cells leave the replicative pool in ever-increasing numbers, owing to shedding or lack of nutrients, by differentiating and by reversion to the resting phase of the cell cycle, G_0. Thus, by the time the tumour is clinically detectable, most cells are not in the replicative pool (and so are relatively resistant to the effects of chemoradiotherapy). The growth fraction is usually 4 per cent to 80 per cent, with an average of less than 20 per cent. Even in some rapidly growing tumours, the growth fraction is only approximately 20 per cent. Indeed, some normal tissues, such as bone marrow and alimentary mucosa, have larger growth fractions and shorter mitotic cycle times than many cancers, even cancers of those tissues. Ultimately the progressive growth of tumours and the rate at which they grow are determined by the excess of cell production over cell loss.

It is very important to recognize that the clinical phase of a tumour – that is, the time from it becoming clinically apparent until it causes the death of the patient (assuming no treatment) – is short in comparison to the preclinical phase. Thus, by the time a solid tumour is detected, it has already completed a major portion of its life cycle. During the long preclinical phase there is time for invasion and metastasis to occur. In addition, there is time for cell heterogeneity to develop within the tumour. This means that over and above the initial mutations, further genetic events occur in sub-populations of the tumour, leading to variation and the outgrowth of sub-populations with different patterns of differentiation and properties (a form of Darwinian evolution).

121. **D: It is stimulated to contract by cholecystokinin**

The gallbladder has three main functions: it stores bile, concentrates bile (5- to 20-fold), and adds mucus to the bile secreted by the liver. It has a capacity of about 50 mL. Its mucous membrane is a lax areolar tissue lined with simple columnar epithelium. Under the epithelium there is a layer of connective tissue, followed by a muscular wall that contracts in response to cholecystokinin, a peptide hormone secreted by the duodenal mucosa in response to the entry of fatty foods into the duodenum.

The gallbladder is supplied by the cystic artery, usually a branch of the right hepatic artery. It runs across the triangle formed by the liver, common hepatic duct, and cystic duct to reach the gallbladder (Calot's triangle). Calot's triangle reliably contains the cystic artery, the cystic lymph node (of Lund), connective tissue, and lymphatics. It is important to dissect out this triangle at laparoscopic cholecystectomy in order to successfully identify and ligate the cystic artery prior to removal of the gallbladder.

The gallbladder is not essential for life. Indeed, rats and horses manage perfectly well without gallbladders. Patients who have had their gallbladder removed lead a normal life and can expect a normal life expectancy. Removal of the gallbladder (cholecystectomy) is a common operation. Indications usually relate to gallstone disease, but rarely it may be performed for conditions such as carcinoma of the gallbladder. It may be performed open but is mostly performed nowadays by the laparoscopic (keyhole) route.

122. **D: The low blood flow in the vasa recta assists in the formation of concentrated urine**

In a normal adult human, the combined blood flow through both kidneys is about 1200 mL/min, or about 20 per cent of the cardiac output. Considering that the kidneys constitute only about 0.4 per cent of the total body weight, they receive an extremely high blood flow compared with other tissues. The high flow to the kidneys greatly exceeds their metabolic demands (the kidneys account for only 6 per cent of total oxygen consumption). The purpose of this additional flow is to supply enough plasma for the high rates of glomerular filtration that are necessary for precise regulation of body fluid volumes and solute concentrations. Organic para-aminohippuric acid has traditionally been used to measure renal blood flow.

The kidneys have effective mechanisms for maintaining the constancy of renal blood flow and GFR over an arterial pressure range between 70 and 170 mmHg, a process called autoregulation. This helps to maintain a normal excretion of metabolic waste products, such as urea and creatinine, that depend on GFR for their excretion. Autoregulation is an intrinsic property of the kidney; therefore, transplanted kidneys will autoregulate. There are two main theories to explain how renal autoregulation of blood flow occurs: tubuloglomerular feedback and the myogenic mechanism.

Angiotensin II preferentially constricts the efferent more than the afferent arteriole. This has the effect of raising glomerular filtration pressure, while reducing renal blood flow. Under the circumstances of decreased arterial blood pressure (when angiotensin II is released) this helps to prevent decreases in GFR (tubuloglomerular feedback method of autoregulation); at the same time by reducing renal blood flow it causes increased reabsorption of sodium and water. In cases of renal artery stenosis, maintenance of the glomerular filtration pressure is dependent on the angiotensin II-dependent vasoconstriction of the efferent arteriole. Administration of ACE inhibitors abolishes the vasoconstriction of the efferent arteriole, resulting in an abrupt fall in the glomerular filtration rate. This explains why ACE inhibitors are contraindicated in renal artery stenosis.

Flow to the renal medulla is supplied by long capillary loops called the vasa recta. These descend into the medulla in parallel with the loops of Henle. The blood flow in them is very low compared with flow in the renal cortex. This helps to maintain the hyperosmotic medullary interstitial gradient, thereby assisting in the formation of a concentrated urine.

123. **B: It is highly dependent on vascular endothelial growth factor (VEGF)**

As soon as tumours grow to more than about 1–2 mm^3 they require the development of new blood vessels to sustain them, a process called angiogenesis (not to be confused with apoptosis which is programmed cell death). This is because the 1–2 mm zone represents the maximum distance across which oxygen and nutrients can diffuse from blood vessels. Beyond 1–2 mm the tumour fails to enlarge without blood vascularization because hypoxia induces apoptosis by activation of p53. Neovascularization has a dual effect on tumour growth: perfusion supplies nutrients and oxygen to the growing tumour, and newly formed endothelial cells stimulate the growth of adjacent tumour cells through the secretion of cytokines.

Tumour cells elaborate angiogenic factors that induce new blood vessel formation. Of the dozen or so tumour-associated angiogenic factors that have been discovered, the two most important are vascular endothelial growth factor (VEGF) and basic fibroblast growth factor (bFGF). Much attention has focused on the use of angiogenesis inhibitors to cure cancer since angiogenesis is critical for the growth and metastasis of tumours. Whether this theoretical benefit translates into clinical practice is another matter and clinical trials are currently in progress.

Angiogenesis is also a hallmark of granulation tissue. It plays an important physiological role in wound healing by assisting in the delivery of oxygen and nutrients to healing tissue, where it is required for growth and repair. Granulation tissue produces a rich 'cytokine soup', including secretion of VEGF and bFGF which stimulates angiogenesis.

124. **B: It may refer pain to the right shoulder tip**

The surface marking of the gallbladder is opposite the tip of the right ninth costal cartilage; that is, where the lateral edge of the right rectus sheath crosses the costal margin. This is an important landmark as it is the site of maximal abdominal tenderness in gallbladder disease.

Gallstone disease may refer pain to the right shoulder tip (Kehr's sign). There is an important anatomical explanation underlying this phenomenon. An inflamed or distended gallbladder may irritate the diaphragm which is supplied by the phrenic nerve ('C3, C4, C5, keeps the diaphragm alive!'). These very same nerve roots also provide sensation to the right shoulder tip by way of the supraclavicular nerves (C3, 4, 5). The body misinterprets the signals that it receives and interprets the pain signals as coming from the right shoulder tip. This is the concept of referred pain (pain felt remote from the site of tissue damage). The very same phenomenon may occur in a ruptured ectopic pregnancy, or splenic rupture, but in this instance the diaphragmatic irritant is free blood within the peritoneal cavity. Indeed, anything that irritates the diaphragm may cause referred pain to the right shoulder tip.

Courvoisier's law states that, in the presence of obstructive jaundice, a palpable gallbladder is unlikely to be due to gallstones. The reason is that gallstones cause chronic inflammation, fibrosis, and a shrunken gallbladder. Rather, the law implies that a palpable gallbladder is more likely to be caused by carcinoma of the head of the pancreas causing an obstruction to biliary outflow. Note, however, that the law is not true the other way around (i.e., in the presence of obstructive jaundice an impalpable gallbladder is always due to gallstones) as 50 per cent of dilated gallbladders cannot be palpated on clinical examination, due to either the patient's obesity or because of overlap of the liver.

Cholelithiasis (the presence of gallstones) is a common condition. Often, they are picked up incidentally on ultrasound scan. The stones are of two types: calcium bilirubinate and cholesterol. In Europe and the United States, 85 per cent are cholesterol stones. Three factors seem to be involved in the formation of cholesterol stones: bile stasis, supersaturation of bile with cholesterol (lithogenic bile), and nucleation factors. Crucially, however, 80 per cent of patients with gallstones remain asymptomatic throughout their life. Therefore, in a patient with proven gallstones on ultrasound scan a good history is imperative in order to assess whether or not the patient's symptoms are really due to the gallstones. If not, they are unlikely to benefit from having the gallbladder removed.

125. **D: The glomerular filtration barrier comprises three layers**

In the normal adult human, the GFR (or normal renal clearance) averages 125 mL/min, or 180 L a day. The entire plasma volume (about 3 L) can therefore be filtered and processed by the kidney approximately 60 times each day. The rate of urine production in humans is dominated by tubular function and not by GFR. The GFR remains relatively constant through autoregulation.

After 35 years of age, GFR falls at about 1 mL/min each year. By the age of 80, GFR has fallen to about 50 per cent of its youthful level. GFR can decrease by as much as 50 per cent before plasma creatinine rises beyond the normal range. Consequently, a normal creatinine does not necessarily imply normal renal function, although a raised creatinine does usually indicate impaired renal function.

A substance used to measure the GFR must be freely filtered at the glomerulus, not be secreted by the tubules, not be reabsorbed, not be metabolized or synthesized in the body, not alter the renal function/GFR, be non-toxic, and be soluble in plasma. Such a substance is the polyfructose molecule, inulin. However, it is too cumbersome to use in routine clinical practice. Instead, GFR is more commonly quantified by measuring the 24-hour urinary creatinine excretion. Para-aminohippuric acid is used to measure renal blood flow and not GFR.

The glomerular filtration barrier comprises 3 layers:

- The capillary endothelium
- Basement membrane
- A layer of epithelial cells (podocytes)

From the anatomy of the glomerulus, it is clear that the 'actual filter' (and the primary restriction point for proteins) is the basement membrane layer.

126. **D: Hepatocellular carcinoma and polyvinyl chloride exposure**

A carcinogen is a substance, form of energy, or organism capable of inducing a cancer. The following carcinogens have been strongly associated with the workplace:

- Scrotal cancer (Pott's cancer) in chimney sweeps
- Mesotheliomas in people exposed to asbestos (workers in the building industry, ship construction, and demolition)
- Transitional cell bladder carcinoma in rubber and dye workers, due to exposure to β-naphthylamine
- Angiosarcomas in workers exposed to polyvinyl chloride

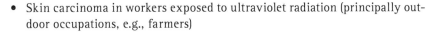

- Skin carcinoma in workers exposed to ultraviolet radiation (principally outdoor occupations, e.g., farmers)

127. **B: Exercise**

Exercise promotes glucose utilization and increased insulin sensitivity. All other options tend to exacerbate insulin resistance.

128. **E: The right subhepatic space or hepatorenal pouch (of Rutherford–Morison) is the most dependent part of the peritoneal cavity**

The liver capsule is composed of two adherent layers: a thick fibrous inner layer called Glisson's capsule (note Gerota's fascia surrounds the kidney) and an outer serous layer that is derived from the peritoneum. Glisson's capsule covers the entire surface of the liver and the serous layer covers most of the liver surface, excluding the 'bare' area of the liver near the diaphragm, the porta hepatis, and the area where the gallbladder is attached to the liver. So tough is Glisson's capsule that a subcapsular haematoma occurring as a result of liver parenchymal injury may be effectively contained by the capsule. The capsule is richly innervated by autonomic fibres, so capsular stretching as a result of malignancy, for example, may be intensely painful.

The liver receives a dual blood supply, from the hepatic artery and the portal vein. The portal vein provides 75 per cent of the total hepatic blood flow, the hepatic artery 25 per cent. The portal vein contains blood from the gut, rich in products of digestion, but is only approximately 85 per cent saturated with oxygen. The hepatic artery oxygen concentration, however, is approximately 99 per cent. Each vessel therefore supplies approximately equal amounts of oxygen to the liver.

The ligamentum venosum is a remnant of the ductus venosus (a channel that shunts blood from the left umbilical vein directly into the inferior vena cava, during gestation, thereby bypassing the liver and preserving oxygenated blood for the head and neck region). The ligamentum teres (or round ligament), in the free edge of the falciform ligament, is a remnant of the left umbilical vein.

Within the peritoneal cavity proper there are various spaces that are potential sites in which pus may collect (forming an abscess). The most important spaces to recognize are the right and left subphrenic (subdiaphragmatic) spaces, the pelvis, the right and left paracolic gutters, and the right subhepatic space (also known as the hepatorenal pouch of Rutherford–Morison). When lying supine, the latter space is the most dependent part of the peritoneal cavity and hence is an area where intraperitoneal fluid is likely to accumulate in the form of an abscess (or 'collection'). The left subhepatic space is the lesser sac.

129. **E: The maximum concentrating ability of the human kidney is 1200 mOsm/L**

The filtered load of glucose normally undergoes complete reabsorption in the proximal convoluted tubule (remember the most important substances for survival are generally absorbed first). Therefore, no glucose is usually found in the urine. However, when the filtered load exceeds the capacity of the tubules to reabsorb glucose (as in uncontrolled diabetes mellitus), urinary excretion of glucose occurs (glycosuria).

Seventy per cent of sodium reabsorption takes place in the proximal convoluted tubule, 20 per cent takes place in the ascending limb of the loop of Henle, and only 10 per cent takes place in the distal convoluted tubule and collecting ducts. It is only the latter which is aldosterone-dependent.

The maximum concentration of urine that can be excreted by the human kidney is 1200 mOsm/L, four times the osmolality of plasma. This is primarily a function of the length of the loop of Henle, the hyperosmotic medullary interstitial gradient, and the concentration of ADH. A counter-current multiplication system sets up an osmotic gradient in the renal medulla which allows an efficient way for urine to be concentrated over a relatively short distance along the nephron with minimal energy expenditure. The descending limb of the loop of Henle is permeable to water (but only slightly permeable to salt and urea). Therefore, water is progressively absorbed down the limb, becoming more concentrated (up to 1200 mOsm/L). The ascending limb is impermeable to water but permeable to sodium chloride. The tubular fluid is therefore hypotonic by the time it reaches the distal convoluted tubule and collecting ducts. In the presence of a high concentration of ADH, by the time the urine is excreted it has a high osmolality (up to 1200 mOsm/L).

The limited ability of the human kidney to concentrate urine to a maximal concentration of 1200 mOsm/L helps to explain why severe dehydration occurs on drinking seawater. The osmolality of seawater averages 2400 mOsm/L, so drinking one litre of seawater would give a total solute concentration of 2400 mOsm. If the maximal urine concentrating ability of the human kidney is 1200 mOsm/L, 2 litres is required to rid the body of these solutes. This would result in a net loss of 1 litre for every litre of seawater drunk, explaining the rapid dehydration that occurs in shipwreck victims who drink seawater. In short, if lost at sea, you are better off drinking nothing than drinking seawater.

130. **C: Burkitt's lymphoma**

Oncogenic microorganisms are capable of producing tumours. Most are viral. However, *Helicobacter pylori* is a good example of a bacterium that has been associated with gastric carcinoma and gastric lymphoma, while *Schistosoma haematobium* is a good example of a parasitic infection that is capable of pro-ducing squamous cell carcinoma of the bladder.

Viruses are obligate intracellular parasites that rely on the host cell's replicative machinery to reproduce themselves. Oncogenic viruses have therefore evolved to induce host-cell replication by activating genes for cell growth. This confers a survival advantage on the virus. However, it is when proliferation becomes uncoordinated and excessive that carcinoma results. Epstein–Barr (DNA) virus has been implicated in the pathogenesis of 3 human cancers:

- Burkitt's lymphoma
- Nasopharyngeal carcinoma
- Hodgkin's disease

Other well-described oncogenic viruses, besides EBV, include 2 RNA viruses:

- Human T-cell leukaemia virus (HTLV-1)
- Hepatitis C virus, leading to hepatocellular carcinoma

and three DNA viruses:

- Hepatitis B virus, leading to hepatocellular carcinoma
- Human herpes virus type 8 (HHV-8), leading to Kaposi's sarcoma in HIV individuals
- Human papilloma virus, leading to cervical carcinoma or anal carcinoma

There are several *mechanisms* by which viruses can induce malignancy:

- Directly, by becoming integrated into a cell's genome and by activation of cellular oncogenes
- Indirectly, through processes (e.g., chronic inflammation) which predispose to malignancy – the mitotically active tissue presumably provides a fertile soil for mutations
- By the production of proteins that inactivate tumour suppressor proteins, such as p53

131. **C: Papillary thyroid cancer**

In the UK, the most common primary thyroid cancer seen is the papillary variant which typically affects young women. Risk factors include previous radiation exposure (e.g., Chernobyl) and previous radiotherapy. Secondary thyroid cancers (metastases) are rare but can arise secondary to renal cell carcinomas. In the developing world, the follicular variant is most common and is associated with iodine deficiency and longstanding goitres. Medullary thyroid tumours (associated with multiple endocrine neoplasia type 2) and lymphomas are less common.

132. **B: They feature at the lower end of the oesophagus**

Portosystemic anastomoses are important sites in the body at which the portal venous circulation meets the systemic venous circulation. There are 5 principal sites where this takes place:

- Lower end of the oesophagus
- Upper end of the anal canal

- Periumbilical region of the anterior abdominal wall
- Bare area of the liver
- Retroperitoneum

In liver failure (cirrhosis), fibrosis of the liver takes place with obliteration of the blood vessels within it. Blood from the portal vein is then unable to drain through the liver into the inferior vena cava. As a result, 80 per cent of the portal blood flow is shunted into collateral channels, so that only 20 per cent reaches the liver. The portosystemic anastomoses open up in liver failure (but not in renal failure) and act as collateral channels, allowing an alternative path for blood to flow. Nevertheless, the opening up of the collaterals does not decrease the level of pressure within the portal system, and portal hypertension ensues. The consequence of this is splenomegaly as a result of portal hypertension. However, the spleen *per se* is not a site of portosystemic anastomosis.

The most important area to remember as a site of portosystemic anastomosis is the lower end of the oesophagus, because of its clinical significance. The veins from the lower third of the oesophagus drain downwards to the left gastric vein (portal system) and above this level oesophageal veins drain into the azygous and hemiazygous systems (systemic system). Subsequently in portal hypertension, dilatation of the veins within the lower end of the oesophagus may take place. These are known as oesophageal varices. The same effect also takes place at the other sites of portosystemic anastomosis. However, there is one key difference between the lower oesophagus and these other sites – that is, oesophageal varices have thin walls and are prone to rupture, as predicted by LaPlace's law. Rupture of oesophageal varices may result in a catastrophic upper gastrointestinal bleed that is often fatal.

Dilatations of veins within the anterior abdominal wall (also a site of portosystemic anastomosis) are known as caput medusae, because of their resemblance to the hair of the Greek mythological character, Medusa. Venous dilatations within the upper end of the anal canal in portal hypertension may lead to the formation of haemorrhoids. However, in practice, they rarely lead to problems and the presence of oesophageal varices is far more significant.

133. A: They behave in a dominant fashion

Cancer is a genetic disease. Oncogenes are growth-promoting genes that are expressed in normal cells (the correct name for its normal precursor is proto-oncogene). They encode for oncoproteins (growth factors, growth receptor molecules, signal transducing molecules, nuclear transcription factors, regulators of the cell cycle) that positively regulate growth and are involved in the growth and differentiation of normal cells. Transcription of oncogenes is tightly regulated in normal cells.

Over-expression of oncoproteins, or mutations of oncogenes resulting in the inappropriate activation of oncoproteins, leads to abnormal cell growth and survival (i.e., tumourigenesis). Mutations in oncogenes that result in tumours are generally gain-of-function mutations, so oncogenes behave in a dominant manner to promote cell transformation; that is, only one copy of the defective gene is sufficient to cause cancer.

Proto-oncogenes are converted into oncogenes through a variety of mechanisms that include:

- Point mutations
- Chromosomal rearrangements
- Gene amplification
- Incorporation of a new promoter (by viruses)
- Incorporation of enhancer sequences (by viruses)

The last two mechanisms are also referred to as insertional mutagenesis.

BRCA-1 is a tumour suppressor gene that accounts for a small proportion of breast cancers.

134. B: GABA

Axons of the Purkinje neurones have GABA as the neurotransmitter, which is inhibitory in nature.

135. E: Splenectomized patients are at high risk of post-splenectomy sepsis

The spleen, the largest of the lymphoid organs, lies under the diaphragm on the left side of the abdomen. It may be summarized by 1, 3, 5, 7, 9, 11. That is, it measures $1 \times 3 \times 5$ inches, weighs 7 oz. (200 g), and lies beneath the 9th to 11th ribs. The spleen lies at the far-left margin of the lesser sac below the diaphragm. Thus, if one's hand is placed in the lesser sac (via the epiploic foramen of Winslow) the spleen is the most laterally placed structure palpable.

Accessory spleen (splenunculi) represent congenital ectopic splenic tissue and are found in up to 20 per cent of individuals. One or several may be found, usually along the splenic vessels or in the peritoneal attachments. They are rarely larger than 2 cm in diameter.

Two 'pedicles', the gastrosplenic and lienorenal ligaments, connect the hilum of the spleen to the greater curvature of the stomach and the anterior surface of the left kidney, respectively. The splenic vessels and pancreatic tail lie in the lienorenal ligament. The short gastric and left gastroepiploic vessels run in the gastrosplenic ligament.

The functions of the spleen may be summarized by FISH:

- Filtration and removal of old blood cells and encapsulated microorganisms
- Immunological functions (production of IgM and opsonins)
- Storage function (30 per cent of the total platelets within the spleen)
- Haematopoiesis (in the developing fetus)

It has recently been evoked that the spleen has an endocrine function through the production of an immuno-potentiating peptide called tuftsin. The kidney, rather than the spleen, is the major site of erythropoietin secretion. Note that the spleen only acts as a site of haematopoiesis in the adult in diseased states where extramedullary haematopoiesis is a feature, such as thalassaemia.

Splenectomy (i.e., removal of the spleen) may be performed as an emergency procedure when the spleen has ruptured through trauma, or as an elective (i.e., scheduled) procedure, usually for haematological disorders where hypersplenism has caused an abnormality in one or more blood parameters. It is essential to understand the anatomical relations of the spleen (e.g., the pancreatic tail, stomach, splenic flexure of the colon, left kidney, diaphragm) in order to prevent inadvertent injury to these at splenectomy. Splenectomized patients are at high risk of post-splenectomy sepsis, especially from encapsulated organisms such as *Haemophilus, Meningococcus,* and *Streptococcus.* Prophylaxis consists of the relevant vaccinations and lifelong penicillin.

136. **E: Parietal cells**

Goblet cells are mucus-secreting cells widely distributed in epithelial surfaces, but especially dense in the gastrointestinal and respiratory tracts.

Kupffer cells have phagocytic properties and are found in the liver. They participate in the removal of ageing erythrocytes and other particulate debris.

The gastric mucosa contains many cell subtypes including acid-secreting cells (also known as parietal or oxyntic cells), pepsin-secreting cells (also known as peptic, chief, or zymogenic cells), and G-cells (gastrin-secreting cells). Peptic cells synthesize and secrete the proteolytic enzyme, pepsin. Parietal cells actively secrete hydrochloric acid into the gastric lumen accounting for the acidic environment encountered in the stomach. However, parietal cells are also involved in the secretion of the glycoprotein, intrinsic factor.

Intrinsic factor plays a pivotal role in the absorption of vitamin B_{12} from the terminal ileum. Autoimmune attack against parietal cells leads to a lack of intrinsic factor and hydrochloric acid, leading to vitamin B_{12} deficiency and achlorhydria. This is known as pernicious anaemia.

137. **D: Inflammation is intimately connected with the clotting system**

Acute inflammation is a stereotyped, non-specific response to tissue injury. It occurs in response to a variety of different tissue insults (both exogenous or endogenous) and not just from infection. For example, it also occurs after ischaemia (hypoxic injury), physical trauma, or in response to noxious chemicals, such as insect bites. Inflammation is fundamentally a protective response, the ultimate goal of which is to rid the organism of both the initial cause of cell injury (e.g., microbes, toxins) and the consequences of such injury (e.g., necrotic tissues). In some situations, however, inflammation may be harmful to the host (a good example is meningitis).

The four cardinal features of acute inflammation are redness (rubor), swelling (tumour), heat (calor), and pain (dolor). Some also add a fifth, such as loss of function (functio laesa) or increased secretion (fluor). Acute inflammation is part of the innate immune response occurring prior to the development of any adaptive immune response that may later occur. In this way acute inflammation acts as a 'danger signal' augmenting the adaptive immune response. The inflammatory response is immediate, but non-specific, whereas the adaptive immune response is slower to develop but is highly specific and acquires memory.

Acute inflammation is initiated by a variety of chemical mediators, all of which interact in a synergistic manner to produce inflammation. These include bacterial-derived products, histamine, serotonin, arachidonic acid metabolites, cytokines, and members of the complement, kinin, clotting, and fibrinolytic systems. The clotting system and inflammation are intimately connected. Therefore, bleeding at the site of injury can initiate acute inflammation.

There are 3 main phases of acute inflammation:

- Widespread vasodilatation (hyperaemia)

- Increased vascular permeability

- Leucocyte extravasation and phagocytosis

The predominant cell type in acute inflammation is the neutrophil (the macrophage predominates in chronic inflammation). Acute inflammation is of relatively short duration, lasting for minutes, several hours or a few days. If it persists for longer then it is generally regarded as chronic inflammation.

138. E: Sixth cervical vertebra

C6 is the critical boundary of the root of the neck. To enter the neck from the chest, the vascular structures pass through a ring-like opening bounded by the scalene muscles laterally, the sternum and 1st rib anteriorly and the vertebra (C6).

139. D: It contains the pampiniform plexus

The contents of the spermatic cord are easily remembered using the 'rule of 3's':

- '*3 constituents*': Vas deferens (the round ligament is the female equivalent), lymphatics, obliterated processus vaginalis

- '*3 nerves*': Genital branch of the genitofemoral nerve (motor to cremaster, sensory to cord), ilioinguinal nerve (within the inguinal canal but outside the spermatic cord), autonomics

- '*3 arteries*': Testicular artery, artery to the vas (from the superior or inferior vesical artery), cremasteric artery (from the inferior epigastric artery)

- '*3 veins*': Pampiniform plexus, vein from the vas, cremasteric vein
- '*3 fascial coverings*': Internal spermatic fascia, external spermatic fascia, cremasteric muscle, and fascia (not dartos muscle which is contained within the wall of the scrotum)

140. **B: Gastric acid assists in the absorption of iron**

Every day 7–10 L of water enter the alimentary canal. Most of this is absorbed by the end of the small intestine so that only 500–600 mL enters the colon. Further reabsorption occurs in the colon so that only about 100 mL are lost from the body in the faeces.

Glucose absorption is dependent on sodium absorption, via a sodium (secondary active) cotransport mechanism. Conversely, the presence of glucose in the intestinal lumen facilitates the absorption of sodium. Water follows by osmosis. This is the physiological basis for the treatment of sodium and water loss in diarrhoea by oral administration of solutions containing sodium chloride and glucose (oral rehydration therapy). Most of the ingested sodium is reabsorbed (normally less than 0.5 per cent of intestinal sodium is lost in the faeces) because of its rapid absorption through the intestinal mucosa. If absorption is greater than the body requirements, the excess is excreted by the kidneys.

A good way to think about the order of absorption of substances throughout the gastrointestinal tract is to remember that the most important substances for survival are generally absorbed first, followed by the less important ones. Thus, glucose takes place mainly in the upper small intestine (duodenum and jejunum), but vitamin B_{12} is absorbed further down, in the terminal ileum (since bodily stores of vitamin B_{12} can last up to 2 years in the complete absence of vitamin B_{12} intake). Iron is absorbed more readily in the ferrous state (Fe^{2+}), but most of the dietary iron is in the ferric (Fe^{3+}) form. Gastric acidity releases iron from the food and favours the ferrous form which is absorbed more easily. The importance of this function in humans is indicated by the fact that iron deficiency anaemia is a troublesome and relatively frequent complication of partial gastrectomy.

141. **D: Amyloidosis**

The 4 possible outcomes of acute inflammation are:

- Resolution (with the complete restoration of normal tissue architecture and function)
- Abscess formation (a localized collection of pus surrounded by granulation tissue; pus is a collection of neutrophils in association with dead and dying organisms)
- Progression to chronic inflammation
- Death (a good example being meningitis)

Amyloidosis follows chronic inflammation, rather than acute inflammation.

142. **D: It is supplied by T10 sympathetic nerves**

The testis is supplied by the testicular artery which arises directly from the descending abdominal aorta at the level of approximately L2. Although at first glance this may seem illogical, when the testis is in closer proximity to other blood vessels such as the internal iliac, the explanation lies in the fact that the testis develops high up on the posterior abdominal wall early in embryonic life. As it descends into the scrotum during development, the testis carries with it the same blood supply that it received whence it was positioned on the posterior abdominal wall (i.e., from the aorta).

The testis drains by way of the pampiniform plexus into the inferior vena cava on the right side, but into the left renal vein on the left side. This may account for the fact that varicoceles (varicosities of the pampiniform plexus secondary to incompetent venous valves) are more common of the left compared with the right. The accumulation of serous fluid around the testis is known as a hydrocele.

As a general rule regarding lymphatic drainage, superficial lymphatics (i.e., in subcutaneous tissues) tend to run with superficial veins, whereas deep lymphatics run with arteries. The testis thus drains lymph to the para-aortic set of lymph nodes, since the testicular artery arises from the aorta. The testis never drains to the inguinal group of lymph nodes, although the scrotum may. The clinical consequence of this is that a testicular carcinoma never results in inguinal lymphadenopathy unless the scrotum is also involved. A scrotal carcinoma, on the other hand, would be expected to produce inguinal lymphadenopathy and this holds true in clinical practice.

The testis is supplied by T10 sympathetic nerves. The consequences of this are two-fold. First, it results in testicular pain (trauma, testicular torsion, etc.) being referred to the umbilicus (T10 dermatome). Second, the ureters are also supplied by T10 sympathetics. Thus, a renal calculus may refer pain down to the testis, as is seen in classical renal colic.

143. **D: Protein is spared until relatively late**

Starvation is a chronic state resulting from inadequate intake of energy. Four main metabolic processes occur during starvation: glycogenolysis, gluconeogenesis, lipolysis, and ketogenesis. No significant hypoglycaemic episodes occur until the end stage of starvation is entered.

During the immediate phase of starvation (0–24 hours), reserves of glycogen from liver and skeletal muscle are utilized. Glucose produced from glycogen lasts only 24 hours. The blood glucose is maintained after glycogen is depleted by gluconeogenesis for which the main substrates are amino acids, lactic acid, and glycerol.

In general, fats spare nitrogen so that protein is preserved until relatively late in starvation. During prolonged starvation, ketone bodies (acetone, acetoacetate, β-hydroxybutyrate) derived from fats are used by the brain and other tissues (such as heart muscle). Although the brain is usually heavily dependent on glucose as its energy source, during starvation it adapts to using ketones.

When fat stores are finally used up, protein catabolism increases and death follows from proteolysis of vital muscles (cardiac muscle, diaphragm). The average time to death is about 60 days.

144. B: It usually heals by organization and repair

Chronic inflammation is inflammation of prolonged duration (weeks or months) in which active inflammation, tissue destruction, and attempts at repair are occurring simultaneously. It may follow acute inflammation (secondary chronic), or it may occur *de novo* in the absence of a preceding acute inflammatory phase (primary chronic).

Chronic inflammation arises in situations where the injurious stimulus persists, as when:

- The injurious agent is endogenous (e.g., acid in stomach and peptic ulceration)
- The injurious agent is non-degradable (e.g., dust particles in pneumoconiosis)
- The injurious agent evades host defence mechanisms (e.g., many intracellular organisms such as tuberculosis)
- The host attacks components of self (e.g., autoimmunity)
- Host resistance (immunity) is suppressed (e.g., malnutrition, HIV)

Neutrophils are a feature of acute, rather than chronic, inflammation. Chronic inflammation is characterized by more extensive tissue destruction than acute inflammation owing to the lengthy nature of the process and the greater lysosomal rupture with the release of numerous lytic enzymes. The destroyed tissue is replaced by granulation tissue. Healing occurs by organization and repair (with fibrosis leaving a scar), rather than through resolution (which is typical of acute inflammation).

The pathological consequences of chronic inflammation include:

- Tissue destruction and scarring
- Development of cancer – The mitotically active tissue provides a fertile ground for the accumulation of mutations
- Amyloidosis – The extracellular deposition of abnormal and insoluble, β-pleated proteinaceous deposits

Amyloid causes its pathological effects by accumulating in body tissues.

145. A: Proximal convoluted tubule

The concentration of glucose is highest in the proximal convoluted tubule and therefore most reabsorption takes place here. The concentration of glucose in the other portion of the nephron is close to zero (Figure 7).

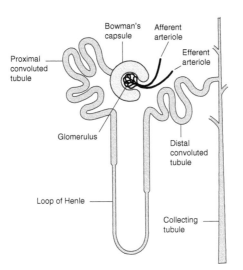

Figure 7   The nephron.

146. **B: It lies medial to the obturator nerve and anterior to the ureter**

The ovary is ovoid in shape, measuring about 3 cm long, 2 cm wide, and 1 cm thick (smaller than the testis), being smaller before menarche and postmenopausally. The anterior border of the ovary is attached to the posterior leaf of the broad ligament by a double fold of peritoneum, the mesovarium. The ovary is thus an intraperitoneal structure and the surface of the ovary, covered with cuboidal epithelium faces the peritoneal cavity. Therefore, ova extruded from the ovary actually pass into the peritoneal cavity. One consequence of this is that an ectopic pregnancy may occur within the peritoneal cavity, in addition to occurring within the fallopian tube.

The ovary flops laterally to lie in the ovarian fossa on the lateral pelvic wall. Immediately behind the fossa is the ureter which may be damaged while operating on the ovary and lateral to the ovary is the obturator neurovascular bundle. A diseased ovary may therefore cause referred pain along the cutaneous distribution of the obturator nerve on the inner side of the thigh. Nerve supply to the ovary is sympathetic originating at T10 and therefore ovarian pain may also be referred to the peri-umbilical region.

The suspensory ligament of the ovary transmits the ovarian artery, vein, and lymphatics. As a general rule regarding lymphatic drainage, superficial lymphatics (i.e., in subcutaneous tissues) tend to run with superficial veins, whereas deep lymphatics run with arteries. As the artery starts from the aorta, lymph drainage therefore passes to the para-aortic lymph nodes. The same applies with the testis in the male.

147. Thyroid-stimulating hormone (TSH)

The pituitary gland (hypophysis) is the conductor of the endocrine orchestra. It is divided into an anterior part and a posterior part. The anterior pituitary (adenohypophysis or pars distalis) secretes 6 hormones:

- *FSH* and *LH*: Reproduction
- *ACTH*: Stress response
- *TSH*: Basal metabolic rate
- *GH*: Growth
- *Prolactin*: Lactation

The posterior pituitary (neurohypophysis or pars nervosa) secretes only 2 hormones:

- *ADH* (*vasopressin*): Osmotic regulation
- *Oxytocin*: Milk ejection and labour

Testosterone is produced from Leydig cells in the testis and from the adrenal glands. CRH is produced by the median eminence of the hypothalamus.

148. C: Tuberculosis

Granulomatous inflammation is a distinctive pattern of chronic inflammation characterized by granuloma formation. It usually occurs in response to the presence of indigestible matter within macrophages. Histologically, a granuloma consists of a microscopic aggregation of activated macrophages that are transformed into epithelium-like cells (epithelioid macrophages), surrounded by a collar of mononuclear leucocytes, principally lymphocytes and occasionally plasma cells. Epithelioid cells may coalesce to form multinucleate giant cells. Their nuclei are often arranged around the periphery of the cell – Langhans giant cells. Do not confuse the term *granuloma* with granulation tissue; the latter is a wound-healing phenomenon and does not contain granulomas.

Tuberculosis is the archetypal granulomatous disease, but it can also occur in other disease states such as other infections (e.g., leprosy, schistosomiasis) or foreign bodies, which may be endogenous (bone, adipose tissue, uric acid crystals) or exogenous (e.g., silica, suture materials). Some causes are idiopathic, such as Crohn's disease and sarcoidosis. Note that Crohn's disease, but not ulcerative colitis, is associated with the presence of granulomas. Lobar pneumonia and bronchopneumonia do not characteristically form granulomas.

If the granuloma is large it may outstrip its own blood supply, resulting in central necrosis. Tuberculosis is characteristically associated with caseating granulomas, with central caseous necrosis. Other conditions such as Crohn's disease and sarcoidosis are associated with non-caseating granulomas.

149. D: Tricuspid

Clinically this patient has bacterial endocarditis. In drug abusers, it usually affects the tricuspid valve because contamination from dirty needles drains into the right side of the heart. It is usually caused by *Staphylococcus aureus.*

150. A: It is drained by tributaries of both the inferior mesenteric and internal iliac veins

The rectum is 12 cm long, starting at the level of S3 and ending at the puborectalis (levator ani–pelvic floor). It is lined by typical columnar intestinal epithelium with many mucous secreting cells (transitional epithelium is almost exclusively confined to the urinary tract of mammals where it is highly specialized to accommodate a great deal of stretch and to withstand the toxicity of the urine).

The rectum has no mesentery and is therefore regarded as retroperitoneal. It is covered by peritoneum on its front and sides in its upper third, only on its front in its middle third and the rectum lies below the peritoneal reflection in its lower third. Do not be confused; although the rectum has no mesentery, the visceral pelvic fascia around the rectum is often referred to by surgeons as the mesorectum. The pararectal lymph nodes are found within the mesorectum, which is removed together with the rectum as a package during rectal excision for carcinoma.

Blood supply is by way of the superior rectal (inferior mesenteric), middle rectal (internal iliac), and inferior rectal (internal pudendal) arteries. The importance of understanding the blood supply of the rectum lies in its vulnerability during the resection of a rectal carcinoma and the formation of a join (anastomosis) from the two remaining ends of the bowel. If blood supply to the anastomosis is tenuous, then the anastomosis may break down in the postoperative period with disastrous consequences. The venous drainage is as for the arteries. Note, however, that there is a portosystemic anastomosis in the lower rectal and upper anal canal walls, as branches of the superior rectal (portal) and inferior/middle rectal veins (systemic) meet in the external and internal venous plexuses. This poses a site where haemorrhoids may form in portal hypertension.

The rectum receives parasympathetic fibres from the pelvic splanchnic nerves, or nervi erigentes, originating from S2 to S4. It functions to relax the internal sphincter, contract the bowel, and transmit a sense of fullness. Note that the vagus nerve only supplies the bowel up to two-thirds along the transverse colon. The whole of the rest of the bowel inferior to this level (the so-called hindgut) receives parasympathetic fibres by way of the pelvic splanchnic nerves. Remember parasympathetic outflow from the spinal cord is craniosacral, whereas sympathetic outflow is thoracolumbar. Sympathetic supply to the rectum is through the lumbar splanchnics and superior hypogastric plexus. Sympathetics contract the internal sphincter, relax the bowel, and transmit pain.

151. D: Identical twins show 90 per cent concordance

In type 1 diabetes mellitus identical twins have 50 per cent concordance, whereas in type 2 there is 90 per cent concordance. Type 1 is associated with HLA DR 3/4, whereas type 2 has no HLA association. Type 1 is a disorder of insulin deficiency and therefore presentation is with weight loss and ketone production, usually early in life in the teenage years. Type 2, which commonly presents after the age of 40, is associated with obesity and insulin resistance rather than insulin deficiency *per se*.

152. A: Granulation tissue actively contracts

The stages of wound healing are as follows:

- Coagulation/haemostasis (immediate)
- Inflammation (0–4 days) – Initially neutrophils and then macrophages which remove tissue debris
- Fibroplasia and epithelialization (4 days to 3 weeks) – Neovascularized tissue is known as granulation tissue
- Contraction, maturation, and remodelling (3 weeks to 18 months) – Fibroblasts differentiate into myofibroblasts which are responsible for active wound contraction

Maximal wound tensile strength is achieved at about day 60, when it is 80 per cent of normal. Resolution is the most favourable outcome of the healing process because it refers to the complete restitution of normal tissue architecture and function. It can occur only if tissue damage is slight, followed by rapid removal of debris. No scar tissue forms in pure resolution.

Repair, on the other hand, is the replacement of damaged tissue by fibrosis or gliosis, which fills or bridges the defect, but has no intrinsic specialized function relevant to the organ in which repair occurs. It occurs when there is substantial damage to the specialized connective tissue framework and/or the tissue lacks the ability to regenerate specialized cells. The result of repair is a scar.

Tissue repair occurs through the formation of granulation tissue. It derives its name from the granular appearance seen by early military surgeons in the bases of wounds that were about to heal, hence the association with a favourable outcome. The granules are caused by the sprouting of endothelial buds as a result of angiogenesis. Granulation tissue replaces a disorganized mess with orderly new fibrous tissue, a process called organization. Granulation tissue should not be confused with granulomas (aggregates of activated macrophages), which are not an integral part of granulation tissue.

Granulation tissue is defined by the presence of 3 cell types:

- *Macrophages*: Responsible for removing tissue debris
- *Fibroblasts*: Responsible for laying down the collagen in fibrous tissue that aids wound contraction
- *Endothelial cells*: Responsible for the formation of new blood vessels (angiogenesis)

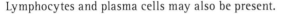

Lymphocytes and plasma cells may also be present.

Healing by primary intention refers to incised wounds where the edges can be apposed. *Healing by secondary intention* is where there has been tissue loss and the edges cannot be suitably apposed. Healing by secondary intention is slower since granulation tissue has to form from the base of the wound and re-epithelialization has to occur from the edges to cover this. The granulation tissue eventually contracts, resulting in scar formation.

153. **E: Transitional cell carcinoma**

Ninety per cent of bladder cancers are transitional cell carcinomas derived from the bladder urothelium. Risk factors include industrial chemicals, smoking, and infection. Schistosomiasis and bladder stones predispose to the squamous cell variety.

154. **E: The ureter is closely related to the lateral fornix of the cervix**

The supports of the uterus are extremely important. The lateral (or transverse) cervical ligaments condense around the uterine artery and run to the lateral pelvic wall. The uterosacral ligaments are primarily condensations of fascia running backwards from the cervix of the uterus past the rectum and attaching to the sacrum. The round ligament of the uterus is the female remnant of the embryonic gubernaculum which guides the testis to the scrotum in the male. It is a continuation of the ovarian ligament which is in the broad ligament attaching the ovary to the uterus. The round ligament then continues from the wall of the uterus in the anterior leaf of the broad ligament to the pelvic wall and then through the deep inguinal ring and inguinal canal to fade out into the labium majorum. It is important only in helping to hold the uterus in its usual anteverted, anteflexed position (i.e., the uterus tends to lie tipped forwards over the female bladder).

Some support is also offered by the anterior pubocervical ligaments. Similarly, the broad ligament holds the uterus in that position but it does not contribute a great deal to preventing uterine prolapse (procidentia). The latter is a condition where the pelvic floor is so weakened, usually following multiple childbirth, that the uterus tends to prolapse through the vagina. This can adversely affect the base of the bladder or even obstruct the ureters and therefore may lead to urinary infections, incontinence, or renal failure.

The blood supply comes mainly from the uterine artery, which takes a very tortuous course up the uterus (to allow for expansion in uterine hypertrophy, e.g., pregnancy). It is a branch of the internal iliac. In so reaching the uterus, the uterine artery must pass across and above the ureter which is heading past the uterus to the bladder. During hysterectomy, this relationship is enormously important as the uterine arteries must be ligated and cut. Clearly, one must recognize the difference and realize the close proximity of the ureter and uterine artery.

The ureters lie adjacent to the lateral fornix of the cervix. Consequently, a ureteric calculus may be felt in the lateral fornix on vaginal examination. The posterior fornix actually has overlying it the peritoneum of the recto-uterine pouch of Douglas, which is normally occupied by coils of small intestine or sigmoid colon and lies between the uterus anteriorly and the rectum posteriorly. The pouch of Douglas is the most dependent part of the pelvis. Consequently, blood may collect here in a ruptured ectopic pregnancy. A needle may be passed into this space (in an attempt to aspirate blood) in order to diagnose the condition (culdocentesis). Furthermore, the instrument used in illegal abortions, if missing the cavity of the uterus, could actually penetrate the posterior fornix and subsequently the peritoneal cavity, often leading to fatal peritonitis and sepsis.

155. **D: von Willebrand factor**

von Willebrand disease is common inherited bleeding disorder caused by deficiency of von Willebrand factor (vWf). The most important function of vWF *in vivo* is to promote the adhesion of platelets to sub-endothelial matrix. It also acts as a carrier for factor VIII and is important for its stability. Hence these patients have a prolonged bleeding time despite a normal platelet count. Clinically, deficiency leads to spontaneous bleeding from mucous membranes, excessive bleeding from wounds and menorrhagia.

156. **A: X-ray crystallography**

Amyloid is a pathologic proteinaceous substance, deposited between cells in various tissues and organs of the body in a wide variety of clinical settings. Amyloidosis results from abnormal folding of proteins, which are deposited as fibrils in extracellular tissues and disrupt normal function. X-ray crystallography demonstrates the characteristic cross-β-pleated sheet conformation. Common organs involved are the kidneys, gastrointestinal tract, and heart. Symptoms can be non-specific initially but may later present with uraemia, malabsorption, or congestive heart failure.

157. **C: Pepsin**

Pepsin is a peptic enzyme of the stomach. It is most active at a pH of 2.0–3.0 and is inactive at a pH above about 5.0. One of the important features of pepsin digestion is its ability to digest the protein collagen, an albuminoid type of protein that is relatively unaffected by other digestive enzymes. Pepsin initiates the process of protein digestion, usually providing only 10–20 percent of the total protein digestion to convert the protein to proteoses, peptones, and a few polypeptides.

158. **E: Membranous bones**

The bone marrow of essentially all bones produces red blood cells until a person is 5 years old. The marrow of the long bones, except for the proximal portions of the humeri and tibiae, becomes fatty and produces no more red blood cells after about age 20 years. Beyond this age, most red cells continue to be produced in the marrow of the membranous bones, such as the vertebrae, sternum, ribs, and ilia. Even in

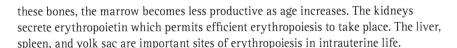

these bones, the marrow becomes less productive as age increases. The kidneys secrete erythropoietin which permits efficient erythropoiesis to take place. The liver, spleen, and yolk sac are important sites of erythropoiesis in intrauterine life.

159. **C: Magnesium**

Hartmann's solution contains sodium 131 mmol/L, chloride 111 mmol/L, potassium 5 mmol/L, lactate 29 mmol/L, and calcium 2 mmol/L. The Ca^{2+} content of Hartmann's is important as it can result in clotting in the tubing if blood is given slowly before or after it in the same line. Hence, the traditional practice, 100 mL of normal saline was given before and after each bag of blood.

160. **D: Factor VII**

The initial reaction in the intrinsic pathway is conversion of inactive factor XII to active factor XII (XIIa). This activation, which is catalysed by high molecular weight kininogen and kallikrein, can be brought about *in vivo* by exposure of blood to collagen fibres underlying the endothelium. Active factor XII then activates factor XI, and active factor XI activates factor IX. Activated factor IX forms a complex with active factor VIII, which is activated when it is separated from von Willebrand factor (vWF). The complex of IXa and VIIIa activates factor X. Phospholipids from aggregated platelets (PL) and Ca^{2+} are necessary for full activation of factor X. The extrinsic pathway is triggered by the release of tissue thromboplastin, a protein–phospholipid mixture that activates factor VII. Factor X can be activated by either of the two systems.

161. **B: The binding of one oxygen molecule increases the affinity of binding of other oxygen molecules**

The oxygen–haemoglobin dissociation curve relates percentage saturation of the oxygen (O_2) carrying power of haemoglobin (Hb) to the saturation of oxygen (Po_2). This curve has a characteristic sigmoid shape. Combination of the first haem in the Hb molecule with O_2 increases the affinity of the second haem for O_2, and oxygenation of the second increases the affinity of the third, and so on, so that the affinity of Hb for the fourth O_2 molecule is many times that for the first. This is known as co-operativity. The decrease in O_2 affinity of Hb when the pH of blood falls is called the Bohr effect.

162. **C: NO**

NO is especially secreted by nerve terminals in areas of the brain responsible for long-term behaviour and for memory. It is synthesised instantly as needed then diffuses out of the presynaptic terminals over a period of seconds rather than being released in vesicular packets. It is also released by the endothelium of blood vessels as endothelium-derived relaxing factor (EDRF). It diffuses into postsynaptic neurons nearby. In the postsynaptic neuron it usually does not greatly alter the membrane potential but instead changes intracellular metabolic functions that modify neuronal excitability.

163. D: Bicarbonate

The solubility of CO_2 in blood is about 20 times that of O_2; therefore, considerably more CO_2 than O_2 is present in simple solution at equal partial pressures. The CO_2 that diffuses into red blood cells is rapidly hydrated to H_2CO_3 because of the presence of carbonic anhydrase. The H_2CO_3 dissociates to H^+ and HCO_3^-, and the H^+ is buffered, primarily by haemoglobin, while the HCO_3^- enters the plasma. There is 49 mL of CO_2 in each decilitre of arterial blood (2.6 mL is dissolved, 2.6 mL as carbamino compound and 43.8 mL as HCO_3^-). Therefore, CO_2 is primarily transported in the arterial blood as bicarbonate.

164. C: Posterior descending coronary artery

The coronary artery anatomy is variable, as are the relative territories of myocardium supplied by each of the arteries. ST-segment depression across all leads implies ischaemia (angina), whereas isolated ST-segment depression in leads V1 and V2 may indicate a posterior myocardial infarction. The most likely artery involved in this case is therefore the posterior descending artery. Either the right coronary or circumflex arteries can supply the posterior descending artery, but it is not possible to identify which from the ECG alone. Left main stem and left anterior descending artery lesions would cause changes over a much larger area.

165. B: Cord Infarction

Cord infarction can occur during thoraco-abdominal aneurysm repair, as the aorta is clamped and a graft is inserted. The arteria radicularis magna supplies the lower part of the spinal cord and may be the dominant artery supplying the lower spinal cord. Disruption can cause infarction of the lower cord, resulting in paraplegia.

166. A: Pre-aortic

Colonic lymphatic drainage terminally reaches superior and inferior mesenteric lymph nodes, which belong to the pre-aortic lymph nodes. Lymph from colon passes through four sets of lymph nodes: Epicolic (lie on the serosal wall of gut) → Paracolic (on medial side of ascending/descending colon and mesenteric border of transverse/sigmoid colon) → Intermediate (on named branches of colonic vessels) → Pre-terminal/pre-aortic (on inferior/superior mesenteric vessels). The efferents from the pre-aortic lymph nodes drain into the coeliac lymph nodes (terminal), which also belong to the pre-aortic category. Coeliac lymph nodes then drain into the intestinal trunks, which ultimately join the cisterna chyli.

167. A: Foramen transverserium

The seven cervical vertebrae are characterised by their small size and by the presence of a foramen in each transverse process. These foramen transverserium are trough-shaped. The five lumbar vertebrae are distinguished from vertebrae in other regions by their large size. They also lack facets for articulation with ribs.

168. E: The lateral cutaneous nerve of the thigh

Meralgia paraesthetica is a painful mononeuropathy of the lateral femoral cutaneous nerve, commonly caused by focal entrapment of this nerve as it passes through the inguinal ligament. Treatment is based on symptoms. Weight reduction, less compressive clothing, non-steroidal anti-inflammatory drugs (NSAIDs), local anaesthetic infiltration, and surgical release have been described as treatment modalities.

169. B: Neck of the fibula

The common peroneal nerve is relatively unprotected as it traverses the lateral aspect of the neck of the fibula and is easily compressed at this site (e.g., by fracture, tight plaster casts, or ganglia). Patients with such an injury present with foot drop, which is usually painless. Examination reveals weakness of ankle dorsiflexion, extensor hallucis longus, and eversion of the foot, but inversion and plantar flexion are normal and the ankle reflex is preserved.

170. E: Palmaris longus

The carpal tunnel is formed anteriorly at the wrist by a deep arch formed by the carpal bones and the flexor retinaculum. The four tendons of the flexor digitorum profundus, the four tendons of the flexor digitorum superficialis, and the tendon of the flexor pollicis longus pass through the carpal tunnel, with the median nerve. The palmaris longus lies superficial to the flexor retinaculum.

171. A: Prevertebral fascia

Fascia around the brachial plexus is called the axillary sheath and is a derivative of the prevertebral fascia. This covers the anterior vertebral muscles and lies on the anterior aspect of scalenus anterior and medius, thus forming the floor of posterior triangle of the neck. The brachial plexus and subclavian artery emerge between scalenus anterior and medius in the neck and pass behind the clavicle to reach the axilla. In the process, they carry an extension of prevertebral fascia over them as a cover (the axillary sheath) towards the axilla. Most of the nerves in the neck are behind the prevertebral fascia but the spinal accessory nerve lies superficial to it and is susceptible to damage.

172. B: Radial nerve

The radial nerve runs in the spiral groove and injury at that level will affect the extensors of the wrist and fingers resulting in 'wrist drop'. Sensory loss will be localised to the back of the radial side of the hand.

173. D: The costovertebral ligament

The costovertebral ligament is a strong fascial attachment between the transverse process of the 1st and 2nd lumbar vertebrae and the inferior margin of the 12th rib. It is encountered only in posterior approaches to the kidney and it can be incised to produce a greater degree of mobility of the 12th rib, thus providing greater exposure and access to the structures that reside within the upper portion of the retroperitoneum.

174. **E: The patient is unable to deviate his right eye laterally**

The abducens nerve innervates the lateral rectus muscle of the eye exclusively; the sole effect of damage to this nerve is that the patient is unable to abduct (laterally deviate) the eye. Ptosis results from lesion of occulomotor nerve. Pupillary light reflex tests function of optic and occulomotor nerves.

175. **D: Inability to extend the knee and numbness over the anterior thigh**

The femoral nerve is the largest branch of the lumbar plexus (L2–4). It forms in the abdomen within the substance of the psoas major muscle and descends posterolaterally through the pelvis to the midpoint of the inguinal ligament. It supplies the anterior thigh muscles (the quadriceps group extends the leg at the knee); it also supplies other anterior thigh muscles (iliacus and sartorius) which allow flexion of the thigh at the hip joint. The femoral nerve also gives several cutaneous branches to the skin on the anteromedial side of the lower limb (saphenous nerve).

176. **A: Flexes the thigh at the hip joint**

The psoas major muscle joins the iliacus muscle, which originates broadly over the inner aspect of the iliac wing of the pelvis. This becomes the iliopsoas muscle and inserts on the lesser trochanter of the femur and thus flexes the thigh at the hip joint. The action of this muscle results in the leg becoming shortened and externally rotated following a fracture of the neck of the femur.

177. **D: External urethral orifice**

The male urethra is approximately 20 cm long and the narrowest parts are the external urethral orifice, bladder neck, and just proximal to navicular fossa. The seminal colliculus is present in the prostatic urethra at the verumontanum. The prostatic urethra is the widest and most dilatable part of the entire male urethra.

178. **D: Weakness of opposition of the thumb**

The history described earlier is typical of carpal tunnel syndrome. Entrapment of the median nerve at the carpal tunnel affects the muscles of the thenar eminence. These are abductor pollicis brevis, flexor pollicis brevis, and opponens pollicis. The nerve supply of flexor pollicis brevis is extremely variable, however, so the best test to perform would be to see if opposition is affected. In addition, the motor branch of the median nerve after the level of the carpal tunnel also innervates the radial (lateral) two lumbricals.

179. **C: There would be no dorsiflexion of the foot**

The common peroneal nerve can be compressed by a below-knee cast at the level of the neck of the fibula. It supplies the muscles of the anterior and lateral compartments of the leg, producing dorsiflexion of the foot, ankle, and toes, as well as eversion of the foot. The superficial peroneal nerve gives sensory supply to most of the dorsum of the foot. The deep peroneal nerve supplies the first web space.

180. **A: Lateral cutaneous nerve of the thigh lesion**

The lateral cutaneous nerve of the thigh supplies the anterolateral aspect of the thigh. It has no motor branches. Meralgia paraesthetica is a condition where there is irritation of the nerve causing sensory changes in the distribution of the lateral cutaneous nerve of the thigh without any motor changes. L2 and L3 supply part of the dermatome described but both have motor branches. The femoral nerve supplies the quadriceps muscle, and the saphenous nerve runs with the saphenous vein to supply an area of skin below the knee on the medial aspect of the leg.

181. **B: C5/C6 root**

A C5/C6 lesion, Erb's palsy, produces sensory loss over the lateral aspect of the upper arm (deltoid paralysis), with loss of shoulder abduction, and paralysis of the biceps, brachialis, and coracobrachialis. In addition to loss of elbow flexion, the biceps are also a powerful supinator of the forearm, so the forearm assumes a pronated position. A T1 lesion produces a claw hand (Klumpke's palsy). Sympathetic chain injury results in Horner's syndrome, with ptosis of the upper eyelid, constriction of the pupil (miosis), and anhidrosis on the affected side.

182. **E: The patient has varicosities of the short saphenous system**

The short saphenous system passes posterior to the lateral malleolus and ascends the leg lateral to the Achilles tendon. It usually perforates the popliteal fossa and terminates in the popliteal vein. The incompetent valve is likely to be at this junction.

183. **D: Tendency for food and fluids to collect in the buccal sulcus after meals**

The facial nerve supplies all the muscles needed for facial expression including the occipitofrontalis, which wrinkles the forehead. A distressing feature is paralysis of the buccinator muscle, which acts to empty the buccal sulcus during mastication. There are no cutaneous sensory fibres in the facial nerve. The levator palpebrae superioris is supplied by the oculomotor nerve, so the patient can still raise their upper lid. The chorda tympani fibres, which transmit taste from the anterior two-thirds of the tongue, pass from the lingual nerve to the facial nerve just below the skull, and therefore remain intact in more distal injuries of the facial nerve.

184. **A: Anteriorly the hepatic artery**

The epiploic foramen of Winslow forms the boundary between the greater and lesser sacs of the abdominal cavity. The boundaries are: anteriorly, the portal triad (portal vein, hepatic artery, and bile duct, all in the free edge of the lesser omentum); posteriorly, the inferior vena cava and right crus of the diaphragm; superiorly, the caudate lobe of the liver; and inferiorly, the superior part of the 1st part of the duodenum. Medially and laterally are the lesser and greater sacs respectively.

185. **A: Thymus**

     The anterior mediastinum is bordered anteriorly by the sternum and posteriorly by the great vessels. It contains the thymus, lymph nodes, fat, and vessels. Disorders of the anterior mediastinum are generally thymic, thyroid (substernal goitre), teratoma (and other germ cell tumours), and lymphomas (Hodgkin disease, non-Hodgkin lymphoma).

186. **C: Femoral nerve, femoral artery, femoral vein, long saphenous vein**

     From lateral to medial, the femoral triangle contains the femoral nerve and its branches; the femoral artery and its branches, including the profunda femoris; and the femoral vein with its main tributary, the long saphenous vein.

187. **D: Pushing to standing from an armchair**

     Triceps attaches to the olecranon and is responsible for extension of the elbow. If olecranon fractures are treated conservatively, an excellent range of movement can be achieved; however, functional outcome is impaired because of a lack of power of extension. This would be most apparent pushing up against gravity, as one has to do when pushing out of a chair. Brushing hair, reaching into cupboards, and pouring kettles are functions mainly achieved by movements of the shoulder, while fastening buttons requires dexterity and may be adversely affected by injuries to the wrist or hand.

188. **B: Numbness of the lower lip on the injected side**

     The inferior alveolar nerve, a branch of the mandibular division of the trigeminal nerve (V), traverses the inferior alveolar, or dental canal of the mandible, to supply all the teeth of that hemimandible; all the teeth on that side are therefore anaesthetised. The mental branch of the nerve emerges through the mental foramen to supply the lower lip, which becomes numb in a successfully performed block. The muscles of the tongue, of mastication and of facial expression are not affected.

189. **A: Deep peroneal nerve**

     The sural nerve arises from the tibial nerve. It is purely sensory and supplies the lateral border of the leg and the lateral border of the foot. It lies approximately 1 cm posterior to the distal fibula and may be damaged during operations on the distal fibula. The saphenous nerve supplies the medial aspect of the leg up to the medial malleolus. The deep peroneal nerve supplies the first web space while the superficial peroneal nerve usually supplies the rest of the dorsum of the foot. The tibial nerve supplies the heel and branches into the medial and lateral plantar nerves to innervate the sole of the foot.

190. **E: Right lower lobe bronchus**

     The right main bronchus is wider, shorter, and runs more vertically than the left main bronchus. Consequently, foreign bodies small enough to be inhaled more commonly enter the right lung. As a result of gravity, the right lower lobe is more likely to receive such foreign bodies.

191. **E: Sodium ions outwards**

Resting membrane potential is maintained between –70 and –95 mV for different types of cells by the prevention of the free movement of certain types of ions. This potential difference is maintained by the Na^+/K^+ ATPase pump, and the repulsion of negative ions from the outside of the membrane because of the high intracellular negative charge on protein molecules. During an action potential depolarisation, voltage-gated sodium channels open, causing a large influx of sodium ions neutralising the resting membrane potential.

192. **D: B-Negative**

When classified according to the ABO system, blood cells from Group A contain type A surface antigen on the red cell membranes and anti-B antibodies in the serum; similarly, Group B red cells have type B surface antigen and anti-A serum antibodies, Group O red cells have no surface antigens and both anti-A and anti-B serum antibodies, Group AB red cells have type A and type B surface antigens and no serum antibodies.

Thus, if the patient's blood agglutinates with antisera anti-A then the red cells must carry the type A surface antigen, making it either Group A or AB. The patient's serum agglutinates with red cells from Group B blood; therefore, it must carry anti-B antibodies; therefore, the patient cannot be AB, which carries no serum antibodies.

The Rhesus blood grouping system consists of 50 different surface antigens of which D is the most significant and immunogenic. A D-positive person has D antigens on the red cells, and no antibodies, while a D-negative person has no antibodies unless previously exposed (either during transfusion or placentally). Since this patient's blood cells agglutinate with antisera anti-D, they carry the D antigen making them D positive. Therefore, this patient's blood type is A positive. In the UK, approximately 85 per cent of the population are RhD positive.

193. **A: Patients on warfarin have a decreased PT**

Warfarin is a synthetic derivative of dicoumarol, which is derived from coumarin, a chemical found naturally in many plants. It decreases blood coagulation by inhibiting vitamin K epoxide reductase, an enzyme that recycles oxidized vitamin K to its reduced form after it has participated in the carboxylation of several blood coagulation proteins, mainly prothrombin and factor VII.

Warfarin is prescribed to people with an increased tendency for thrombosis, or as secondary prophylaxis in those individuals that have already formed a thrombus. Thus, common clinical indications for warfarin use are atrial fibrillation, the presence of artificial heart valves, deep venous thrombosis, and pulmonary embolism. Warfarin is also used in antiphospholipid syndrome.

Warfarin is contraindicated in pregnancy, as it passes through the placental barrier and is teratogenic (causing warfarin embryopathy).

The only common side-effect of warfarin is haemorrhage (bleeding). The risk of severe bleeding is small but definite and any benefit needs to outweigh this risk when warfarin is considered as a therapeutic measure. The risk of bleeding is augmented if the international normalized ratio (INR) is out of range (owing to accidental or deliberate overdose or from interactions), and may cause haemoptysis (coughing up blood), excessive bruising, bleeding from nose or gums, or blood in urine or stool.

Warfarin is slower-acting than heparin, although it has a number of advantages. Heparin must be given by injection, whereas warfarin is available orally. Warfarin has a long half-life and need only be given once a day. Heparin can also cause heparin-induced thrombocytopenia (an antibody-mediated decrease in platelet levels), which increases the risk for thrombosis (through platelet activation), as well as osteoporosis.

Warfarin inhibits the vitamin K-dependent synthesis of biologically active forms of the calcium-dependent clotting factors II, VII, IX, and X, as well as the regulatory factors protein C, protein S, and protein Z. When warfarin is initially commenced, it may promote clot formation temporarily. This is because the level of protein C and protein S are also dependent on vitamin K activity. Warfarin causes a decline in protein C levels in the first 36 hours. Thus, when warfarin is loaded rapidly at greater than 5 mg per day, it is beneficial to co-administer heparin, an anticoagulant that acts upon antithrombin and helps reduce the risk of thrombosis, with warfarin therapy for 4–5 days. The effects of warfarin can be reversed with vitamin K or, when rapid reversal is needed (such as in case of severe bleeding), with prothrombin complex concentrate (e.g., Octaplex) – which contains only the factors inhibited by warfarin – or fresh frozen plasma (depending upon the clinical indication) in addition to intravenous vitamin K.

194. **C: Increased heat production in skeletal muscle**

Malignant hyperthermia (MH) is a rare life-threatening condition that is triggered by exposure to certain drugs used for general anaesthesia (specifically all volatile anaesthetics), nearly all gas anaesthetics, and the neuromuscular blocking agent succinylcholine. In susceptible individuals, these drugs can induce a drastic and uncontrolled increase in skeletal muscle oxidative metabolism, which overwhelms the body's capacity to supply oxygen, remove carbon dioxide, and regulate body temperature, eventually leading to circulatory collapse and death if not treated quickly.

Susceptibility to MH is often inherited as an autosomal dominant disorder due to mutations in the ryanodine receptor in the sarcoplasmic reticulum of skeletal muscle. It is usually revealed by anaesthesia, or when a family member develops the symptoms. When MH develops during a procedure, treatment with dantrolene sodium is usually initiated; dantrolene (a post-synaptic muscle relaxant that lessens excitation–contraction coupling in muscle cells) and the avoidance of anaesthesia in susceptible people have markedly reduced the mortality from this condition.

Characteristic signs are muscular rigidity, followed by a hypercatabolic state with increased oxygen consumption, increased carbon dioxide production, tachycardia, and an increase in body temperature (hyperthermia) at a rate of up to around 2°C/hour; temperatures up to 42°C are not uncommon. Rhabdomyolysis (breakdown of muscle tissue) may develop, as indicated by red-brown discolouration of the urine and cardiological or neurological evidence of electrolyte disturbances. Anaesthesia for known MH-susceptible patients requires avoidance of triggering agents (all volatile anaesthetic agents and succinylcholine). All other drugs are safe (including nitrous oxide), as are regional anaesthetic techniques.

195. **C: A voluntary control**

Both cardiac muscle and smooth muscle are involuntary. Smooth muscle is non-striated whereas cardiac and smooth muscle, are both striated. Smooth muscle is fusiform and cardiac muscle is branching.

196. **B: Bypass lungs in the fetus**

Foetal blood is oxygenated by the placenta and not the lungs. Blood passes from the right atrium through the foramen ovale to the left atrium and some blood flows into the right ventricle and pulmonary trunk and then through the ductus arteriosus into the aorta, bypassing the lungs.

197. **D: Psoas major**

75 per cent of appendices are retrocaecal and lie adjacent to the psoas major muscle. Extension or external rotation moves the muscle and causes pain due to irritation by the inflamed appendix.

198. **B: Fibular neck**

The common peroneal nerve lies lateral to the fibular neck and supplies the peroneal muscles, which control foot dorsiflexion and eversion.

199. **D: Avulsion of flexor digitorum profundus**

Flexor digitorum profundus inserts into the base of the distal phalanx and bends the distal interphalangeal joint. Flexor digitorum superficialis inserts at the base of the middle phalanx and bends the proximal interphalangeal joint.

200. **B: Inferior belly of omohyoid**

The posterior triangle of the neck is bounded by the clavicle, sternocleidomastoid and trapezius. This triangle is divided by the inferior belly of the omohyoid muscle into the supraclavicular triangle inferiorly and the occipital triangle superiorly.

The omohyoid is innervated by a branch of the cervical plexus, the ansa cervicalis, and mostly acts to stabilise the hyoid bone. The inferior belly of the omohyoid is innervated by the three cervical branches (C1-C3) that make up the ansa cervicalis. The superior belly of omohyoid is innervated by the superior root of ansa cervicalis which contains only fibers from the first cervical spinal nerves (C1).

SECTION 3: SINGLE BEST ANSWER QUESTIONS

1. A 19-year-old man returns from holiday in Tenerife. Four weeks later, he develops a swollen, hot, painful, red knee joint, with an effusion.
   - A Acute gout
   - B Enteropathic arthritis
   - C Pseudogout
   - D Reiter's syndrome
   - E Septic arthritis

2. An 18-year-old presents with jaundice. On questioning he admits that the last time he had a cold he went a slightly yellow colour. His brother has had a past episode of jaundice. Liver function tests reveal: bilirubin 80 µmol/L; ALT 25 IU/L; ALP 150 IU/L. Select the likely diagnosis.

   (*Normal ranges are: bilirubin 3–17 µmol/L; ALT 3–35 IU/L; ALP 30–300 IU/L.*)
   - A Autoimmune hepatitis
   - B Gilbert's syndrome
   - C Hepatitis A
   - D Hepatitis B
   - E Hepatitis C

3. A 55-year-old woman presents with painless jaundice and pruritus. On direct questioning, she admits to having dark urine and pale stools.

   (*Normal ranges are: bilirubin 3–17 µmol/L; ALT 3–35 IU/L; ALP 30–300 IU/L.*)
   - A Autoimmune hepatitis
   - B Carcinoma of the head of pancreas
   - C Cholangiocarcinoma
   - D Gallstones
   - E Primary biliary cirrhosis

4. A 22-year-old student has just returned from an uneventful holiday in Africa. He is jaundiced and has moderate hepatomegaly. Liver function tests reveal: bilirubin 110 µmol/L; ALT 250 IU/L; ALP 350 IU/L. Also detected are specific IgM antibodies. Select the likely diagnosis.

   (*Normal ranges are: bilirubin 3–17 µmol/L; ALT 3–35 IU/L; ALP 30–300 IU/L.*)
   - A Hepatitis A
   - B Hepatitis B
   - C Hepatitis C
   - D Malaria
   - E Primary sclerosing cholangitis

5. A 42-year-old female is involved in a motorcycle accident with a Glasgow Coma Scale (GCS) score of 7 following a severe head injury. A left-sided pneumothorax was treated with a chest drain insertion and her pulse is now 150 beats/min and blood pressure 120/75 mmHg after 2 L of crystalloid. Her abdomen is soft but difficult to assess. Select the best appropriate investigation.

A Emergency laparotomy
B Abdominal ultrasound (FAST scan)
C CT abdomen
D Angiography
E Observation

6. A 42-year-old woman has a 1.5 cm swelling above the outer canthus of the eye. On examination, it is soft, deep to the skin, with no deep attachments. Select the likely diagnosis.

A Neurofibroma
B Lipoma
C Ganglion
D Sebaceous (epidermoid) cyst
E Dermoid cyst

7. A 52-year-old man has a 1 cm cutaneous lump on the anterior aspect of the lower limb which followed an insect bite one year earlier. Select the likely diagnosis.

A Neurofibroma
B Lipoma
C Histiocytoma
D Sebaceous (epidermoid) cyst
E Dermoid cyst

8. A 45-year-old patient with familial adenomatous polyposis presents with severely dysplastic changes in the sigmoid colon. Select the appropriate management.

A Anterior resection
B Subtotal colectomy
C Panproctocolectomy
D Abdominoperineal excision
E Restorative proctocolectomy

9. A 19-year-old female has long-standing ulcerative colitis affecting the whole colon. She is found to have a malignancy on a biopsy taken 5 cm from the anal verge and severe dysplasia on other biopsies from the colon. Select the appropriate management.

A Anterior resection
B Subtotal colectomy
C Panproctocolectomy
D Abdominoperineal excision
E No treatment required

10. A melanoma invading the papillary dermis. Select the correct cancer staging.

A Clarke's level I
B Clarke's level II
C Clarke's level III
D Clarke's level IV
E Clarke's level V

11. A 42-year-old African male has recently been diagnosed with malaria and is taking quinine. He presents with fatigue, dark urine, and shortness of breath. Select the likely diagnosis.

A Sickle cell disease
B Beta-thalassaemia
C Pernicious anaemia
D Glucose-6-phosphate dehydrogenase deficiency
E Sideroblastic anaemia

12. An 11-year-old Scottish, Caucasian girl presents with mild anaemia and jaundice. Her blood tests reveal a normal MCV, but her red cell osmotic fragility test is increased. Select the likely diagnosis.
    A Iron-deficiency anaemia
    B Hereditary spherocytosis
    C Vitamin B_{12} deficiency anaemia
    D Sickle cell disease
    E Beta-thalassaemia

13. A 25-year-old African man presents with severe lumbar back pain and jaundice. His blood tests demonstrate a normocytic, normochromic anaemia, high reticulocyte count. His ESR is low. Select the likely diagnosis.
    A Iron-deficiency anaemia
    B Hereditary spherocytosis
    C Vitamin B_{12} deficiency anaemia
    D Sickle cell disease
    E Beta-thalassaemia

14. A 72-year-old male has a blood transfusion for an acute gastrointestinal bleed. Thirty minutes later he develops a temperature of 39.5°C, tachycardia, and hypotension. There is no evidence of haemolysis on blood film. Select the likely diagnosis.
    A Immediate haemolytic reaction
    B Febrile reaction
    C Allergic reaction
    D Viral hepatitis
    E Septicaemia

15. A 65-year-old woman presents one week post-transfusion with anaemia, jaundice, and fever. Select the likely diagnosis.
    A Febrile reaction
    B Allergic reaction

C Viral hepatitis
D Septicaemia
E Delayed haemolytic reaction

16. A 13-year-old boy falls while playing football. He has an abrasion over the site of tenderness and an X-ray shows a fracture through one of the cortices.
    A Spiral
    B Stress
    C Pathological
    D Open
    E Incomplete

17. An 84-year-old woman presents with a painful right tibia. Her X-ray shows abnormal cortical thickening, a visible fracture, and thickening in a bowed tibia.
    A Transverse
    B Spiral
    C Stress
    D Pathological
    E Comminuted

18. A 15-year-old girl refuses to have an appendicectomy. Single most likely person from the options listed from whom to take consent.
    A Patient
    B Parents
    C Surgeon
    D Judge
    E Hospital management

19. An unconscious stabbed patient needs an emergency thoracotomy. Single most likely person from the options listed from whom to take consent.
    A Patient
    B Partner
    C Surgeon

D Judge

E Hospital management

20. A diabetic patient with chronic, stable schizophrenia presents with a gangrenous toe which requires an amputation. He understands the implications but refuses surgery. Who is the single most likely person from the options listed from whom to take consent.

A Patient

B Partner

C Surgeon

D Psychiatrist

E Judge

21. The patient is complaining of tingling in the tips of their fingers. Select the single most likely structure from the options listed that was likely to have been injured.

A Phrenic nerve

B Stellate ganglion

C Parathyroid glands

D Recurrent laryngeal nerve

E External laryngeal nerve

22. An opera singer complains that her voice is becoming weak after singing for a short period of time. Select the single most likely structure from the options listed that was likely to have been injured.

A Phrenic nerve

B Stellate ganglion

C Parathyroid glands

D Recurrent laryngeal nerve

E External laryngeal nerve

23. A smoker presents with unilateral ptosis and a small pupil. Select the single most likely structure from the options listed that was likely to have been injured.

A Phrenic nerve

B Stellate ganglion

C Parathyroid glands

D Recurrent laryngeal nerve

E External laryngeal nerve

24. Which nerve supplies the tibialis anterior muscle?

A Saphenous nerve

B Femoral nerve

C Tibial nerve

D Superficial peroneal nerve

E Deep peroneal nerve

25. Which nerve supplies the quadratus femoris muscle?

A Obturator nerve

B Saphenous nerve

C Femoral nerve

D Tibial nerve

E Sural nerve

26. Which nerve supplies the adductor magnus muscle?

A Obturator nerve

B Saphenous nerve

C Femoral nerve

D Tibial nerve

E Sural nerve

27. A healthy full-term baby was born 5 hours ago after a prolonged labour. The child's right arm is medially rotated with the palm of the hand facing backwards. Select the root value related to this injury?

A C5

B C5-6

C C5-7

D C7

E C8-T1

28. While the patient is holding on to the overhead railing, the bus suddenly stops. The patient

presents with weakness of the small muscles of the hand and sensory loss over the medial aspect of the hand and forearm. Select the root value related to this injury?

A C5
B C5-6
C C7
D C8-T1
E C5-8, T1

29. Arising in the upper, inner thigh. Select the single most likely diagnosis.

A Direct inguinal hernia
B Indirect inguinal hernia
C Obturator hernia
D Femoral hernia
E Pantaloon hernia

30. Arising from the umbilicus in the adult. Select the single most likely diagnosis.

A Inguinal hernia
B Epigastric hernia
C Paraumbilical hernia
D Umbilical hernia
E Pantaloon hernia

31. Arising below and lateral to the pubic tubercle. Select the single most likely diagnosis.

A Direct inguinal hernia
B Indirect inguinal hernia
C Obturator hernia
D Femoral hernia
E Epigastric hernia

32. What tumour marker is associated with ovarian carcinoma?

A CA-125
B CA19-9
C CEA
D LDH
E Alpha-fetoprotein

33. What tumour marker is associated with hepatocellular carcinoma?

A CA-125
B CA19-9
C CEA
D LDH
E Alpha-fetoprotein

34. What tumour marker is associated with colorectal cancer?

A CA-125
B CA19-9
C CEA
D LDH
E Alpha-fetoprotein

35. A 16-year-old girl presents with a history of asthma and epilepsy with anterior chest pain. Select the likely diagnosis.

A Pneumonia
B Pulmonary embolus
C Pneumothorax
D Tietze's syndrome (costochondritis)
E Oesophageal spasm

36. A 32-year-old woman presents 3 weeks post-partum with pleuritic chest pain, breathlessness, and haemoptysis. Select the likely diagnosis.

A Myocardial infarction
B Pneumonia
C Pulmonary embolus
D Pneumothorax
E Dissecting aortic aneurysm

37. Concerning the course of the thoracic duct:

A It arises at L3
B It passes through the left crus of the diaphragm
C It ascends anterior to the oesophagus

D It crosses the midline from right to left at T5

E It drains into the right internal jugular vein

38. Concerning the diaphragm:
    A The central portion obtains its sensory supply from the lower six intercostals nerves
    B The oesophageal hiatus opens at T12
    C The left phrenic nerve pierces the central tendon
    D The inferior vena cava opening is at T10
    E The sympathetic chain passes through the median arcuate ligament

39. Concerning the blood supply of the oesophagus:
    A The arterial supply to the upper third is derived from the superior thyroid artery
    B The arterial supply to the lower third is derived from the left gastric artery
    C The thoracic oesophagus drains into the hemi-azygous vein
    D The abdominal oesophagus drains via the splenic vein
    E The arterial supply to the middle third is derived from the inferior thyroid artery

40. Which of the following structures is found at the transpyloric plane of Addison?
    A Fundus of stomach
    B Tail of pancreas
    C Inferior mesenteric artery branching from aorta
    D Upper border of L3
    E Duodenojejunal flexure

41. Concerning blood supply of the stomach:
    A The right gastric artery is derived from the splenic artery
    B The cystic artery is derived from the left gastric artery
    C The gastroduodenal branch of the hepatic artery gives off the left gastroepiploic artery
    D The splenic artery gives off the superior pancreaticoduodenal artery
    E The short gastric arteries are derived from the splenic artery

42. Concerning the parathyroid glands:
    A Approximately 30 per cent are aberrant
    B The upper parathyroid glands are 4th branchial pouch derivatives
    C The upper parathyroid glands are supplied by the superior thyroid artery
    D The lower parathyroid glands are 2nd branchial pouch derivatives
    E The upper parathyroid glands develop in association with the thymus gland

43. Concerning the blood supply to the femoral head:
    A The arterial supply from the ligamentum teres contributes more significantly in adulthood
    B The main blood supply is derived from the obturator artery in the adult
    C Lateral and medial circumflex femoral arteries supply the femoral head via retinacula
    D Vessels from the diaphysis of cancellous bone provide an insignificant arterial blood supply in adulthood

E Fractures that are extracapsular have a high risk of avascular necrosis

44. **Concerning the femoral canal:**
    A It is bound laterally by the pectineal ligament
    B It is bound medially by the femoral vein
    C It is bound posteriorly by the lacunar ligament
    D It is bound anteriorly by the inguinal ligament
    E It transmits the spermatic cord

45. **Concerning the adrenal cortex:**
    A The zona glomerulosa is the most superficial layer
    B The zone fasciculata is the most superficial layer
    C The most superficial two layers produce glucocorticoids, oestrogens, and androgens
    D The most superficial layers produce adrenaline
    E Mineralocorticoid production occurs in the zona reticularis

46. **Concerning stomach secretions:**
    A G-cells secrete hydrochloric acid (HCl) and pepsinogen
    B HCl secretion is inhibited by secretin
    C Chief cells produce intrinsic factor
    D Parietal cells produce gastrin
    E Gastric secretion is approximately 2–3 L per day

47. **Concerning abscesses:**
    A They are enclosed in a pyogenic membrane composed of fibrotic connective tissue
    B *Staphylococcus aureus* is most often the cause of a pilonidal abscess
    C Coliforms are most often the cause of a psoas abscess
    D A sterile abscess may contain bacteria
    E Pus contains a mixture of dead and live neutrophils

48. **Concerning Dukes classification of colorectal cancer:**
    A In class B, there is breach of muscularis propria
    B In class A, the 5-year survival rate is approximately 75 per cent
    C In class C2, the apical node is negative
    D In class C1, the 5-year survival rate is approximately 65 per cent
    E In class D, the 5-year survival rate is approximately 25 per cent

49. **Concerning staging of malignant melanoma:**
    A Clarke's levels give a better indication of prognosis than Breslow thickness
    B Clarke level IV involves invasion into the subcutaneous tissue
    C A Breslow thickness of <0.75 mm confers a 90 per cent 5-year survival rate
    D Breslow thickness is measured in millimetres from the epidermis
    E Clarke level II only involves the epidermis

50. **Concerning multiple endocrine neoplasia (MEN) syndromes:**
    A Type I is characterised by medullary thyroid carcinoma
    B Type IIa is characterised by pancreatic adenoma
    C Type I is characterised by pituitary adenoma

D Type IIa is characterised by submucosal neurofibromas

E Type I but not type II is characterised by parathyroid hyperplasia

51. Concerning actinomycosis:
    A Actinomyces meyeri is the most commonly implicated pathogen
    B It is easily differentiated from malignancy by history and clinical examination
    C 'Sulphur granules' found at the time of surgery are pathognomonic
    D Serology may help to confirm/refute the diagnosis
    E It has been linked to the usage of the intrauterine contraceptive device

52. During fracture healing, what type of bone makes up the provisional callus?
    A Cortical bone
    B Cancellous bone
    C Cartilage
    D Woven bone
    E Lamellar bone

53. A woman has a pleomorphic adenoma. She is undergoing a total parotidectomy. Which important vascular structure should the surgeon be most aware of?
    A Facial artery
    B Facial vein
    C External carotid artery
    D Retromandibular vein
    E Internal jugular vein

54. What is the cardiac index?
    A Stroke volume × heart rate
    B Mean arterial pressure × systemic vascular resistance
    C Cardiac output divided by body weight
    D Cardiac output divided by heart rate
    E Cardiac output divided by body surface area

55. A patient is known to have exposure to beta-naphthylamine. What is he/she at increased risk of developing?
    A Small-cell lung carcinoma
    B Bladder cancer
    C Breast cancer
    D Chemical pneumonitis
    E Lymphoma

56. When does the heart rate decrease?
    A After a meal
    B On inspiration
    C Pressure on the eyeball
    D Pressure on the sinoatrial node
    E Exercise

57. Which of the following suggests that respiratory failure is chronic rather than acute?
    A Plasma bicarbonate of 39 mmol/L
    B Pao_2 of 9 kPa
    C Pao_2 of 7 kPa
    D Arterial pH of 7.2
    E Hypoventilation

58. A 12-year-old boy develops acute tonsillitis. He starts to complain of pain in the ear. What nerve is likely to be involved?
    A Superior laryngeal
    B Glossopharyngeal
    C Facial
    D Hypoglossal
    E Lesser palatine

59. A man undergoes an open inguinal hernia repair. During the procedure the spermatic cord is

visualized. What structures does this contain?

A Dartos muscle

B Femoral branch of the genitofemoral nerve

C Ilioinguinal nerve

D Inferior epigastric artery

E Pampiniform plexus

60. **Which statement applies to the original Dukes classification for colorectal carcinoma?**

A Is a tumour grading scale

B Accurately defines the number of lymph nodes involved

C Distinguishes tumours that penetrate the muscularis mucosa from those that are confined by the mucosa

D Does not take into account the presence of metastases

E Highlights the improved prognosis in those patients with villous rather than tubular carcinoma

61. **In acute osteomyelitis of a long bone, which statement applies?**

A If blood-borne, is usually caused by streptococci

B Acute inflammation causes a rise in intraosseous pressure

C The involucrum is a focus of dead bone

D Early radiographs will demonstrate rarefaction and periosteal new bone formation

E *Pseudomonas* tends to occur in patients with sickle cell disease

62. **In intestinal anastomatic leaks, which statement applies?**

A Are apparent 10–14 days after surgery

B Abdominal pain, pyrexia, and tachycardia are suggestive of a leak

C The appearance of bowel contents through the abdominal wound is proof of an anastomatic leak

D Early leaks are best tested by local surgical repair

E Late leaks are treated by urgent laparotomy, abdominal washout, and repair

63. **Complications of an above-knee amputation include which of the following?**

A Joint contractures affecting the hip joint

B Sudek's atrophy

C Myoglobinuria

D Neuroma formation

E Amyloid deposition

64. **Which statement applies to the cephalic vein?**

A Begins in the region of the anatomical snuffbox

B At the elbow is deep to the lateral cutaneous nerve of the forearm

C Ends by joining the brachial vein

D Is medial to the biceps muscle in the arm

E Has no valves

65. **Thyrotoxicosis is characterized by which of the following?**

A Weight gain

B Proximal myopathy

C Enopthalmos

D Hypertrophy of the vascular elastic lamina

E Nose bleeds

66. **Which is a feature of a cervical rib?**

A A cause of brachial artery aneurysm

B Best diagnosed by posteroanterior (PA) chest radiograph

C Compresses the upper trunk of the brachial plexus

D A cause of thoracic outlet syndrome

E Most commonly symptomatic in the 50–60 years age group

67. **Which statement applies to the hepatic portal vein?**

A Is formed by the union of the splenic and superior mesenteric veins

B Runs behind the epiploic foramen

C Lies anterior to the common hepatic artery

D Originates behind the body of the pancreas

E Approximately 25 per cent of hepatic blood flow is derived from the hepatic portal vein

68. **Which statement regarding Hodgkin's disease is true?**

A Typically seen in the gastrointestinal tract

B May be classified using the Rappaport classification

C Is characterized by Reed–Sternberg cells

D The lymphocyte-depleted type is associated with a more favourable prognosis

E Usually presents with painful lymphadenopathy

69. **What is supplied by the facial nerve?**

A Palatoglossus muscle

B Medial pterygoid muscle

C Masseter muscle

D Temporalis

E Parasympathetic fibres to the submandibular gland

70. **Which is a feature of the submandibular duct?**

A Lies between mylohyoid and hyoglossus muscle

B Is 10 cm long

C Develops from the endoderm

D Is closely related to the facial nerve

E Opens into the mouth at the side of the cheek

71. **In intussusception in children, which statement applies?**

A Occurs more commonly in girls

B The most common form is ileo-ileal

C Is characterized by severe colicky abdominal pain with pain-free intervals

D There is an association with Henoch–Schönlein purpura

E Usually occurs in the 2–3 years age group

72. **Which statement is true of Sjögren's syndrome?**

A Is a condition in which the patient has wet eyes and mouth

B Is most commonly seen in young men

C Is characterized by beta-pleated sheets

D Is associated with autoimmune diseases

E Predisposes to adenocarcinoma

73. **Which of the following is associated with hyperparathyroidism?**

A Paravertebral ossification

B Peptic ulcer

C Retinal haemorrhages

D Aortic stenosis

E Hoarse voice

74. **Which statement applies to the posterior triangle of the neck?**

A Is bounded by the lateral third of the clavicle inferiorly

B Has a roof formed by the prevertebral fascia

C Has a roof pierced by the external jugular vein

D Is bounded by the anterior border of sternocleidomastoid

E Contains the carotid sheath

75. **Which statement applies to the tongue?**

A Develops from the 1st and 3rd branchial arches

B Has taste buds supplied by the hypoglossal nerve

C Is supplied by the facial artery

D Has a profuse anastomosis of blood vessels across the midline

E Deviates to the left in lesions of the left glossopharyngeal nerve

76. **Which statement is true of postcricoid carcinoma?**

A Is more common in patients with Plummer–Vinson syndrome

B Is highly radiosensitive

C Is associated with workers exposed to iron

D Has a 5-year survival rate of more than 60 per cent

E Is more common in males

77. **Which of the following statements is true of Colles' fracture?**

A Is a cause of carpal tunnel syndrome

B Results in palmar displacement of the distal fractured fragment

C Extends into the wrist (radiocarpal) joint

D Is typically associated with compression of the ulnar nerve

E Involves the ulnar styloid process

78. **When a person lifts his right leg and stands unaided with only his left foot on the ground, the iliac** crest on the right side does not descend (negative Trendelenburg sign) provided that one of the following applies. Which?

A The right gluteus medius muscle is actively contracted

B The left hip joint is not congenitally dislocated

C The right superior gluteal nerve is intact

D The left psoas muscle is actively contracted

E The neck of the right femur has not been shortened by a healed fracture

79. **Which of the following describes laminar flow in a blood vessel?**

A Has maximum velocity in the centre

B Is a flow regime characterized by low momentum diffusion and high momentum convection

C Produces the highest concentration of cells at the periphery of the vessel

D Reynolds numbers of greater than 2300 are generally considered to be of a laminar type

E Is considered to be 'rough' whereas turbulent flow is considered to be 'smooth'

80. **Which is true of umbilical hernias in children?**

A Are a rare problem (1 in 10,000)

B Are commonly associated with incarceration of the bowel

C Are most commonly found in Caucasian children

D Are typically associated with a patent vitello-intestinal duct

E Have small orifices and characteristically close spontaneously before the age of 5 years

81. A patient is suspected of having a haemolytic transfusion reaction. How should the patient best be managed?
    A Removal of inessential foreign body irritants (nasogastric tube, Foley's catheter)
    B Fluid restriction
    C 0.1 M HCl infusion
    D Steroids
    E Fluids and mannitol

82. Which of the following statements concerning access to the abdomen is true?
    A Muscle-splitting incisions are more painful than cutting incisions
    B Failure to close the peritoneum increases the incidence of adhesions
    C Collagenase dissolves sutures near wound edges
    D The Veress needle in laparoscopic surgery is inserted under direct vision
    E Burst abdomen is preceded by serosanguinous discharge

83. Which of the following is true of pseudomembranous colitis?
    A Does not cause colonic bleeding
    B Is caused by *Clostridium perfringes*
    C Is the result of metronidazole administration
    D Is a cause of toxic dilation of the stomach
    E Responds to treatment with vancomycin

84. The diagnosis of acute cholecystitis can be reliably confirmed by which of the following?
    A Ultrasound
    B Plain radiograph
    C Abdominal radiograph
    D Oral cholecystography
    E Liver function tests

85. According to the modified Glasgow scoring system, indices of poor prognosis in severe pancreatitis at 48 hours include which of the following?
    A Albumin of 30 g/L
    B Urea of 10 mmol/L
    C Corrected serum calcium of 2.98 mmol/L
    D Arterial Po_2 of 10 kPa
    E Blood glucose of 6 mmol/L

86. Which statement is true of the rectum?
    A Has a venous drainage into the superior mesenteric vein
    B Has a lymphatic drainage to the superficial inguinal nodes
    C Is supplied by the superior mesenteric ganglia
    D Is anteriorly bounded by the seminal vesicles and prostate
    E Receives its main arterial blood supply from the middle rectal artery

87. The germinal centre of a lymph node:
    A Contains mainly T-lymphocytes
    B Contains Langerhans dendritic cells
    C Generates immunoglobulin-producing plasma cells
    D Is characteristically enlarged in established infectious mononucleosis
    E Contains the cords and sinuses

88. All eukaryotic cells have membrane- bound organelles. Which one of the following organelles is self-replicating?
    A Golgi body
    B Ribosome

C Rough endoplasmic reticulum

D Mitochondria

E Lysosome

89. **With regard to antidiabetic agents, which drug stimulates release of insulin from the pancreas?**

A Actrapid

B Gliclazide

C Metformin

D Rosiglitazone

E Acarbose

90. **With regard to development of the kidney:**

A It is derived from endoderm

B The transcription factor WT-1 is necessary for the competence of the mesenchyme to be induced

C There are two phases of kidney development

D The kidneys descend during development to their final site

E The metanephric blastema gives rise to the collecting ducts

91. **With regard to cerebrospinal fluid (CSF):**

A It is produced by arachnoid granulations

B It is produced at a rate of 30 mL/min

C It is situated within the subdural space

D It flows between the lateral ventricles and third ventricle via the foramen of Magendie

E It turns over approximately 4–5 times daily

92. **With regard to antibodies (immunoglobulins):**

A They are produced by mast cells

B The antigen binding region is located in the constant region

C Antibody class is defined by the structure of the light chain

D Diversity is partly achieved through somatic hypermutation

E They are composed of one heavy chain and two light chains

93. **A patient is diagnosed as having iron deficiency anaemia. Which of the following is the peripheral blood film likely to show?**

A Macrocytic anaemia

B Microcytic anaemia

C Ring sideroblasts

D Sickle-shaped cells

E Howell–Jolly bodies

94. **With regard to diaphragmatic development:**

A Is formed by the fusion of two separate elements

B Develops in the thoracic region

C The left pleuroperitoneal canal is larger and closes later than the right

D The central tendon arises from the pleuroperitoneal membranes

E The septum transversum migrates cranially (rostrally) in development

95. **With regard to CSF composition:**

A CSF is produced through a passive process

B The composition of CSF is identical to that of plasma

C The protein content of CSF is 0.5 per cent that of plasma

D The potassium content of CSF is higher than that of plasma

E The pH of CSF is heavily buffered

96. **With regard to IgM antibodies:**

A They cross the placenta

B They are characteristically produced in a secondary immune response

C They can activate complement

D They are usually found lining mucosal surfaces

E They are usually monomeric

97. **Which antibiotic acts by inhibiting protein synthesis?**
    A Penicillin
    B Erythromycin
    C Cefuroxime
    D Trimethoprim
    E Co-trimoxazole

98. **The speed of nerve conduction decreases with:**
    A Increasing axonal diameter
    B Increasing membrane capacitance
    C Decreasing axonal resistance
    D Myelination by Schwann cells
    E Increasing temperature

99. **The human major histocompatibility complex (MHC):**
    A Resides on chromosome 11
    B Is composed of six human leukocyte antigen (HLA) genes
    C Codes for three classes of antigens
    D Will be identical in dizygotic twins
    E Codes for blood group antigens

100. **Which one of the following statements regarding von Willebrand's disease is true?**
    A It commonly exhibits an autosomal dominant pattern of inheritance
    B It presents with reduced bleeding times
    C It always has associated reduced factor VIII levels
    D It is associated with reduced or abnormal platelets
    E It is X-linked recessive

101. **With regard to intestinal development:**
    A The gut is a mesodermal derivative
    B The whole of the foregut apart from the stomach undergoes rotation
    C The stomach is a midgut derivative
    D Rupture of the cloacal membrane creates the mouth
    E Midgut development involves herniation of bowel into the umbilicus

102. **With regard to skeletal muscle fibres:**
    A They are each normally innervated by more than one motor neurone
    B They become less excitable as the extracellular ionized calcium levels fall
    C Calcium is taken up by the sarcotubular system when they contract
    D Actin and myosin filaments shorten when they contract
    E They contain intracellular stores of calcium ions

103. **With regard to the MHC:**
    A CD4 (helper) T-cells recognize antigen only in the context of MHC Class I
    B Class II MHC is expressed on all nucleated cells of the body
    C Class II MHC contains β_2-microglobulin
    D Class II MHC presents exogenous antigens
    E Class II MHC is expressed in low levels on the surface of dendritic cells

104. In acute inflammation, which is the predominant cell type involved?
    A Basophil
    B Eosinophil
    C Lymphocyte
    D Monocyte
    E Neutrophil

105. A disease inherited as an autosomal dominant disorder:
    A Requires that both parents carry the abnormality
    B Usually prevents reproduction
    C Affects males and females equally
    D Affects all the children of the affected adult
    E May be transmitted by a carrier who does not manifest the disease

106. With regard to the Palatine tonsil:
    A It lies on the middle pharyngeal constrictor muscle
    B It is supplied by the superior pharyngeal artery
    C It is lined by columnar epithelium
    D Inflammation may cause referred pain to the ear
    E Bleeding after tonsillectomy is usually due to arterial bleeding

107. With regard to coronary blood flow:
    A Blood flow to the left ventricle increases in early systole
    B Local metabolic activity is the chief factor determining rate of blood flow to the heart
    C Coronary blood flow to the left ventricle increases in hypothermia
    D Coronary blood flow is increased in aortic stenosis
    E The myocardium extracts 25 per cent of the oxygen from the coronary blood

108. With regard to bacterial structure and classification:
    A Gram-positive bacteria contain lipopolysaccharide
    B Gram-positive bacteria retain an iodine purple dye complex
    C Gram-negative bacteria possess thicker layers of peptidoglycan than Gram-negative bacteria
    D The endotoxin part of lipopolysaccharide is the O-antigen portion
    E All cocci are Gram-positive

109. Derivatives of the hindgut are typically supplied by the:
    A Coeliac artery
    B Ductus arteriosus
    C Inferior mesenteric artery
    D Superior mesenteric artery
    E Umbilical artery

110. With regard to cardiac conducting tissue:
    A Purkinje fibres lead to contraction of the apex before the base of the heart
    B Sinoatrial node cells are found in both atria
    C Sinoatrial node cells are unable to generate impulses when completely denervated
    D Sinoatrial node cells are connected to the AV node by fine bundles of Purkinje tissue
    E The pacemaker of the heart is the region of the heart that has the slowest intrinsic firing rate

111. Splenectomy increases susceptibility to which of the following organisms?
    A *Streptococcus pyogenes*
    B *Schistosomiasis haematobium*

C Bacteroides fragilis

D Neisseria meningitidis

E Staphylococcus aureus

112. During a cholecystectomy, the cystic artery must be located and ligated. This arterial supply most commonly arises from the:

A Gastroduodenal artery

B Hepatic artery proper

C Right hepatic artery

D Left hepatic artery

E Superior pancreatico-duodenal artery

113. A teenager would like genetic counselling. His mother has phenylketonuria, or PKU (which is inherited as autosomal recessive). He has a brother with PKU. What is the chance that he is a carrier of the disease?

A 0 per cent

B 25 per cent

C 50 per cent

D 75 per cent

E 100 per cent

114. With regard to the parotid gland:

A It contains within it branches of the facial nerve deep to the retro-mandibular vein

B It consists of superficial, middle, and deep lobes

C Secreto-motor innervation is via the glossopharyngeal and auriculotemporal nerves

D Its duct pierces the masseter muscle to enter the mouth opposite the upper second molar tooth

E It produces mainly a mucous secretion

115. With regard to circulating red blood cells (erythrocytes):

A They have a normal lifespan of 6–8 weeks

B They are broken down in the bone marrow

C They contain the enzyme glutal-dehyde anhydrase

D They lack nuclei and mitochondria

E They swell to bursting point when suspended in 0.9 per cent saline

116. With regard to *Helicobacter pylori* (*H. pylori*):

A It is a Gram-positive organism

B It is a known carcinogen

C Approximately 5 per cent of the population are infected with *H. pylori*

D It is destroyed by the acidic environment present within the stomach

E Infection can be prevented through vaccination

117. Cells in the pancreas that secrete glucagon and insulin are:

A A- and B-cells

B Acinar cells

C D cells

D Pancreatic D1 cells

E Pancreatic polypeptide cells

118. Which of the following is true of erythrocytes?

A They travel at slower velocity in venules than in capillaries

B They are normally spherical

C They make little contribution to the buffering capacity of the blood

D Following haemolysis, erythrocytes release erythropoietin which stimulates the production of more erythrocytes

E They deform as they pass through the capillaries

119. Cholera:
    A Is transmitted by the blood-borne route
    B Is caused by infection with *Shigella sonnei*
    C Is usually accompanied by marked mucosal inflammation and ulceration
    D Is caused by a toxin which increases adenylate cyclase activity
    E Is caused by endotoxin

120. Which of the following muscles is *not* a muscle of mastication?
    A Medial pterygoid
    B Buccinator
    C Masseter
    D Lateral pterygoid
    E Temporalis

121. With regard to the thoracic duct:
    A It drains into the confluence of the right internal jugular and subclavian veins
    B It lies anterior to the oesophagus as it passes through the diaphragm
    C It crosses the midline at the level of T5
    D It has no valves
    E If it is injured, a haemothorax may result

122. With regard to the mechanics of respiration:
    A Compliance is defined as the change in pressure per unit volume
    B Compliance is synonymous with elastance
    C Sighing serves no physiological purpose
    D The lung follows the same behaviour in inflation and deflation
    E Emphysema results in increased lung compliance

123. Budd–Chiari syndrome is:
    A A congenital inability to metabolize bilirubin
    B A dietary deficiency of an essential amino acid
    C Agenesis of the hepatic lobe
    D Occlusion of the hepatic venous drainage
    E Malignant transformation of the biliary epithelium

124. Which one of the following is true concerning retrospective and prospective studies?
    A Prospective studies are also known as case-control studies
    B Prospective studies allow direct determination of incidence rates
    C The retrospective approach has the advantage that there is little or no bias
    D In a prospective study, the cohort consists of people who are found to have the disease in question
    E The prospective approach is usually used to determine the aetiology of a rare disease

125. With regard to the lungs:
    A The left lung has three lobes
    B The horizontal fissure is present in the left lung
    C Each lung has eight bronchopulmonary segments
    D A foreign body is more likely to enter the left bronchus than the right
    E The lungs receive a dual blood supply

126. Which one of the following is true of haemoglobin?
    A Most haemoglobin circulates as free protein in plasma
    B Oxygen attaches to the globin chains

C Each haemoglobin molecule combines with eight oxygen atoms

D In normal adult haemoglobin, iron exists in the ferric state

E Normal adult haemoglobin contains two alpha and two gamma chains

127. With regard to metaplasia:
A It is irreversible
B It is most important in the upper oesophagus
C Metaplasia in the bronchus involves a change from columnar to stratified squamous epithelium
D It is harmless
E Barrett's oesophagus involves a change from glandular to stratified squamous epithelium

128. A 52-year-old man presents with episodic hypertension, an adrenal mass, and elevated catecholamines. The most likely diagnosis is:
A Adrenal cortical carcinoma
B Adrenal cortical hyperplasia
C Pheochromocytoma
D Ganglioneuroma
E Neuroblastoma

129. Which one of the following studies is regarded as the gold standard in epidemiological research?
A Cross-sectional study
B Case–control study
C Case report
D Randomized controlled trial
E Non-randomized controlled trial

130. With regard to the pleura:
A The pleura ends level with the 12th rib posteriorly
B It extends above the clavicle superiorly
C The visceral layer is richly innervated

D It extends above the neck of the 1st rib superiorly
E The pleural reflection on the right side matches that on the left side identically

131. Which one of the following is true of erythropoietin?
A It is a polypeptide
B Secretion is decreased at high altitude
C In adults, it is mainly made in the liver
D It acts via a secondary messenger
E Production is decreased by local hypoxia

132. Which of the following is a defining characteristic of a malignant tumour?
A Increase in size with time
B Chromosomal abnormalities
C Presence of a pseudo-capsule
D Invasion beyond the basement membrane
E Well-ordered maturation

133. With regard to the pericardium:
A It is two layers thick
B It is poorly innervated
C It is responsible for the formation of the transverse and oblique sinuses
D Pericardiocentesis may be detrimental in the management of cardiac tamponade
E It is essential in order to maintain a normal cardiac output

134. Which one of the following is true of aldosterone?
A It is a steroid hormone secreted by the adrenal medulla
B Production is decreased by angiotensin-converting enzyme inhibitors

C Secretion results in increased potassium reabsorption from the nephron

D Secretion results in a rise in urinary pH

E Production ceases following the removal of the kidneys and their juxtaglomerular cells

135. Which of the following are cytological features of malignancy?

A Hyperchromatism

B Pyknosis

C Karyorrhexis

D Decreased nuclear-to-cytoplasmic ratio

E Low mitotic index

136. A 63-year-old male has a progressive history of congestive cardiac failure. At post-mortem, the heart demonstrates extensive replacement of the myocardium by an acellular, eosinophilic material. This material is most likely to be:

A Cholesterol

B Calcium salt deposits

C Myocyte fibrinoid necrosis

D Post-infarctive cicatrix (scar)

E Amyloid

137. Which one of the following statements is true?

A The standard error provides a measure of the spread of observations around the mean

B The standard deviation is equal to the standard error divided by the square-root of the sample size

C The standard error is generally larger than the standard deviation

D In a positively skewed distribution, the median is greater than the mode, but greater than the mean

E The mean and standard deviation of a random sample will generally be different from the mean and standard deviation of the true population

138. Which of the following regarding the coronary arteries is correct:

A The sinoatrial node is supplied by the left coronary artery in most cases

B The atrioventricular node is supplied by the left coronary artery in most cases

C The circumflex artery is a branch of the right coronary artery

D Occlusion of the anterior interventricular artery (left anterior descending artery) results in an anterior myocardial infarction

E Angina is always due to atherosclerosis of the coronary vessels

139. With regard to the renin–angiotensin system:

A Angiotensinogen is secreted by the juxtaglomerular apparatus

B The lung catalyses the conversion of angiotensinogen to angiotensin I

C Activation results in the stimulation of aldosterone release

D Angiotensin II is a potent vasodilator

E Angiotensin-converting enzyme is found principally in the liver

140. Carcinomas most often metastasize by which of the following routes?

A Bloodstream

B Lymphatics

C Trans-coelomic

D Peri-neural

E Implantation

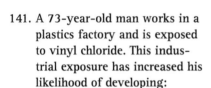

141. A 73-year-old man works in a plastics factory and is exposed to vinyl chloride. This industrial exposure has increased his likelihood of developing:
    A Focal nodular hyperplasia
    B Hepatic adenoma
    C Hepatic angiosarcoma
    D Hepatic fibroma
    E Hepatocellular carcinoma

142. With regard to tumour suppressor genes:
    A They encode proteins that positively regulate growth
    B They behave in a dominant fashion
    C Gain-of-function of tumour suppressor genes results in neoplastic growth
    D p53 and Rb-1 are tumour suppressor genes
    E p53 normally functions as an anti-apoptotic factor

143. Which one of the following muscles is innervated by the facial nerve?
    A Temporalis
    B Anterior belly of digastric
    C Buccinator
    D Masseter
    E Lateral pterygoid

144. With regard to the transpyloric plane (of Addison):
    A It is halfway between the suprasternal notch and umbilicus
    B It lies at the level of T12
    C It lies at the origin of the inferior mesenteric artery
    D It lies level with the hilum of the kidneys
    E It is the point at which the aorta bifurcates

145. With regard to gastric acid secretion:
    A It is inhibited by gastrin
    B It is potentiated by histamine
    C It commences only when food enters the stomach
    D It is stimulated by the glossopharyngeal nerve
    E It is stimulated by somatostatin

146. With regard to the adrenal gland (suprarenal gland):
    A The suprarenal vein on each side drains into the corresponding renal vein
    B The adrenal gland is situated within the same fascial compartment as the kidney
    C The zona glomerulosa forms the innermost layer of the adrenal cortex
    D The anterior surface of the right adrenal gland is overlapped by the inferior vena cava
    E The adrenal medulla is derived from embryonic mesoderm

147. Which one of the following is true of gastrin?
    A It is secreted in the body of the stomach
    B It is stimulated by low pH
    C It stimulates gastric acid production
    D It inhibits gastric motility
    E Decreased secretion results in the Zollinger–Ellison syndrome

148. Lung carcinoma:
    A Is the third most common cause of death from neoplasia in the UK
    B Has rarely metastasized at the time of presentation
    C May produce paraneoplastic syndromes

D Is most commonly due to small-
cell (oat-cell) carcinoma

E Is most commonly caused by
asbestos exposure

149. Prokaryotes differ from eukaryotes
in that prokaryotes have:

A Peptidoglycan

B Sterols in their membranes

C 2–6 chromosomes

D An endoplasmic reticulum

E Larger 80S ribosomes

150. With regard to the vermiform
appendix:

A It is most often situated in a
pelvic position

B It receives blood via the right
colic branch of the superior
mesenteric artery

C It lies at McBurney's point
(halfway between the anterior
superior iliac spine and umbilicus)

D It is unimportant in humans

E It is a retroperitoneal structure

151. With regard to the exocrine
pancreas:

A It secretes digestive juices with a
pH of 4–5

B It develops from a single ventral
pancreatic bud

C Secretion is inhibited by
cholecystokinin

D The main stimulation for secretion
occurs during the intestinal phase

E It produces secretin

152. A 67-year-old male undergoes
an elective right colectomy for
adenocarcinoma of the caecum.
If distant non-nodal metastases
are discovered, which organ would
likely be affected first?

A Brain

B Lung

C Adrenal

D Liver

E Bone

153. With regard to acute appendicitis:

A It is most common at the
extremes of age

B It may result in thrombosis of the
appendicular artery (endarteritis
obliterans)

C It often resolves with conservative management such as
antibiotics

D If untreated it is rarely
life-threatening

E Classically it refers pain to the
epigastric region

154. Which one of the following is true
of pancreatic enzymes:

A Trypsin is a powerful activator
of other pancreatic proteolytic
enzymes

B The pancreas secretes enterokinase (enteropeptidase)

C Chymotrypsinogen activates trypsinogen to form trypsin

D The pancreas secretes proteases in
their activated form

E The pancreas normally contains a
trypsin activator

155. Which one of the following is the
most common malignant tumour
of bone?

A Chondroblastoma

B Giant-cell tumour

C Osteosarcoma

D Chondrosarcoma

E Secondary carcinoma

156. A research assistant is studying
the production of an anthrax
vaccine. He must destroy all
vegetative cells and spores of

Bacillus anthracis that have contaminated the pipette. What agent should he use?

A Boiling

B Ethanol alcohol

C Oxidizing agents

D Autoclaving

E Anionic detergents

157. **With regard to the greater omentum:**

A It has no surgical importance

B It is supplied by the right and left gastric arteries

C It is two layers thick

D It provides a route of access to the lesser sac

E The anterior layers descend from the lesser curvature of the stomach

158. **With regard to the endocrine pancreas:**

A It secretes hormones into a highly branched ductal system

B Glucagon is secreted from β-islet cells

C Islets of Langerhans make up only 2 per cent of the volume of the gland

D Somatostatin is secreted from α-islet cells

E Glucagon stimulates glycogenesis

159. **Apoptosis:**

A Is always a pathological event

B Involves the death of large contiguous areas of cells

C Is usually accompanied by inflammation

D May be seen in histological section

E Leaves a permanent clump of cellular debris

160. **The virus responsible for causing acquired immunodeficiency syndrome (AIDS) has which one of the following features?**

A A double-stranded genome

B Lacks a viral envelope

C Lacks reverse transcriptase

D Is a member of the adenovirus group

E Destroys CD4 T-lymphocytes

161. **With regard to the ureters:**

A They are lined by stratified squamous epithelium

B They enter the bladder obliquely, forming a flap valve

C The point of narrowest calibre is at the pelviureteric junction

D The arterial supply of the lower third of the ureter is by way of the descending abdominal aorta

E In the female, the ureters are crossed below by the uterine arteries in the broad ligament

162. **Which one of the following is true of bile?**

A Bile salts are derived from the waste products of haemoglobin

B It is actively concentrated in the gallbladder

C Thirty per cent is reabsorbed by the enterohepatic circulation

D Bile contains enzymes required for the digestion of fat

E Accumulation of bile salts is responsible for causing jaundice

163. **Which one of the following tissues is likely to regenerate following damage?**

A Cerebral cortex

B Peripheral neurones

C Skeletal muscle

D Cardiac muscle

E Spinal cord

164. Deficiencies of which of the following factors usually predispose to thrombosis rather than bleeding?
    A Factor V
    B Factor VIII
    C Factor IX
    D Factor X
    E Factor XII

165. With regard to the blood supply of the stomach:
    A The right half of the lesser curvature is supplied by the right gastoepiploic artery
    B The left half of the greater curvature is supplied by the left gastric artery
    C The fundus of the stomach is supplied by the left gastric artery
    D The gastroduodenal artery is a branch of the common hepatic artery
    E The right gastric artery is most commonly implicated in a bleeding duodenal ulcer

166. Which one of these statements regarding insulin is true?
    A Insulin receptors use cAMP as their signal transducer
    B It is secreted by alpha-cells of the pancreas
    C Secretion is stimulated by somatostatin
    D It is an anabolic hormone
    E Release is inhibited by the ingestion of amino acids

167. With regard to necrosis:
    A It is a physiological or pathological process
    B Single cells are involved
    C Liquefactive necrosis classically occurs in the brain
    D Necrotic cells are phagocytosed by adjacent cells
    E Caseous necrosis is the most common type

168. A Swan–Ganz catheter is inserted into a patient with acute respiratory distress syndrome (ARDS). His pulmonary artery pressure is 6 mmHg. The same pressure would be expected in which of the following structures?
    A Aorta
    B Left atrium
    C Left ventricle
    D Right atrium
    E Systemic veins

169. With regard to the femoral triangle, which of the following is correct?
    A The femoral vein lies lateral to the femoral artery
    B The femoral nerve lies within the femoral sheath
    C The femoral artery lies at the mid-point of the inguinal ligament
    D The femoral nerve is the most medially placed structure
    E Cloquet's node lies most medially within the femoral canal

170. With regard to the hypothalamo-pituitary axis:
    A Oxytocin is synthesized in the posterior pituitary gland
    B Prolactin is under dominant inhibitory regulation
    C Thyroxine is a steroid hormone
    D Thyroid-stimulating hormone (TSH) acts via tyrosine kinase receptors
    E GH binds to intracellular receptors

171. Which one of the following is the best definition of gangrene?
    A Digestion of living tissue by saprophytic bacteria
    B Digestion of dead tissue by saprophytic bacteria
    C Gas production in dead tissue
    D Necrosis of tissue caused by bacterial toxins
    E Necrosis of tissue caused by ischaemia

172. A woman has episodic abdominal pain which is worse after fatty meals. Which hormone is responsible for her post-prandial worsening of symptoms?
    A Somatostatin
    B Secretin
    C Pepsin
    D Cholecystokinin
    E Gastrin

173. With regard to the shoulder (glenohumeral) joint:
    A It is a ball-and-socket fibrocartilaginous joint
    B It has high mobility at the expense of stability
    C It is supported mainly by way of ligaments
    D It lies in close relation to the musculocutaneous nerve
    E It most commonly dislocates posteriorly

174. Which one of the following is true of cortisol?
    A It is a protein
    B It lowers blood glucose
    C It is an anabolic hormone
    D It is stimulated by renin
    E It has a peak hormonal concentration in the morning

175. Which one of the following increases the risk of thrombosis?
    A Immobility
    B Thrombocytopenia
    C Reduced blood viscosity
    D An intact endothelium
    E Heparin

176. With regard to the hip joint, which of the following is true?
    A The blood supply to the femoral head arises from a single source
    B It may refer pain to the knee
    C It is the most commonly dislocated joint in the body
    D It lies deep to the sciatic nerve
    E The fibrous capsule is strengthened by two ligaments

177. With regard to calcium homeostasis:
    A The active form of vitamin D is 25-hydroxycholecalciferol
    B PTH secretion is stimulated by the pituitary gland
    C Activated vitamin D decreases calcium absorption from the intestine
    D PTH acts directly on osteoblasts in bone
    E In the kidney, PTH increases calcium excretion and increases phosphate reabsorption from the urine

178. With regard to an embolus:
    A It most often arises from a thrombus formed within arteries
    B It is the same as a thrombus
    C Embolus due to thrombus is impossible to distinguish from post-mortem clot
    D Embolus is always due to thrombus
    E It generally has a worse outcome than thrombus

179. Which of the following veins empties into the left renal vein?
    A Hepatic
    B Left suprarenal
    C Right gonadal
    D Left phrenic
    E Right renal

180. With regard to the anatomical snuffbox:
    A Tenderness at its base is indicative of a fractured hamate
    B It is bounded medially by the abductor pollicis longus
    C The basilic vein begins in its roof
    D The skin overlying it is supplied by cutaneous branches of the median nerve
    E The pulsation of the radial artery may be felt at its base

181. With regard to thyroxine:
    A The thyroid gland produces more T3 than T4
    B TRH directly results in thyroxine release from the thyroid gland
    C Thyroxine promotes the growth and development of the brain
    D Thyroxine decreases basal metabolic rate
    E Thyroxine acts on cell surface receptors

182. Ischaemia:
    A Refers to generalized tissue death due to toxins, trauma, or vascular occlusion
    B Is synonymous with the term 'infarction'
    C Is an abnormal reduction of the blood supply to, or drainage from, an organ or tissue
    D Is always due to vascular occlusion
    E Leads to a worse outcome in tissues with a collateral circulation

183. The Brunner glands secrete an alkaline product that helps maintain an optimal pH for pancreatic enzyme activity. Where are these glands located?
    A At the base of the villi throughout the small intestine
    B Epithelium of the ampulla of Vater
    C Submucosa of the ileum
    D Submucosa of the jejunum
    E Submucosa of the duodenum

184. With regard to the knee joint:
    A It is a synovial, pivot joint
    B The cruciate ligaments are intracapsular and intrasynovial
    C The suprapatellar bursa (pouch) communicates with the knee joint
    D Inflammation of the prepatellar bursa is known as 'clergyman's knee'
    E The menisci play an important role in the locking and unlocking mechanism of the knee joint

185. During diabetic ketoacidosis:
    A The pH of the blood is high
    B Cheyne–Stokes breathing is characteristic
    C Hyperkalaemia occurs
    D Blood glucose levels are typically low
    E Volume status is euvolaemic

186. With regard to acute myocardial infarction:
    A It usually results from an embolus
    B It always causes chest pain
    C It induces acute inflammatory changes, maximal at 1–3 days post-infarct
    D Infarcts less than 12 hours old are clearly visible on macroscopic examination
    E The infarcted tissue is replaced by new cardiac muscle

187. A woman sprains her ankle while running down a flight of stairs. Which ligament did she most likely injure?
    A Deltoid
    B Anterior talo-tibial
    C Medial collateral
    D Calcaneo-fibular
    E Calcaneo-tibial

188. With regard to the brachial plexus:
    A It has principal root values C6–T2
    B The serratus anterior muscle is innervated by the subscapular nerve
    C A lesion involving the lower roots of the brachial plexus results in a classic Erb–Duchenne palsy
    D Cords lie in relation to the third part of the axillary artery
    E Roots lie in the neck between the scalenus anterior and medius muscles

189. With regard to adrenal gland disorders:
    A Adrenal insufficiency results in hypokalaemia and hypernatraemia
    B Conn's syndrome results in hyperkalaemia
    C Cushing's disease is due to a cortisol-producing tumour of the adrenal cortex
    D Pheochromocytoma is due to oversecretion of cortisol by a tumour of the adrenal medulla
    E Congenital adrenal hyperplasia (adrenogenital syndrome) results in virilization and salt wasting

190. Atherosclerosis:
    A Is irreversible
    B Most commonly occurs at branching points within the circulation
    C Is a disease that primarily affects the tunica media of arteries
    D Is accompanied by acute inflammation
    E Is accelerated by hypocholesterolaemia

191. What structure is involved in tarsal tunnel syndrome with heel pain?
    A Anterior tibial artery
    B Deep peroneal nerve
    C Peroneal artery
    D Superficial peroneal nerve
    E Tibial nerve

192. With regard to the brachial plexus:
    A The ulnar nerve arises from the posterior cord
    B The radial nerve arises from the lateral cord
    C The musculocutaneous nerve arises from the lateral cord
    D The median nerve arises from the anterior cord
    E The axillary nerve arises from the lateral cord

193. Which one of the following is true of testosterone?
    A Secretion occurs only in males
    B It is secreted from the Sertoli cells of the testis
    C It is a peptide hormone
    D It is essential for spermatogenesis
    E It depends on FSH for secretion

194. Which of the following regarding local anaesthetics is true?
    A Cocaine is an amide
    B Addition of adrenaline increases systemic absorption of the local anaesthetic
    C One of the first signs of toxicity is perioral paraesthesia

D They work by blocking potassium channels in the nerve endings

E They inhibit the propagation of impulses in Aß fibres first

195. A surgeon's finger is placed in the epiploic foramen of Winslow. The superior margin is:

A Common bile duct

B First part of the duodenum

C Head of pancreas

D Hepatic veins

E Caudate lobe of the liver

196. With regard to the carpal tunnel:

A It is a fibro-osseous tunnel containing the extensor tendons

B It contains within it the ulnar nerve and artery

C Entrapment of the median nerve within it is known as cubital tunnel syndrome

D It contains ten tendons within it

E It contains within it the palmar cutaneous branch of the median nerve

197. Which femoral fracture is at risk of developing avascular necrosis?

A Subcapital neck fracture

B Intertrochanteric fracture

C Subtrochanteric fracture

D Spiral shaft fracture

E Medial condylar fracture

198. Why is the internal vertebral venous plexus important in cancer metastases?

A It is devoid of valves

B It drains tumour tissue

C It has high flow velocity

D It has low flow velocity

E It has retrograde flow

199. The rotator cuff muscles of the shoulder include:

A Latissimus dorsi

B Rhomboid major

C Serratus anterior

D Infraspinatus

E Deltoid

200. Heberden and Bouchard's nodes are typically seen in which form of joint disease?

A Osteoarthritis

B Rheumatoid arthritis

C Psoriatic arthritis

D Crystal arthritis

E Septic arthritis

SECTION 3: SBA ANSWERS AND EXPLANATIONS

1. **E: Septic arthritis**

   The diagnosis is septic arthritis until proven otherwise. The organism responsible in this particular instance is *Neisseria gonorrhoeae* (gonococcal arthritis), although the most common organism implicated in septic arthritis over all age groups is *Staphylococcus aureus*. Gonococcal arthritis may cause a septic arthritis (as illustrated here with the presence of organisms within joint aspirate), or a reactive arthritis with sterile joint fluid. The treatment consists of oral penicillin, ciprofloxacin or doxycycline for 2 weeks, and joint rest.

2. **B: Gilbert's syndrome**

   The diagnosis is Gilbert's syndrome, which affects some 2–3 per cent of the population. The clinical features are mild, fluctuant unconjugated hyperbilirubinaemia.

   The jaundice is typically mild and presents only intermittently, often noticed after an infection or a period of fasting. This is possibly because fasting increases plasma concentrations of free fatty acids which compete with bilirubin for transport by albumin and uptake into liver cells. Bilirubin rarely exceeds 100 µmol/L. There may be mild malaise and hepatic tenderness, but there are no other abnormal physical signs. The liver is histologically normal and individuals have a normal lifespan.

   The hyperbilirubinaemia is due to a defect in the regulatory part of the gene coding for bilirubin UDP-glucuronyl transferase; in some cases, there is also decreased hepatic uptake of bilirubin. In cases where there is a family history, the pattern of inheritance is autosomal dominant.

3. **E: Primary biliary cirrhosis**

   The symptoms, signs, and liver function tests are consistent with a mixed cholestatic/obstructive and hepatocellular picture. A high titre of antimitochondrial antibodies is characteristic of primary biliary cirrhosis, which is an autoimmune condition that typically affects middle-aged women.

   Antimitochondrial antibodies are found in the serum of over 95 per cent of patients with primary biliary cirrhosis, and of the mitochondrial proteins involved, the antigen M2 is specific to the condition. Diagnosis can be confirmed by liver biopsy.

The course and prognosis is very variable, although the median survival is only 7–10 years. Once jaundice develops, survival is below 2 years. Liver transplantation should therefore be offered when the serum bilirubin reaches 100 µmol/L. Post-transplantation 5-year survival is above 75 per cent.

4. **A: Hepatitis A**

The history and liver function tests are characteristic of acute hepatitis, with a predominantly raised ALT reflecting hepatocellular damage ('transaminitis'). The travel history and the timing of the events make viral hepatitis A the most likely cause in this particular case.

Serum transaminases rise 22–40 days after exposure, IgM rises from day 25 and signifies recent infection; IgG remains detectable for life. Infection with hepatitis A virus never progresses to chronic liver disease and only rarely causes fulminant hepatitis, so the mortality rate associated with hepatitis A infection is about 0.1 per cent.

5. **B: Abdominal ultrasound (FAST scan)**

The patient is stable enough to undergo a FAST scan, but not to be transferred to the radiology department for a CT scan ('doughnut of death').

6. **E: Dermoid cyst**

A dermoid cyst is a subcutaneous lump that develops mostly in the midline along the lines of fusion in the face and neck. It is a result of the inclusion of epidermal cells deep to the skin, which can be congenital or secondary to trauma.

7. **C: Histiocytoma**

This is also known as a dermatofibroma. They often occur on the lower limbs and like implantation dermoid cysts, often follow trauma. They are skin-coloured in appearance and woody-hard in consistency.

8. **E: Restorative proctocolectomy**

This operation involves excision of the entire colon and rectum, with an ileo-anal anastomosis. It is a complex operation, but aims to preserve continence.

9. **C: Panproctocolectomy**

It is not possible to establish adequate clearance distally and preserve the anal sphincter. The whole of the colon is required to be excised to avoid potential future malignancy.

10. **B: Clarke's level II**

Clarke's levels are defined as:

- I: Confined to the epidermis
- II: Extends to the papillary dermis

- III: Extends to the papillary-reticular junction
- IV: Extends to the reticular dermis
- V: Invades the subcutaneous tissue

11. D: Glucose-6-phosphate dehydrogenase deficiency

Glucose-6-phosphate dehydrogenase deficiency is a hereditary condition in which red blood cells (RBCs) break down, or haemolyse, when the body is exposed to certain drugs, stress, or infection. Risk factors include: aspirin, antimalarials, and non-steroidal anti-inflammatory drugs; and it is more common in patients of African American or Middle Eastern descent, with a male predominance.

12. B: Hereditary spherocytosis

This condition is inherited in an autosomal dominant pattern, mostly seen in northern Europeans. The defect in the cell membrane leads to premature cell destruction.

13. D: Sickle cell disease

The diagnosis is sickle cell crisis. The definitive diagnosis is made through haemoglobin electrophoresis.

14. E: Septicaemia

The risk is highest in blood maintained in suboptimal conditions where the blood is not stored properly prior to transfusion.

15. E: Delayed haemolytic reaction

The patient is usually immunized to the antigen at previous transfusion, but the concentration of the antibodies is too low to produce an immediate reaction. Production of a further IgG usually one week later leads to delayed haemolysis.

16. E: Incomplete

This is an incomplete, or 'greenstick', fracture because it involves one of the cortices.

17. D: Pathological

The patient has Paget's disease as evidenced by thickening of the bone and a bowed tibia. It is associated with an isolated elevated alkaline phosphatase, in the presence of normal calcium, phosphate, and aminotransferases. A bone scan is useful for determining the activity and extent of this condition.

18. B: Parents

An adolescent has the right to accept surgery, but those under 18 cannot refuse life-saving surgery and the parents can consent for this procedure.

19. C: Surgeon

The surgeon has a legal and moral duty to treat the patient in an emergency under these circumstances.

20. **A: Patient**

    Even those 'under section' to receive psychiatric treatment cannot be forced to have a surgical procedure for a physical condition if they are deemed to be competent.

21. **C: Parathyroid glands**

    Acral paraesthesia is a common manifestation of hypocalcaemia secondary to damage to the parathyroid glands.

22. **E: External laryngeal nerve**

    Injury to the external laryngeal nerve, which supplies the important cricothyroid muscle (that controls voice pitch), produces this deficit.

23. **B: Stellate ganglion**

    These are the manifestations of Horner's syndrome.

24. **E: Deep peroneal nerve**

    The deep peroneal nerve is also known as the anterior tibial nerve. It supplies the muscles of the anterior compartment of the leg, extensor hallucis longus, extensor digitorum longus, extensor digitorum brevis, peroneus tertius and, most importantly, tibialis anterior.

25. **C: Femoral nerve**

    Quadratus femoris is composed of three vastus muscles and the rectus femoris. The femoral nerve also innervates iliacus, pectineus, and sartorius.

26. **A: Obturator nerve**

    The obturator nerve supplies the muscles of the medial compartment of the thigh.

27. **B: C5-6**

    This is an Erb's palsy, caused by injury to the upper trunk of the brachial plexus (C5-6). The hand takes on the 'waiter's-tip' position.

28. **D: C8-T1**

    This is Dejerine–Klumpke palsy, caused by injury to the lower roots of the brachial plexus (C8, T1). It gives the typical appearance of a 'claw-hand'.

29. **C: Obturator hernia**

    Obturator hernias protrude through the obturator foramen which is bounded by the superior pubic ramus, anterior acetabular wall, and ischio-pubic ramus. Irritating the obturator nerve can lead to referred knee pain, or paraesthesia in the inner thigh.

30. **C: Paraumbilical hernia**

    Umbilical hernias in the adult population are rare. They are secondary to increased intra-abdominal pressure. A paraumbilical hernia is seen more commonly.

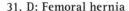

31. **D: Femoral hernia**

Femoral hernias pass through the femoral canal, which is below and lateral to the pubic tubercle. The femoral canal is medial to the femoral vein and contains fat and lymphatics ('Cloquet's lymph node').

32. **A: CA-125**

CA-125 is used for the diagnosis, response to treatment, and follow-up for recurrence in ovarian tumours.

33. **E: Alpha-fetoprotein**

Alpha-fetoprotein is often raised in hepatocellular carcinoma. It is the most widely used tumour marker for the condition and is an independent prognostic indicator.

34. **C: CEA**

Carcino-embryonic antigen (CEA) is the tumour marker of choice for patients with colorectal cancer. It is used for monitoring colorectal cancer, especially when the disease has metastasized.

35. **D: Tietze's syndrome (costochondritis)**

Tietze's syndrome, or costochondritis, presents with pain and swelling over the sternocostal junction. It is usually evident on palpation and perceived pain is exacerbated with respiration.

36. **C: Pulmonary embolus**

The symptoms of a pulmonary embolus include sudden-onset dyspnoea, tachypnoea, pleuritic chest pain, cough, and haemoptysis. On clinical examination, a pleural friction rub may be auscultated. Risk factors are attributed to Virchow's triad. Her risk factors include recent pregnancy which changes blood flow dynamics and increases the risk of a pulmonary embolus developing.

37. **D: It crosses the midline from right to left at T5**

The thoracic duct arises between L1 and L2 as the cysterna chyli and passes through the right crus of the diaphragm. It ascends posterior to the oesophagus, crosses the midline from right to left at T5, and drains into the left brachiocephalic vein (at the confluence of the internal jugular and subclavian veins).

38. **C: The left phrenic nerve pierces the central tendon**

The diaphragm's motor innervation is obtained from the phrenic nerve (C3, 4, 5). This nerve also conveys sensation to the central portion of the diaphragm, but the lower six intercostals nerves supply sensation to the periphery. The following relate to structures passing through the diaphragm at specific vertebral levels:

- *T8*: Right phrenic nerve, inferior vena cava
- *T10*: Vagus nerve, left gastric vein/artery, oesophagus
- *T12*: Azygous vein, aorta, thoracic duct

The left phrenic nerve pieces the central tendon.

39. **B: The arterial supply to the lower third is derived from the left gastric artery**

    The arterial supply to the oesophagus is:

    Cervical portion: Inferior thyroid

    Thoracic portion: Descending aorta

    Abdominal portion: Left gastric

    The venous drainage of the oesophagus is:

    Cervical portion: Inferior thyroid

    Thoracic portion: Azygous

    Abdominal portion: Left gastric (and part of azygous)

40. **E: Duodenojejunal flexure**

    The transpyloric plane of Addison is a perpendicular plane found midway between the pubic symphysis and the jugular notch. Structures found at this level include:

    - L1 vertebral body
    - Tip of the 9th costal cartilage
    - Duodenojejunal flexure
    - Hilum of kidneys
    - Hilum of spleen
    - Origin of portal vein formed from anastomosis of splenic and superior mesenteric vein
    - Attachment of transverse mesocolon
    - Termination of spinal cord
    - Fundus of the gallbladder
    - Superior mesenteric artery branching off the aorta
    - Neck of pancreas
    - Pylorus of stomach

41. **E: The short gastric arteries are derived from the splenic artery**

    The blood supply to the stomach may be summarised as follows:

    - Coeliac plexus (T12):
        - Left gastric artery
        - Splenic artery:
            - Short gastric arteries
            - Left gastro-epiploic artery

- Hepatic artery:
  - Right gastric artery
  - Cystic artery
  - Gastroduodenal artery: superior pancreaticoduodenal artery, right gastroepiploic artery

42. B: The upper parathyroid glands are 4th branchial pouch derivatives

About 90 per cent of parathyroid glands are closely related to the thyroid, the majority lying anteriorly; approximately 10 per cent are aberrant and are invariably the lower/inferior glands. Aberrant glands may be found in the mediastinum, behind the oesophagus, and anterior to the trachea; in rare situations, parathyroid glands may be found within the thyroid (intra-thyroidal). Superior parathyroid glands are 4th branchial (pharyngeal) pouch derivatives, whereas inferior glands are 3rd pouch derivatives, developing along with the thymus. Therefore, when the thymus descends from its embryological origin, it drags the inferior parathyroid glands inferiorly with it. Hence, the propensity for inferior parathyroid glands to end up in the mediastinum together with the thymus.

43. C: Lateral and medial circumflex femoral arteries supply the femoral head via retinacula

The arterial supply from the ligamentum teres contributes more significantly in childhood. The obturator artery gives off a branch via the ligamentum teres, which provides a negligible blood supply to the femoral head in adults. Lateral and medial circumflex femoral arteries supply the femoral head via retinacula, which reflect back in longitudinal bands over the hip capsule. Vessels from the diaphysis of cancellous bone provide a significant arterial blood supply in adulthood. Fractures that are intracapsular have a high risk of resultant avascular necrosis of the femoral head, as it is separated from the trochanteric anastomosis; peritrochanteric fractures leave this anastomosis undisturbed, and thus avascular necrosis is less likely. Slipped femoral epiphysis in children may disrupt the ligamentum teres, which provides a significant arterial blood supply to the femoral head in this age group – this is seen in Perthes disease.

44. D: It is bound anteriorly by the inguinal ligament

The boundaries of the femoral canal, which is a small gap at the medial aspect of the femoral sheath, can be summarised as:

Anterior: Inguinal ligament

Posterior: Pectineal ligament

Medial: Lacunar ligament

Lateral: Femoral vein

The canal contains fat and Cloquet's lymph node; the canal has two primary functions: as a lymphatic drainage for the lower limb and a space to accommodate femoral vein distension during increased venous return, as in exercise.

45. **A: The zona glomerulosa is the most superficial layer**

The zona glomerulosa is involved in the production of mineralocorticoids and is the most superficial layer of the adrenal cortex. The zona fasciculata and reticularis (middle and deepest layers, respectively) produce glucocorticoids, oestrogens, and androgens; progestogens are produced as precursors to the synthesis of other hormones. The adrenal medulla produces adrenaline.

46. **B: HCl secretion is inhibited by secretin**

G-cells secrete gastrin and are found in the glands of the pylorus. Gastrin stimulates HCl production by parietal cells. Parietal cells, which are found in the glands on the fundus, also secrete intrinsic factor. The secretion of HCl is inhibited by secretin (produced by the duodenum), cholecystokinin (CCK), and somatostatin. Chief cells secrete pepsinogen (precursor of pepsin). Daily gastric secretion amounts to 1–1.5 L per day.

47. **E: Pus contains a mixture of dead and live neutrophils**

An abscess is a localised tissue collection of pus, surrounded by a 'pyogenic membrane', which itself is not a true membrane, rather a wall of fibrin, capillaries, neutrophils, and fibroblasts. Pus contains a mixture of dead and live neutrophils, fibrin, lipid, coagulation, and complement factors. A pre-existing pilonidal sinus gives rise to a pilonidal abscess; coliforms are the most frequently implicated organism. A psoas abscess is most frequently caused by *S. aureus*, tuberculosis, and other rare microorganisms. A sterile abscess is defined as an abscess devoid of microorganisms; this may occur following sterilisation of a septic abscess (i.e., with antibiotics), or following intramuscular injection of paraldehyde.

48. **A: In class B, there is breach of muscularis propria**

- *Class A*: 5-year survival = 90–100 per cent; disease limited to muscularis propria
- *Class B*: 5-year survival = 75 per cent; disease breaches muscularis; no lymph node involvement
- *Class C1*: 5-year survival = 30–40 per cent; lymph node involvement, but not the apical node
- *Class C2*: 5-year survival = 25 per cent; apical lymph node involvement
- *Class D*: 5-year survival = <15 per cent; distant metastases

49. **A: Breslow thickness of <0.75mm confirms 90 percent 5-year survival**

Breslow thickness gives a better indication of prognosis than Clarke's levels because the thickness of the papillary and reticular dermis varies in different bodily locations. Breslow thickness is measured vertically in millimetres from the base of the granular layer. The survival rates are:

<0.75 mm: 90 per cent 5-year survival

0.76–1.5 mm: 80 per cent 5-year survival

1.5–4 mm: 65 per cent 5-year survival

>4 mm: 35 per cent 5-year survival

Clark's level is a related staging system, used in conjunction with Breslow's depth, which describes the level of anatomical invasion in the skin:

I: Epidermal involvement only

II: Papillary dermis invasion

III: Fills papillary dermis

IV: Reticular dermis invasion

V: Subcutaneous tissue involvement

50. **C: Type I is characterised by pituitary adenoma**

Multiple endocrine neoplasia is inherited in an autosomal dominant fashion and can be classified as Type I, Type IIa, or Type IIb.

The features of Type I can be memorised by the 3 P's:

- Pancreas (adenoma/carcinoma islet cells, e.g., gastrinoma)
- Pituitary (adenoma, rarely carcinoma)
- Parathyroids (hyperplasia)

The features of Type IIa are:

- Thyroid (medullary carcinoma)
- Adrenal (phaeochromocytoma)
- Parathyroids (hyperplasia)

The features of Type IIb are:

- Thyroid (medullary carcinoma)
- Adrenal (phaeochromocytoma)
- Mucosal neuromas
- Marfanoid-type habitus

51. **E: It has been linked to the usage of the intrauterine contraceptive device**

Actinomyces israelii is the most commonly implicated pathogen. The characteristic cause is progressive and indolent; patients present with pain, fever, weight loss, and a palpable mass – as a result, actinomycosis is commonly misdiagnosed as malignancy. Tissue injury precedes development to actino-mycosis (e.g., dental procedures leading to cervical actinomycosis; aspiration leading to pulmonary actinomycosis; the intrauterine contraceptive device has been implicated in the development of genital actinomycosis). Diagnosis is based on clinical diagnosis, accompanied with fine-needle aspiration – serology is not useful. 'Sulphur granules' are seen in less than 50 per cent of cases at surgery. Although characteristic of the infection they are not pathognomonic as they may also be seen in other infections such as those caused by Nocardia.

52. **D: Woven bone**

During fracture healing, provisional callus is composed of woven bone. This is gradually replaced with lamellar bone. Woven bone is characterized by a haphazard organization of collagen fibres and is mechanically weak. Lamellar bone has a regular parallel alignment of collagen into sheets (lamellae) and is mechanically strong.

53. **D: Retromandibular vein**

There are several important structures to be aware of during parotid surgery. From superficial to deep are the following structures:

- Facial nerve (VII cranial nerve)
- Retromandibular vein – Often large and responsible for causing troublesome bleeding
- External carotid artery – Deep and rarely encountered

Also at risk is the great auricular nerve (sensory to the earlobe and angle of mandible) and the risk of Frey's syndrome (gustatory sweating caused by misdirected reinnervation to the sweat glands through injury to the parasympathetic secretomotor fibres of the auriculotemporal nerve).

54. **E: Cardiac output divided by body surface area**

The cardiac index is defined as the cardiac output (CO) relative to body surface area, thus relating heart performance to the size of the individual. The unit of measurement is litres per minute per square metre ($L/min/m^2$). CO is a function of heart rate (HR) and stroke volume (SV): CO = HR × SV. Mean arterial blood pressure (MABP) is a function of CO and total peripheral resistance (TPR): MABP = CO × TPR.

55. **B: Bladder cancer**

Beta-naphthylamine is a carcinogen that increases the risk of transitional cell carcinoma of the bladder. It was commonly used by workers in the aniline dye industry.

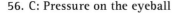

56. **C: Pressure on the eyeball**

Heart rate (HR) increases when physiological demand increases (e.g., increased blood flow to skeletal muscles during exercise, to the gut after a heavy meal). Pressure on the sinoatrial (SA) node results in activation of the Bainbridge reflex (or atrial reflex) whereby an increase in HR occurs as a result of an increase in atrial pressure. During inspiration, intrathoracic pressure decreases. This triggers increased venous return, which causes an increased HR through the Bainbridge reflex and Frank–Starling's law. Various vago-tonic manoeuvres (e.g., Valsalva manoeuvre, carotid sinus massage, pressure on eyeballs, ice-water facial immersion, swallowing of ice-cold water) result in increased parasympathetic tone through the vagus nerve, which results in a decrease in HR. Such manoeuvres may be clinically useful in terminating supraventricular arrhythmias.

57. **A: Plasma bicarbonate of 39 mmol/L**

Respiratory failure is associated with hypoxia and either a normal/low CO_2 (type 1 respiratory failure) or a raised CO_2 (type 2 respiratory failure). Type 2 respiratory failure in the setting of a raised carbon dioxide leads to a respi-ratory acidosis. When respiratory failure is chronic, rather than acute, pH compensation occurs through the kidneys.

Renal compensation occurs whereby the renal tubules act to increase the resorption of bicarbonate thereby normalizing the plasma pH (a normal bicar-bonate range is 22–30 mmol/L, so 39 mmol/L is raised). This is why patients with long-term, stable chronic obstructive pulmonary disease often have a normal pH but a raised plasma CO_2 and bicarbonate on their arterial blood gases. Renal compensation takes several days before it is fully functional (hence it is a sign of chronic respiratory failure, rather than acute).

58. **B: Glossopharyngeal nerve**

The palatine tonsils are closely related to the glossopharyngeal nerve (cranial nerve IX) which is also the same nerve that supplies the middle ear (Jacobson's nerve). Pain from the tonsils is therefore commonly misinterpreted by the body as coming from the ear when it is in fact not. Referred otalgia is common after tonsillectomy and is also commonly seen in patients presenting with tonsillar and/or base of tongue tumours.

59. **E: Pampiniform plexus**

The contents of the spermatic cord may be remembered by the 'Rule of 3's' as follows:

3 constituents: Vas deferens (round ligament uterus in females), lymphatics, obliterated processus vaginalis.

3 arteries: Testicular artery, artery to vas (a branch of the superior/inferior vesi-cal), cremasteric artery (a branch of the inferior epigastric).

3 nerves: Genital branch of the genitofemoral (motor to cremaster muscle, sensory to cord), ilioinguinal nerve (inside the inguinal canal but outside the cord), autonomics.

3 veins: Pampiniform venous plexus, vein from vas, cremasteric vein.

3 fascial coverings: Internal spermatic fascia, external spermatic fascia, cremasteric muscle and fascia.

The ilioinguinal nerve is inside the inguinal canal, but importantly lies outside the spermatic cord. The dartos muscle lies within the scrotal layers and is not to be confused with the cremaster muscle.

60. **D: Does not take into account the presence of metastases**

Dukes classification is a histological staging system (defines how far the tumour has spread). The individual stage gives valuable information for the prognosis and management of the patient. A grading system describes the degree of cellular differentiation. Stage A represents a tumour confined to the wall of the bowel, stage B when the tumour has penetrated the serosal surface and stage C when there is local lymph node involvement. Stage D was added later and represents widespread distant metastases, as this is a histological not a clinical staging system. A more detailed method is the TNM system which addresses many more details about tumour spread.

61. **B: Acute inflammation causes a rise in intraosseous pressure**

Osteomyelitis is an infection of bone caused by pyogenic bacteria. *Staphylococcus aureus* is the most common causative organism. Acute inflammation causes a rise in intramedullary pressure resulting in pain and vessel thrombosis. The classical pathological sequelae are as follows. Bone death results in the formation of a sequestrum, but healing is by new bone formation (the involucrum). A cloacae forms (holes in the involucrum through which pus formed in the medulla discharges). Finally, a tract from drainage from cloaca to the skin is apparent (sinus). Early plain radiographs are often normal, but after 7–10 days bone rarefaction, periosteal new bone and sequestra may be seen. Patients with sickle cell disease are prone to osteomyelitis caused by *Salmonella*.

62. **B: Abdominal pain, pyrexia, and tachycardia are suggestive of a leak**

Anastomoses involving the large bowel are more likely to leak than the small bowel. The small bowel has a better blood supply (perfusion), more fluid contents and lower intraluminal pressure compared to the large bowel. Surgical technique plays an important role in preventing leakage. Anastomatic leaks may be apparent in the immediate postoperative period, but it is more usual for signs and symptoms to develop at day 5/6 when bowel peristalsis commences. Abdominal pain, pyrexia, and tachycardia are all suggestive of a leak. The appearance of bowel contents through the abdominal wound is not proof of a leak. Extensive dissection may be caused by injury to an unrelated portion of bowel, which had necrosed and leaked. In general, early leaks are best treated by exterioration of the anastomatic ends or by creating a proximal defunctioning stoma. Late leaks often result in adhesions, abscesses, or fistulae. Urgent laparotomy is rarely indicated and conservative management should be adopted.

63. **D: Neuroma formation**

    Joint contractures affecting the hip joint are a contraindication to offering a patient an above-knee amputation. Sudek's atrophy is the type I form of complex regional pain syndrome and does not demonstrate nerve lesions. This is not commonly associated with amputation. Myoglobinuria is the presence of myoglobin in the urine and is associated with rhabdomyolysis or muscle destruction. Amputation neuroma is a tumour that may occur near the stump following an amputation. Amyloid is a family of unusual proteins, all characterized by beta-pleated sheets, and associated with chronic infections, chronic inflammatory diseases, and certain neoplasms.

64. **A: Begins in the region of the anatomical snuffbox**

    The cephalic vein is a superficial vein of the upper limb that arises within the anatomical snuffbox. It communicates with the basilic vein by the median cubital vein at the elbow and is located in the superficial fascia along the anterolateral surface of the biceps muscle. At the elbow, it is superficial to the lateral cutaneous nerve of the forearm. Superiorly, the cephalic vein passes between the deltoid and pectoralis major muscles (deltopectoral groove) and through the deltopectoral triangle, where it empties into the axillary vein. As it is a vein, it contains valves.

65. **B: Proximal myopathy**

    The patient is generally a young female and the condition may be familial. The thyroid is usually moderately diffusely enlarged and soft and a bruit may be heard. The patient may be hot, with moist and warm skin due to peripheral vasodilatation. Weight loss may be a feature despite increased food intake. Fine hand tremor with hyperkinesia and increased bowel mobility is also common. Cardiac enlargement and abnormal heart sounds are suggestive of Cushing's syndrome. Eye signs are usual. Menstrual irregularity and infertility are common.

66. **D: A cause of thoracic outlet syndrome**

    A cervical rib is an extra rib, which arises from the 7th cervical vertebra. It is a congenital abnormality that is located above the 1st rib. Thoracic outlet syndrome is caused by compression of the lower trunk of the brachial plexus or subclavian artery. It is associated with the formation of subclavian aneurysms. Chest radiographs with apical lordotic views and cervical spine radiographs are recommended. Onset is from the second to eighth decade with a peak in the fourth decade. It is more common in females.

67. **A: Is formed by the union of the splenic and superior mesenteric veins**

    The hepatic portal vein is the venous drainage from the gastrointestinal tract and spleen into the liver. It is formed by the confluence of the superior mesenteric and splenic veins. The anterior boundaries of the epiploic foramen of Winslow is the hepatic portal vein. The portal vein is posterior to the common hepatic artery. The hepatic portal vein originates behind the neck of the pancreas. Approximately 75 per cent of hepatic blood flow is derived from the hepatic portal vein, while the remainder is from the hepatic arteries.

68. **C: Is characterized by Reed–Sternberg cells**

    Hodgkin's disease often presents with painless enlargement of one or more lymph nodes (usually in the cervical region) and is characterized histologically by the presence of Reed–Sternberg cells. Non-Hodgkin's disease is commonly seen in the gastrointestinal tract. The Ann Arbour system divided Hodgkin's disease into four stages, according to its extent, with A or B subtypes according to absence or presence of constitutional systems. The lymphocyte-depleted type of Hodgkin's disease is associated with the worse prognosis.

69. **E: Parasympathetic fibres to the submandibular gland**

    The facial nerve is the seventh (VII) of twelve paired cranial nerves. It emerges from the brainstem between the pons and the medulla, controls the muscles of facial expression, and provides taste sensations for the anterior two-thirds of the tongue and oral cavity. It also supplies preganglionic parasympathetic fibres to many head and neck ganglia (including the submandibular and sublingual glands via the chorda tympani). The vagus nerve (X) supplies the palatoglossus muscle and the trigeminal nerve (V) supplies the medial pterygoid, masseter, and temporalis muscles.

70. **A: Lies between mylohyoid and hyoglossus muscle**

    The submandibular (Wharton's) duct is 5 cm long. First it lies between mylohyoid and hyoglossus muscles and then between the sublingual gland and geniohyoid muscle. The duct develops in the ectoderm from a groove in the floor of the mouth. It opens into the floor of the mouth adjacent to the frenulum. The facial nerve (CN VII) runs through the parotid gland.

71. **D: There is an association with Henoch–Schönlein purpura**

    Intussusception is an invagination of a portion of bowel into its own lumen. It occurs most commonly in boys aged 3–12 months. The majority of intussusceptions are ileo-colic, but ileo-ileal, ileo-ileocolic, and colo-colic have also been described. Henoch–Schönlein purpura is a systemic vasculitis characterized by deposition of immune complexes containing the antibody IgA into the skin and kidney. There is an association with intussusception.

72. **D: Is associated with autoimmune diseases**

    Sjögren's syndrome is an autoimmune disease characterized by dryness of the mouth and eyes. There is a female predominance with an average age of onset in the late forties. Amyloid comprises a family of unusual proteins, all of which have characteristic beta-pleated sheet structure, and is not directly related to Sjögren's disease. Five per cent of patients with Sjögren's disease will develop lymphoma.

73. **B: Peptic ulcer**

Parathyroid hormone (PTH) increases serum calcium levels at the expense of phosphate. In 70 per cent of cases the condition is asymptomatic. Symptomatic forms are described as 'stones' (nephrolithiasis and nephrocalcinosis), 'bones' (bone pain and arthralgia), 'groans' (peptic ulcer disease and pancreatitis), and 'psychic overtones'. Calcium may increase gastrin secretion, which in turn may lead to peptic ulcer disease. The calcium may deposit in the eye leading to cataract formation. Hoarseness due to laryngeal spasm is associated with hypoparathyroidism.

74. **C: Has a roof pierced by the external jugular vein**

The boundaries of the posterior triangle of the neck are: posterior border of sternocleidomastoid, anterior border of trapezium, and the medial third of the clavicle. The roof is formed by investing fascia, platysma, and the external jugular vein. The floor is composed of prevertebral fascia covering muscles, subclavian artery, trunks of the brachial plexus, and cervical plexus. The carotid sheath is contained in the anterior triangle of the neck.

75. **A: Develops from the 1st and 3rd branchial arches**

The tongue is a branchial arch derivative and is derived from the 1st and 3rd branchial arches. Special taste to the anterior two-thirds of the tongue is from the chorda tympani nerve (a branch of the facial nerve, VII) and special taste sensation to the posterior one-third of the tongue derives from the glossopharyngeal nerve (IX). Somatic touch to the anterior two-thirds of the tongue is by way of the lingual nerve (Va) and to the posterior one-third is by way of the glossopharyngeal nerve (IX), as is the case with special taste.

The hypoglossal nerve (XII) supplies all the intrinsic muscles of the tongue, with the exception of palatoglossus which is supplied by the pharyngeal plexus of nerves (IX, X, sympathetics). A left hypoglossal nerve palsy will result in a deviated tongue to the left on tongue protrusion (but note the question says glossopharyngeal nerve!).

The tongue receives its blood supply primarily from the lingual artery, a branch of the external carotid artery. The fibrous septum dividing the two halves of the tongue prevents any significant anastomosis of blood vessels across the midline. In contrast, a significant feature of the tongue's lymphatic drainage is that lymph from one side, especially of the posterior part, may reach nodes on both sides of the neck (in contrast to the blood supply which remains unilateral). Because the lymphatic plexus freely communicates across the midline, cancer of the tongue frequently metastasizes bilaterally.

76. **A: Is more common in patients with Plummer–Vinson syndrome**

Postcricoid tumours are more common in females. They are associated with iron deficiency anaemia and patients with Plummer–Vinson syndrome (also known as George–Paterson–Brown–Kelly syndrome) are at higher risk of developing such tumours. Such tumours require multimodal (combination) therapy (radiotherapy, chemotherapy, and surgery). If surgically operable, they can be safely resected and reconstructed with a good chance of cure with minimal morbidity.

Postcricoid tumours are highly lethal with a poor prognosis and a 5-year survival generally ranging from 15 to 20 per cent.

77. **A: Is a cause of carpal tunnel syndrome**

Colles' fracture is a distal fracture of the radius that is a known cause of carpal tunnel syndrome (compression of the median nerve in the carpal tunnel). It rarely results in ulnar nerve compression. A Colles' fracture is extra-articular by definition and does not extend into the wrist joint, otherwise this would make it an intra-articular fracture (Barton's fracture). The distal fragment in a Colles' fracture is displaced dorsally, unlike in a Smith's fracture where the distal fragment is displaced volarly (ventrally). Associated fracture of the ulnar styloid process may occur in more than 60 per cent of cases, although this does not form part of the true Colles' fracture (especially as it may not occur in all cases) and is a common associated injury.

78. **B: The left hip joint is not congenitally dislocated**

The Trendelenburg test is a favourite of examiners, so it is worth spending a moment discussing it. Put simply, the test is an assessment of insufficiency of the hip abductor system.

Ask the patient to stand on his or her good leg and flex the other leg at the knee. The opposite side of the pelvis should rise to help to balance the trunk on the leg by bringing the centre of gravity over the weight-bearing foot. This involves the use of the hip abductors – the gluteus medius and minimus. This manoeuvre is then repeated by asking the patient to stand on the bad leg. The test is positive if the opposite side of the pelvis falls and the patient has difficulty standing. You may notice that the patient throws the upper part of the body over the affected hip in order to compensate for the loss of balance due to the pelvic dip on the contralateral side (Trendelenburg lurch).

In this scenario the left gluteal abductors (and left superior gluteal nerve), but not the psoas muscle, are working.

A Trendelenburg test can be positive for two main reasons: neurological or mechanical. Neurological causes can be due to generalized motor weakness as seen with myelomeningocele and spinal cord lesions, or more specific problems, such as superior gluteal nerve dysfunction/injury (e.g., following hip surgery).

The mechanical causes include conditions that affect the abductor muscle lever arm, such as:

- Congenital dislocation of the hip
- Coxa vara
- Fractures of the femoral neck
- Dislocation or subluxation of the hip joint
- Neuromuscular diseases (e.g., poliomyelitis)
- Pain arising in the hip joint, inhibiting the gluteal muscles

These conditions shorten the length of the muscle from its origin to its insertion, and significantly reduce its strength.

It should be noted that the test is not valid in children below the age of 4 years, and that it has a 10 per cent false-positive rate due to pain, generalized weakness, poor cooperation, or bad balance.

79. **A: Has maximum velocity in the centre**

In a vessel, laminar flow is governed by Poiseuille's law. Flow is maximal in the centre of a tube, with the highest concentration of cells in the centre. For flow in a pipe, laminar (smooth) flow occurs when the Reynold's number is less than 2300 and turbulent (rough) flow occurs when it is greater than 4000. Turbulent flow is a fluid regime characterized by chaotic, stochastic property changes. This includes low-momentum diffusion, high-momentum convection, and rapid variation of pressure and velocity in space and time.

80. **E: Have small orifices and characteristically close spontaneously before the age of 5 years**

Congenital umbilical hernia is a congenital malformation, common in infants of African descent. Among adults, it is three times more common in women than in men; among children, the gender ratio is roughly equal. Umbilical hernias in children are common with an incidence of 1 in 10. Obstruction and strangulation of the underlying hernia is rare because the underlying defect in the abdominal wall is larger compared to inguinal hernia of the newborn. The size of the base of the herniated tissue is inversely correlated with risk of strangulation (i.e., narrow base is more likely to strangulate). A persistence of a patent vitelline duct permits an intermittent discharge of enteric contents from the umbilicus. It is a very rare abnormality and may be associated with umbilical polyps. When the hernia's orifice is small (<2 cm), 90 per cent close by 5 years.

81. **E: Fluids and mannitol**

Haemolytic transfusion reactions lead to hypotension and oliguria. The increased haemoglobin in the plasma will be cleared via the kidney, which leads to haemoglobinuria. Inserting a urinary catheter with subsequent demonstration of oliguria and haemoglobinuria not only confirms the diagnosis, but is also useful in monitoring therapy. Treatment commences with discontinuation of the transfusion, followed by aggressive fluid resuscitation to support the hypotensive episode and increased urine output. Inducing diuresis through fluid resuscitation and osmotic diuretics is an important step to eliminate the haemolysed red cell membranes and help prevent renal failure. Alkalinisation of the urine (pH >7) helps prevent haemoglobin aggregation and renal failure. Steroids have a limited role in this context.

82. **E: Burst abdomen is preceded by serosanguinous discharge**

Cutting through muscle produces more postoperative pain than muscle splitting incisions where the anatomical planes between muscle fibres are used. There is no evidence that closing the peritoneum reduces the development of adhesions. The release of collagenase near wound edges weakens the skin and there-fore sutures should be placed 1 cm away. The tip of the first trocar cannot be visualized before the camera is inserted unless a small laparotomy incision is made. The 'pink sign' indicates impending wound disruption.

83. **E: Responds to treatment with vancomycin**

Pseudomembranous colitis, also known as antibiotic-associated diarrhoea (AAD), is an infection of the colon. The main causative agent is *Clostridium difficile*. Patients present with diarrhoea, fever, abdominal pain, and rec-tal bleeding. In severe cases, life-threatening complications can develop, including toxic megacolon. A major risk factor for this condition includes recent antibiotic usage. Clindamycin is the antibiotic classically implicated as the causative agent, but any antibiotic can cause the condition. Due to frequent administration, cephalosporin antibiotics (cefazolin and cephalexin) account for a large percentage of cases. Medical treatment of this condition includes metronidazole or vancomycin.

84. **A: Ultrasound**

There are no blood tests that are specific and sensitive to establish the diag-nosis of acute cholecystitis. (Raised alkaline phosphatase, bilirubin, WBC, and CRP are only suggestive of the underlying diagnosis.) However, ultrasound, CT scan, and hepatobiliary scintigraphy with technetium-99m DISIDA (bilirubin) analogue are all sensitive and specific modalities for the diagnosis of acute cholecystitis. Plain radiographs are not beneficial.

85. **A: Albumin of 30 g/L**

The modified Glasgow scoring system is an indicator of prognostic severity (Table 11). One point is scored for each criterion met on admission and again at 48 hours after admission (1–2 points is associated with a mortality of <1 per cent, 3–4 points with 15 per cent, and 6 points with a mortality approaching 100 per cent).

Table 11 Modified Glasgow scoring

Po_2	<8 kPA (60 mmHg)
Age	>55 years
Neutrophils/WCC	>15 × 10⁹/L
Ca (corrected)	<2 mmol/L
Raised urea	>16 mmol/L
Enzymes (LDH)	>600 IU/L
Albumin	<32 g/L
Sugar (glucose)	>10 mmol/L

86. **D: Is anteriorly bounded by to the seminal vesicles and prostate**

The blood supply of the rectum is supplied by the superior rectal artery (first two-thirds of rectum) and the middle rectal artery (last third of rectum). The venous drainage is the superior and middle rectal veins. The nerve supply comprises the inferior anal nerves and inferior mesenteric ganglia. The lymphatic drainage comprises the inferior mesenteric, pararectal, and internal iliac lymph nodes. In males, the anterior border of the rectum comprises the rectovesical pouch, small bowel, Denonvillier's fascia, bladder, vas, seminal vesicles, and prostate.

87. **C: Generates immunoglobulin-producing plasma cells**

The germinal centres of lymph nodes contain mainly B-lymphocytes and follicular dendritic cells. Follicular dendritic cells are able to trap antigen on their cell surface for long periods. They help to initiate a B-cell response to antigens entering the lymph node and play an important role in affinity maturation (a process which results in an increase in the affinity of the antibodies produced during the course of a humoral immune response). Follicular dendritic cells should not be confused with Langerhans' dendritic cells which are professional antigen-presenting cells found in the skin.

The cords and sinuses of a lymph node are situated in the medulla. The medullary cords are rich in plasma cells, whereas the sinuses are rich in macrophages. The paracortical zone (or interfollicular area) is rich in T-lymphocytes.

There is characteristically an expansion of the paracortex, rather than the germinal centres, in infectious mononucleosis (and many other viral infections), so-called reactive hyperplasia. This manifests clinically as lymphadenopathy.

88. **D: Mitochondria**

Mitochondria are found in all eukaryotic cells. They contain their own DNA and are thought to be symbiotic prokaryotes that have been assimilated into eukaryotic cells in our biological past (endosymbiotic theory). They replicate by mitosis to form a clonal population. All the mitochondrial DNA in humans is derived from the clonal population of the ovum and therefore are maternally inherited.

89. **B: Gliclazide**

Sulphonylureas (gliclazide and glibenclamide) are indicated when diet fails to control hyperglycaemia. Sulphonylureas stimulate insulin release from the pancreas and are therefore of use only in patients who still have residual pancreatic islet cell function. Side effects include weight gain and hypoglycaemia.

Metformin increases the sensitivity to insulin at the receptor level, but should be avoided in patients with impaired renal function. Side effects include lactic acidosis, nausea, vomiting, and diarrhoea.

Rosiglitazone is an example of a thiazolidinedione. This class of drugs act by increasing the sensitivity of insulin by binding to a nuclear receptor called PPAR-γ. It is not a first-line treatment and should be used in combination with metformin or a sulphonylurea. Rosiglitazone is currently contraindicated in heart failure as it is thought to worsen this condition.

Acarbose acts by delaying the digestion and absorption of starch and sucrose, through the inhibition of intestinal alpha-glucosidases. Its main side effect is flatulence.

90. **B: The transcription factor WT-1 is necessary for the competence of the mesenchyme to be induced**

The kidney develops from the intermediate column of mesoderm. There are 3 phases of kidney development, the definitive kidney developing in the last phase:

Stage 1: Pronephros – Primitive tubules

Stage 2: Mesonephros – Functional in the embryo, producing a dilute urine important in maintaining the composition of the amniotic fluid. They also contribute to the male genital system

Stage 3: Metanephros – True, hind kidneys

The definitive metanephroi are induced early in the fifth week by the ureteric buds that sprout from the mesonephric ducts. The ureteric bud induces the mesenchymal cells to condense around it, forming the metanephric blastema. The development of the ureteric bud and the metanephric blastema depends on reciprocal induction, neither being able to develop in the absence of the other. The metanephric blastema causes the ureteric bud to grow and bifurcate and the ureteric bud induces the mesenchyme to differentiate into nephrons. If the ureteric bud does not reach/signal properly to the surrounding mesenchyme, or vice versa, a kidney will not form (renal agenesis). If the ureteric bud bifurcates prematurely, a bifid ureter may result. Alternatively, if two ureteric buds develop an ectopic ureter may result.

The ureteric bud branches and gives rise to the collecting ducts and ureters; the metanephric blastema gives rise to the tubules, or nephrons.

The transcription factor and tumour suppressor gene, WT-1, is expressed in metanephric blastema, making it competent to receive signals from the ureteric bud that are essential for its induction. Mutations in the gene are associated with a cancer of the kidney in children known as Wilm's tumour.

The kidneys ascend from their original sacral location to a lumbar site. The mechanism responsible is not understood, but the differential growth of the lumbar and sacral regions of the embryo may play a role. Several anomalies can arise from variations in this process of ascent. A kidney may fail to ascend, remaining as a pelvic kidney. The inferior poles of the two metanephroi may fuse during ascent, forming a U-shaped horseshoe kidney. During ascent this kidney comes caught under the inferior mesenteric artery and therefore does not reach its normal site.

91. E: It turns over approximately 4–5 times daily

Cerebrospinal fluid (CSF), situated within the ventricles and the subarachnoid space, bathes the surface of the brain and spinal cord, supplies nutrients to it, protects it, and reduces its effective buoyancy. It also plays an important homeostatic role and is crucial for maintaining a constant external environment for neurones and glia. In humans, the volume is about 150 mL and its rate of production is 0.5 mL/min (or approximately 30 mL/hour or 600 mL/day). Thus, the CSF turns over about four times daily.

Most of the CSF is produced by the choroid plexus, which is situated in the lateral, third, and fourth ventricles. It flows between the lateral ventricles and third ventricle via the interventricular foramen (of Monro). The third and fourth ventricles communicate via the cerebral aqueduct (or aqueduct of Sylvius). The fourth ventricle communicates with the spinal cord by way of the single median foramen of Magendie and the two laterally placed foramina of Luschka. CSF is absorbed directly into the cerebral venous sinuses through the arachnoid villi, or granulations, by a process known as 'mass or bulk flow'.

Occasionally, the earlier physiology is disrupted and it becomes the centre of a pathological process. Hydrocephalus is an increase in the volume of CSF within the cerebral ventricles. It may arise from the oversecretion of CSF, impaired absorption of CSF, or obstruction of CSF pathways.

92. D: Diversity is partly achieved through somatic hypermutation

Antibodies (immunoglobulins) are a heterogeneous group of proteins produced by plasma cells and B-lymphocytes that react with antigens. All have a similar structure with two heavy chains and two light chains. In addition, antibodies are made up of variable and constant regions. The antigen binding region is located in the variable region, whereas the complement fixing and antibody receptor binding activity is found in the constant region. The structure of the heavy-chain constant region determines the class of the antibody (i.e., IgG, IgM, IgA, IgE, etc.). Although mast cells do not produce antibodies, they contain immunoglobulin receptors on their cell surfaces. As a result mast cells are able to bind pre-formed IgE on their cell surface which plays an important role in allergy and anaphylaxis (Type I hypersensitivity reaction).

Any individual has about 10^{10} different antibodies. This astonishing degree of diversity arises through 4 main processes:

- Pairing of different combinations of heavy and light chains
- Recombination of V, D, and J segments (VJ for light chains)
- Variability in the joins of the recombined segments through imprecise joining by recombinatorial machinery and by the addition of extra random nucleotides by terminal deoxynucleotide transferase
- Somatic hypermutation – A poorly understood mechanism for introducing mutations into V regions of activated B-cells (antigen driven)

A malignant tumour of plasma cells may result in the overproduction of a monoclonal population of immunoglobulins. This is known as multiple myeloma.

93. **B: Microcytic anaemia**

Iron-deficiency anaemia is the most common cause of hypochromic, microcytic anaemia. Iron-deficiency anaemia occurs when the dietary intake or absorption of iron is insufficient and haemoglobin, which contains iron, cannot be formed. The principal cause of iron-deficiency anaemia in pre-menopausal women is blood lost during menses. Iron-deficiency anaemia is characterized by pallor, fatigue, and weakness. Because it tends to develop slowly, adaptation occurs and the disease often goes unrecognized for some time. Hair loss and light-headedness can also be associated with iron-deficiency anaemia.

The blood smear of a patient with iron-deficiency shows many hypochromatic and rather small RBCs, and may also show poikilocytosis (variation in shape) and anisocytosis (variation in size). With more severe iron-deficiency anaemia the peripheral blood smear may show target cells, hypochromic pencil-shaped cells, and occasionally small numbers of nucleated RBCs (reticulocytes). The diagnosis of iron-deficiency anaemia will be suggested by appropriate history (e.g., anaemia in a menstruating woman) and by diagnostic tests such as a low serum ferritin, a low serum iron level, an elevated serum transferrin, and a high total iron-binding capacity (TIBC). Serum ferritin is the most sensitive laboratory test for iron-deficiency anaemia.

If the cause is dietary iron deficiency, then iron supplements, usually with ferrous sulphate or ferrous gluconate, will usually correct the anaemia.

94. **C: The left pleuroperitoneal canal is larger and closes later compared with the right**

    The diaphragm is a composite musculotendinous structure formed in the embryo by the fusion of 4 separate elements:

    - Septum transversum (giving rise to the non-muscular central tendon)
    - Pleuroperitoneal membranes – Closes the primitive communication between the pleural and peritoneal cavities (forms the bulk of the diaphragmatic muscle)
    - A peripheral rim derived from the body wall (paraxial mesoderm)
    - Dorsal oesophageal mesenchyme (forms the left and right crura)

    The septum transversum develops within the cervical region. This explains how the diaphragm derives its innervation from the phrenic nerve ('C3, C4, C5, keeps the diaphragm alive!'). Caudal translocation of the septum transversum is accompanied by elongation of the phrenic nerves and explains the long course of the phrenic nerves (from the cervical roots) through the thoracic cavity.

    In a congenital diaphragmatic hernia, one of the pleuroperitoneal canals (which forms a communication between the pleural and peritoneal cavities, respectively) fails to close off through failure of pleuroperitoneal membrane development. This allows the developing abdominal viscera to bulge into the pleural cavity. If the mass of displaced viscera is large enough, it will stunt the growth of lung on that side, resulting in pulmonary hypoplasia and respiratory insufficiency, which may be fatal. The left side is involved four to eight times more often than the right, primarily because the left pleuroperitoneal canal is larger and closes later than the right, but also because of the liver on the right side.

95. **C: The protein content of cerebrospinal fluid is 0.5 per cent that of plasma**

    The constituents of the CSF are regulated by an active process that takes place within the choroid plexus. Thus the composition of CSF is different from that of plasma. Of importance to mention are the concentrations of K^+, Ca^{2+}, bicarbonate, and protein that are lower in CSF than in plasma. This is to prevent high concentrations of these electrolytes inadvertently exciting neurones present within the brain substance. The potassium content of the CSF in this respect is particularly important. Further buffering of the K^+ content of CSF take place through astrocytes.

    Likewise, the low protein content of the CSF (the CSF protein content is 0.5 per cent that of plasma) is deliberate to prevent some proteins and amino acids acting as 'false neurotransmitters'. The CSF is more acidic than plasma because pH of the CSF plays a critical role in the regulation of pulmonary ventilation and cerebral blood flow. Another reason why the CSF protein is kept deliberately low is to prevent proteins buffering pH. The result is that the pH of the CSF accurately reflects carbon dioxide levels of the blood. In this way changes in pH act as a powerful regulator of the respiratory system (through the action of pH on central chemoreceptors) and on cerebral blood flow.

96. **C: They can activate complement**

    IgM antibodies are usually pentameric, whereas IgG is monomeric and IgA is usually found as a dimer linked by a J-chain. IgM antibodies are characteristic of a primary immune response; IgG antibodies predominate in a secondary immune response. IgM is an effective activator of complement when it has bound specific antigen. IgA, rather than IgM, is found lining mucosal surfaces and is secreted into breast milk; IgA is therefore known as secretory immunoglobulin.

    IgM cannot cross the placenta, whereas IgG can. The consequences of this are three-fold. First, if IgM antibodies directed against infectious organisms are found in the foetal blood, they are an indicator of intra-uterine infection. Second, antibodies to ordinary ABO blood groups (anti-A and anti-B) are usually of the IgM type and hence do not cross the placenta. Third, because IgG can cross the placenta, whereas IgM cannot, it explains why rhesus haemolytic disease of the newborn is uncommon with the first pregnancy (the initial exposure to rhesus antigen evokes the formation of IgM antibodies). Subsequent exposure during a second or third pregnancy generally leads to a brisk IgG antibody response.

97. **B: Erythromycin**

    Penicillins and cephalosporins (which includes cefuroxime, cefotaxime, ceftriaxone) inhibit bacterial cell wall synthesis through the inhibition of peptidoglycan cross-linking. This weakens the cell wall of bacteria and renders them susceptible to osmotic shock. Macrolides (such as erythromycin), tetracyclines, aminoglycosides, and chloramphenicol act by interfering with bacterial protein synthesis. Sulphonamides (e.g., trimethoprim, co-trimoxazole) work by inhibiting the synthesis of nucleic acid (Table 12).

Table 12 Antibotics and their mechanism of action

Mechanism of action	Examples
Inhibition of cell wall synthesis	Penicillins, cephalosporins, vancomycin
Inhibition of protein synthesis	Macrolides, tetracyclines, aminoglycosides, chloramphenicol, clindamycin
Inhibition of nucleic acid synthesis	Sulphonamides, trimethoprim, quinolones, metronidazole, rifampicin
Inhibition of cell membrane synthesis	Lincomycins, polymyxins

98. **B: Increasing membrane capacitance**

The speed of nerve conduction increases with:

- Increasing axonal diameter which decreases axonal resistance
- Myelination (insulation of axons) by Schwann cells in the peripheral nervous system, or oligodendrocytes in the central nervous system
- Increasing temperature
- Decreasing membrane capacitance

Capacitance slows down passive conduction because some of the current has to be used to charge or discharge the capacitance before it can spread further.

The effect of temperature on axonal velocity is easily understood by remembering what happens to one's hands when playing in the snow on a cold day. Most will be able to recall that hands go numb, but retain the ability to feel pain. The reason is straightforward and is based on axonal velocity. Light touch is carried by myelinated, Aβ nerve fibres. As the temperature decreases, the velocity of impulse propagation decreases until a point comes at which the amplitude of impulse is insufficient to regenerate the action potential at the next node of Ranvier. Cooling has the further effect of slowing sodium conductance at the nodes of Ranvier. Saltatory conduction is therefore disrupted; the result being that the hands are numb. Pain, on the other hand, is carried by unmyelinated C fibres. The generation of action potentials is not therefore restricted to the nodes of Ranvier and pain sensation is preserved until far lower temperatures are reached.

The myelin sheath increases velocity by three mechanisms: first, by insulating the axon; second, by decreasing membrane capacitance; and third, by restricting the generation of axon potentials to the nodes of Ranvier. The importance of myelination in increasing the speed of nerve conduction is illustrated by certain disease states where the myelin sheath is absent or lacking. One example is the condition multiple sclerosis which is a chronic, inflammatory, demyelinating condition resulting in multifocal lesions within the white matter of the central nervous system. The equivalent disease process within the peripheral nervous system is known as Guillain–Barré syndrome. Both result in neurological deficits, such as motor weakness and sensory loss as a result of the decreased velocity of impulse propagation down nerve fibres.

99. **B: Is composed of six human leukocyte antigen (HLA) genes**

The human MHC is situated on chromosome 6. There are 6 pairs of allelic genes (A, B, C, DP, DQ, DR). The human MHC will be identical only in monozygotic (identical) twins. There are two classes of MHC antigens: class I antigens are expressed on the surface of all nucleated cells; class II are expressed only on the surfaces of cells such as antigen-presenting cells.

100. **A: It commonly exhibits an autosomal dominant pattern of inheritance**

Von Willebrand disease is the most common hereditary bleeding disorder. It is caused by an abnormality, either quantitative or qualitative, of the von Willebrand factor, which is a large multimeric glycoprotein that functions as the carrier protein for factor VIII. Von Willebrand factor is also required for normal platelet adhesion. Von Willebrand disease can be classified into 3 main types:

- Type 1 accounts for 70–80 per cent of cases. It is characterized by a partial quantitative decrease of qualitatively normal von Willebrand factor and factor VIII. An individual with type 1 disease generally has mild clinical symptoms, and this type is usually inherited as an autosomal dominant trait; however, penetrance may widely vary in a single family.
- Type 2 accounts for 15–20 per cent of cases. It is a variant with primarily qualitative defects of von Willebrand factor. It can be either autosomal dominant or autosomal recessive.
- Type 3 is the most severe form. In the homozygous patient, it is characterized by marked deficiencies of both von Willebrand factor and factor VIII in the plasma, and the absence of von Willebrand factor from both platelets and endothelial cells. It is characterized by severe clinical bleeding and is inherited as an autosomal recessive trait.

Investigations commonly reveal a normal platelet count and prothrombin time, with a prolonged activated partial thromboplastin time (APTT) and bleeding time.

101. **E: Midgut development involves herniation of bowel into the umbilicus**

The gut is an endodermal derivative created from a midline gut tube through a complex series of rotations. The gut is divided into 3 distinct territories:

- Foregut = mouth up to second part of duodenum
- Midgut = second part of duodenum up to two-thirds along the transverse colon
- Hindgut = two-thirds along the transverse colon up to the anus

This distinction is important developmentally, anatomically, and clinically.

One consequence of the midline development of the gut is that visceral pain arising from the intestine often refers to the midline in the adult. Thus, foregut pain typically refers to the epigastric region, midgut pain to the peri-umbilical region, and hindgut pain to the suprapubic region.

The cranial end of the embryological gut tube is capped by the buccopharyngeal membrane and the caudal end by the cloacal membrane. Both later rupture, forming the orifices of the body (i.e., the mouth and anus, respectively).

The stomach forms the thoracic part of the foregut. The dorsal wall of the stomach grows faster than the ventral wall, resulting in a dorsal 'greater curvature' and a ventral 'lesser curvature'. Subsequently, the stomach rotates 90 degrees about the craniocaudal axis. As a result, the greater curvature lies to the left. This has the consequence that the two vagus nerves that initially flanked the stomach on the left and right now lie posterior and anterior in the region of the stomach (remembered by the mnemonic RIP, or Right Is Posterior). An additional tilting caudally orients the greater curvature so that it lies inferiorly.

Excessive growth of the midgut results in its herniation into the umbilicus, forming the primary intestinal loop. This loop undergoes a 90-degree rotation counterclockwise. Subsequently, the midgut is rapidly retracted into the abdomen. As it does so, it rotates counterclockwise a further 180 degrees. Finally, the caecum moves inferiorly to give the definitive organization of the intestine. If the anterior abdominal wall does not close completely, loops of midgut may remain outside the abdominal cavity at birth, forming a condition known as omphalocele, or gastroschisis. Abnormal rotation of gut can cause a spectrum of anomalies; for example, there may be freely (malrotated) suspended coils of intestine that are prone to volvulus, causing constriction of its blood supply.

102. **E: They contain intracellular stores of calcium ions**

A single motor neurone supplies a group of muscle fibres in what is known as a motor unit. The more precise the movement, the fewer the muscle fibres supplied by one motor neurone. However, each muscle fibre is innervated by only one motor neurone.

Mammalian skeletal muscle is optimally organized for rapid excitation of muscle contraction in a process known as 'excitation–contraction coupling'. Calcium is released from the intracellular stores (sarcotubular system) when skeletal muscle contracts. Calcium reuptake occurs through an active mechanism requiring a calcium pump. During contraction, the actin and myosin filaments do not shorten but slide together over one another (sliding filament theory).

Decreasing extracellular calcium increases excitability and may lead to spontaneous contractions (tetany), possibly by increasing sodium permeability. In hypocalcaemia this may manifest clinically as Chvostek's sign (activation of the facial nerve and muscles by merely tapping the skin) or Trousseau's sign (carpopedal spasm producing the '*main d'accoucheur*'). Fatal spasm of the larynx and seizures may later ensue if calcium levels are not corrected. Hyperventilation (overbreathing) may cause a similar effect through the respiratory alkalosis that it generates. Amino acids buffer the change in pH by losing protons to the plasma and in doing so become negatively charged. This negative charge binds free calcium in the plasma, resulting in hypocalcaemia.

103. **D: Class II MHC presents exogenous antigens**

Two principal classes of MHC exist; both play as important role in antigen presentation and recognition by T-cells. Class I MHC molecules are made up of one heavy chain and a light chain called β_2-microglobulin. Class II molecules do not contain β_2-microglobulin and consist of two chains of similar size.

Almost all nucleated cells of the body express MHC class I molecules on their cell surfaces. Hepatocytes express relatively low levels of class I MHC. This may explain why infection by certain hepatitis viruses (namely hepatitis B and C) or Plasmodium protozoa (the cause of malaria) commonly leads to a chronic carrier state in the host. Non-nucleated cells such as erythrocytes express little or no class I MHC; infection in the interior of red cells (such as malaria) can therefore go undetected. Class II MHC molecules are constitutively expressed only by certain cells involved in immune responses, though they can be induced in a variety of cells. Class II MHC molecules are richly expressed on the surface of dendritic cells.

The two classes of MHC are specialized to present different sources of antigen. MHC class I molecules present endogenously synthesized antigens (e.g., viral proteins). MHC class II molecules present exogenously derived proteins (e.g., extracellular microbes) that are first internalized and processed in the endosomes or lysosomes. Class I MHC molecules present peptides generated in the cytosol to CD8 T-cells, whereas MHC class II molecules present peptides degraded in intracellular vesicles to CD4 T-cells.

104. **E: Neutrophil**

The predominant cell type seen in acute inflammation is neutrophils. These generally infiltrate the area over 24 hours, and after 24–48 hours they are replaced by macrophages.

105. **C: Affects males and females equally**

Autosomal dominant disorders affect males and females equally since there is no involvement of the sex chromosomes and autosomes are similar for males and females. Only one of the parents needs to carry the abnormality for it to be classified as an autosomal dominant disorder; if both parents were required to carry the abnormality it would be an autosomal recessive disorder.

Only half the children of an affected adult would inherit the condition since half would receive the normal autosome. Carriers of an autosomal dominant trait do not exist; carriers of a dominant character exhibit the disease.

Autosomal dominant conditions are commonly transmitted from one generation to the next, either because of their late onset (e.g., Huntington's disease) or because reproduction occurs before death ensues.

106. **D: Inflammation may cause referred pain to the ear**

The palatine tonsils ('tonsils') are a large collection of lymphoid tissue that project into the oropharynx from the tonsillar fossa, between the palatoglossal arch (in front) and the palatopharyngeal arch (behind). They are most prominent in early life and regress in later years as the lymphoid tissue atrophies. The surface marking is medial to the lower masseter. The palatine, lingual, pharyngeal ('adenoids'), and tubal tonsils collectively form an interrupted circle of protective lymphoid tissue at the upper end of the respiratory and alimentary tracts known as Waldeyer's ring. This area has a role in the priming of lymphocytes for antigens during the early years of life.

The floor of the tonsillar fossa (lateral wall) is the lower part of the superior constrictor, with styloglossus on its lateral side. The luminal surface of the tonsil is covered by non-keratinized stratified squamous epithelium which deeply invaginates the tonsil forming blind-ended tonsillar crypts. The tonsillar branch of the facial artery (in turn a branch of the external carotid artery) forms the main arterial supply. It enters the tonsil by piercing the superior constrictor.

The main function of the tonsils is immunological, especially within the early years of life. Since they harbour microbes, this makes them vulnerable to infection and inflammation (tonsillitis). Lymphatic channels pierce the superior constrictor to reach the deep cervical nodes, especially the jugulodigastric (or tonsillar) node below the angle of the mandible. This is the lymph node that is most commonly enlarged in tonsillitis (jugulodigastric lymphadenopathy). The mucous membrane overlying the tonsil is supplied mainly by the tonsillar branch of the glossopharyngeal nerve. The glossopharyngeal nerve also supplies the middle ear through its tympanic branch. This explains why tonsillitis commonly causes referred pain to the middle ear. Ear pain may also feature in the early postoperative period after tonsillectomy.

Tonsillectomy (removal of the tonsils) is indicated for recurrent episodes of tonsillitis or obstructive sleep apnoea. Removal does not appear to compromise immune function. The main complication after tonsillectomy is haemorrhage and the usual cause is venous, rather than arterial bleeding, from the external palatine, or paratonsillar, vein. The close proximity of the internal carotid artery (which lies 2.5 cm posterolateral) to the palatine tonsil must be borne in mind at tonsillectomy in order to prevent inadvertent injury.

107. **B: Local metabolic activity is the chief factor determining rate of blood flow to the heart**

Given that there is a high myocardial oxygen demand at rest (around 20 times that of skeletal muscle), certain functional adaptations ensure that supply adequately meets demand.

- The heart receives 4–5 per cent of the cardiac output (CO)
- There is a high capillary density
- There is a high oxygen extraction ratio. The myocardium extracts around 70 per cent of the oxygen that is delivered to it from the coronary blood. In contrast, the body average is only 25 per cent
- There is efficient metabolic hyperaemia, where local metabolism is the dominant controller of coronary flow. The extra oxygen required at high work rates is supplied chiefly by an increase in blood flow rather than an increase in the oxygen extraction ratio

Unlike other vascular beds, the coronary flow to the left ventricle is greatest in diastole. This occurs because of the mechanical compression of the coronary vessels during systole, such that there is reversal of the transmural pressure gradient across the vessel wall, leading to momentary occlusion. Coronary perfusion is reduced in aortic stenosis (narrowing) because the coronary ostia lie distal to the aortic valve. This is why patients with aortic stenosis get angina.

In hypothermia there is a fall in metabolic rate and CO. This reduces cardiac work, resulting in a decrease in the rate of production of vasodilator metabolites (adenosine, carbon dioxide, etc.). The reduction in coronary artery perfusion pressure explains why angina is commonly triggered by exposure to the cold.

108. **B: Gram-positive bacteria retain an iodine purple dye complex**

Microorganisms can be classified into bacteria, viruses, fungi, protozoa, and parasites. Bacteria can be classified according to their:

- *Staining properties*: Gram-positive, Gram-negative, acid-fast, etc.
- *Morphology*: Round (cocci), rods (bacilli), spiral (spirochaetes), comma-shaped (vibrio), flagellated, possession of a capsule, etc.
- *Oxygen requirements*: Aerobic or anaerobic; obligate or facultative.
- *Ability to form spores*: Spore-forming or non-spore forming.

In Gram-positive bacteria, the peptidoglycan forms a thick (20–80 nm) layer external to the cell membrane. In Gram-negative species the peptidoglycan layer is thinner (only 5–10 nm) but is overlaid by an outer membrane. The principal molecules in the outer membrane of Gram-negative bacteria are lipopolysaccharides (LPSs).

These structural differences form the basis of the Gram stain. Gram-positive bacteria are able to retain an iodine purple dye complex when exposed to a brief alcohol wash. Gram-negative bacteria have a smaller cell wall but a higher lipid content and as a result the alcohol washes away the purple dye. Gram-positive bacteria appear blue and Gram-negative bacteria are counterstained with a pink dye.

As a general rule:

- All cocci are Gram-positive (except *Neisseria* which causes meningitis and gonorrhoea).
- All bacilli are Gram-negative (except *Clostridia,* Mycobacteria, and the organisms that cause anthrax, listeria, diphtheria, and actinomycosis).

The LPS in the outer membrane of Gram-negative bacteria is a complex molecule found nowhere else in nature and is an important factor in bacterial survival in the mammalian host. It consists of 3 portions:

- A lipid portion (lipid A) embedded in the outer membrane (the damaging endotoxin). As it is embedded in the outer membrane it exerts its effects only when bacteria lyse.
- A conserved core polysaccharide.
- The highly variable O-polysaccharide (O-antigen), responsible for antigenic diversity. It has been hypothesized that such structural variability is an attempt by the bacterium to evade host defences.

Endotoxins are not in themselves toxic (unlike exotoxins) but they can induce toxic effects due to their potent activation of the complement cascade, coagulation cascade, and stimulating the release of powerful cytokines (such as TNFα, IL-1, etc.) from leucocytes. In overwhelming infections, the patient is said to suffer from endotoxic shock.

109. C: Inferior mesenteric artery

The artery to the hindgut and its derivatives is the inferior mesenteric artery. The coeliac artery supplies structures derived from the caudal foregut. In the fetus, the ductus arteriosus shunts blood from the pulmonary trunk to the aorta to bypass the lungs. The superior mesenteric artery supplies the structures derived from the midgut. In the fetus, the umbilical artery delivers blood to the placental circulation.

110. A: Purkinje fibres lead to contraction of the apex before the base of the heart

The group of cells that show the highest automaticity (that is, the cells with which the resting membrane potential drifts towards the threshold fastest) dictates the overall heart rate (HR) and is accordingly called the primary intrinsic pacemaker of the heart. These are normally the pacemaker cells from the SA node which discharge at about 60–80 times/min. The SA node is found in the right atrium near its junction with the superior vena cava. The SA node receives a rich innervation from both arms of the autonomic nervous system (sympathetic and parasympathetic). By this means they can exert a powerful extrinsic influence on the heart.

Atrial fibres conduct impulses from the SA node to the atrioventricular (AV) node. The AV node provides the only communication in the normal heart between the atria and ventricles. Conduction through this node is slower than the remaining myocardium; this synchronizes the sequential atrial and ventricular contraction. Purkinje fibres are confined to the ventricles.

Impulse generation is due to spontaneous diastolic depolarization of the cells. The SA node has intrinsic rhythmicity and can generate impulses independently, even when completely denervated.

Purkinje fibres are larger than ventricular myocardial cells and this facilitates the rapid spread of depolarization over the entire ventricular myocardium. Purkinje fibres travel to the apex before proceeding to the base of the heart.

This arrangement enables the activation wave to spread from the apex to the base of the ventricles. The resulting pattern of activation leads to a ventricular contraction from apex to base which optimizes the extrusion of blood from the chambers.

Problems with cardiac conduction are commonly encountered in clinical practice. Arrhythmias are the most common cause of death following a myocardial infarction. In the event that the SA node function is abnormal, as in sick sinus syndrome, or following myocardial ischaemia, other sites with a slower intrinsic rate can substitute the role of the pacemaker, resulting in an escape rhythm.

111. D: *Neisseria meningitidis*

The spleen plays an important role in the removal of dead and dying erythrocytes and in the defence against microbes. Removal of the spleen (splenectomy) leaves the host susceptible to a wide array of pathogens but especially to encapsulated organisms.

Certain bacteria have evolved ways of evading the human immune system. One way is through the production of a 'slimy' capsule on the outside of the bacterial cell wall. Such a capsule resists phagocytosis and ingestion by macrophages and neutrophils. This allows them not only to escape direct destruction by phagocytes but also to avoid stimulating T-cell responses through the presentation of bacterial peptides by macrophages. The only way that such organisms can be defeated is by making them more palatable by coating their capsular polysaccharide surfaces in opsonizing antibody.

The production of antibody against capsular polysaccharide primarily occurs through T-cell independent mechanisms. The spleen plays a central role in both the initiation of the antibody response and the phagocytosis of opsonized encapsulated bacteria from the bloodstream. This helps to explain why following a splenectomy the host is most susceptible to infection by encapsulated organisms, notably *Streptococcus pneumoniae* (Pneumococcus), *Neisseria meningitidis* (Meningococcus), and *Haemophilus influenzae*.

Understanding the earlier, one can quickly envisage what preventative strategies must be employed post-splenectomy. Patients are given relevant vaccinations and are advised to take prophylactic penicillin, in most cases for the rest of their lives. In addition, they are advised to wear a Medic Alert bracelet to warn other healthcare professionals of their condition.

112. C: Right hepatic artery

The cystic artery most commonly arises from the right hepatic artery. In decreasing order of occurrence, it can also arise from the left hepatic artery, gastro-duodenal artery, or hepatic artery proper. The superior pancreatico-duodenal artery is located too inferiorly to contribute to the blood supply to the gallbladder.

113. C: Fifty per cent

The key to this question is to understand that, in order to have a child with an autosomal recessive disease, both parents must carry the gene; so although the mother may have the disease, the father has to be a carrier. The question fails to inform you that he has the disease, so you can safely assume that he carries only one abnormal gene. To be a carrier for an autosomal recessive disease, you will have one normal and one abnormal copy of the gene. As his mother carries both abnormal genes, and his father carries one abnormal gene and one normal gene, there is a 50 per cent chance that the teenager has the disease and a 50 per cent chance that he is a carrier.

Phenylketonuria (PKU) is an inborn error of metabolism. As a result of a specific enzyme deficiency, phenylalanine accumulates. The enzyme block leads to a deficiency of tyrosine, leading to a reduction in melanin; thus children often have blue eyes and blonde hair. Pigmented areas of the brain are affected, such as the substantia nigra. PKU is tested for at birth in children using the Guthrie test. PKU can be treated by removing phenylalanine from the diet. If PKU is detected early enough in childhood, mental retardation can be prevented.

114. **C: Secreto-motor innervation is via the glossopharyngeal and auriculotemporal nerves**

The parotid gland is the largest of the major salivary glands. It is mainly a serous gland, with only a few scattered mucinous acini. This in part explains why salivary stones (calculi) are rarely encountered in the parotid gland and are found more often in the submandibular gland, where the secretion is more mucinous and where the gland lies below the opening of the duct (which impedes drainage and encourages stasis).

Anteriorly, the gland overlaps the masseter. The parotid duct (of Stensen), not to be confused with Wharton's duct (which is the submandibular duct), passes forward over the masseter and turns around its anterior border to pierce the buccinator (not masseter) muscle. The buccinator muscle acts like a sphincter at this point and plays an extremely important role in preventing the reflux of air into the parotid (and hence its insufflation) when the intraoral pressure is raised, as when playing a trumpet. The duct opens on the mucous membrane of the cheek opposite the second upper molar tooth.

The parotid gland consists of two lobes: superficial and deep. Hence the importance of looking in the mouth in cases where a parotid swelling is present, to look for, or exclude, involvement of the deep lobe. There is no middle lobe, although there may be an accessory lobe. The parotid is surrounded by a tough fascial capsule, derived from the investing layer of deep cervical fascia, that is richly innervated. It is the acute swelling of this fibrous envelope that produces the pain of mumps parotitis, a virus infection of the gland.

From superficial to the deep within the parotid lie the following:

- Five terminal branches of the facial nerve (also known as the pes anserinus, or 'goose's foot')
- Retromandibular vein
- External carotid artery

The branches of the facial nerve lie most superficially within the parotid gland and hence are extremely vulnerable to damage in parotid surgery. Thus, if the retromandibular vein comes into view, it is too late; the facial nerve has already been severed! It is important to identify and protect the various branches of the facial nerve, which may be remembered by the mnemonic 'Ten Zulus Baited My Cat' (from top to bottom):

- Ten = Temporal branch
- Zulus = Zygomatic branch
- Baited = Buccal branch
- My = Marginal mandibular branch
- Cat = Cervical branch

The branches of the facial nerve are also likely to be injured by a malignant tumour of the parotid, which is usually highly invasive and quickly involves the facial nerve, causing a facial paralysis.

The secreto-motor supply to the parotid (for secretion of saliva) is by way of parasympathetic fibres of the glossopharyngeal nerve, synapsing in the otic ganglion and relaying onwards to the parotid gland through the auriculotemporal nerve. The importance of knowing this lies in a phenomenon known as Frey's syndrome which may occur, not infrequently, following parotid surgery, or penetrating trauma to the parotid gland. It is caused by misdirected reinnervation of the auriculotemporal nerve fibres to the sweat glands in the facial skin following its injury. The patient may complain of gustatory sweating (i.e., a stimulus intended for saliva production produces sweating instead).

115. **D: They lack nuclei and mitochondria**

Erythrocytes do not contain nuclei (they are anucleate) or mitochondria. This maximizes the haemoglobin-carrying capacity of red cells. The absence of mitochondria precludes aerobic energy production; hence they are very efficient oxygen transporters because they do not consume any O_2 directly. Erythrocytes are thus totally dependent on the anaerobic metabolism of glucose to generate the energy needed to maintain electrochemical gradients across their cell membranes.

Without nuclei, erythrocytes are unable to replace deteriorating enzymes and membrane proteins; this shortens their life expectancy. The average lifespan of a normal erythrocyte is 120 days (or 16–18 weeks). Lifespan may be reduced further as a result of the premature destruction of red cells. This is a feature of haemolysis. Aged red cells are removed from the circulation by the spleen and liver.

Erythrocytes contain the enzyme carbonic anhydrase that catalyses the reaction $CO_2 + H_2O = H^+ + HCO_3^-$ and requires zinc as a cofactor. This plays an important role in carbon dioxide transport and in the buffering of pH.

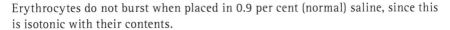

Erythrocytes do not burst when placed in 0.9 per cent (normal) saline, since this is isotonic with their contents.

116. **B: It is a known carcinogen**

    Helicobacter pylori is a Gram-negative, micro-aerophilic, motile, spiral-shaped bacterium which selectively colonizes the mucous layer of the stomach and duodenum. Around 50 per cent of all humans worldwide are infected with the organism. However, it seems to cause disease only in a small proportion of all those infected. It is still unclear at present as to why this is the case but it probably reflects differences in virulence among different strains, along with differences in the background genetics of the host that affects their susceptibility to the organism.

    It is now firmly established that *H. pylori* causes more than 90 per cent of duodenal ulcers and up to 80 per cent of gastric ulcers. The link between *H. pylori* infection and subsequent gastritis and peptic ulcer disease has been established through studies of human volunteers, antibiotic treatment studies, and epidemiological studies. *H. pylori* is also a known risk factor for gastric adenocarcinoma and lymphoma. Indeed, *H. pylori* has been classified as a class 1 (definite) carcinogen for malignancy.

    H. pylori is unique among bacteria in being able to survive within the acidic environment of the stomach. It achieves this by producing a urease enzyme which produces ammonia from endogenous urea, thereby buffering gastric acid in the immediate vicinity of the organism. The elaboration of urease by *H. pylori* forms the basis of the urea breath test that may be used in the diagnosis of *H. pylori* infection.

    H. pylori is treated with antibiotic therapy. *H. pylori* eradication therapy (also known as triple therapy) usually consists of a proton pump inhibitor in conjunction with two antibiotics. At present, there is no known vaccination against *H. pylori*. However, development of a vaccine against *H. pylori* would have the potential to prevent peptic ulcer disease and perhaps even gastric carcinoma.

117. **A: A- and B-cells**

    In the pancreas, A- and B-cells of the islets of Langerhans secrete glucagons and insulin, respectively. Pancreatic D1 cells release a product similar to vasoactive intestinal polypeptide (VIP). Pancreatic polypeptide cells secrete pancreatic polypeptide and D-cells secrete somatostatin. Acinar cells are part of the exocrine, not endocrine, pancreas and are involved in the release of enzymes and digestive juices, rather than hormones.

118. **E: They deform as they pass through the capillaries**

    Unstressed erythrocytes normally appear as biconcave discs. This provides a 20–30 per cent greater surface area than a sphere relative to cell volume, thus significantly enhancing gaseous exchange. This shape, with the fluidity of the plasma membrane, allows the erythrocyte to deform easily thus making them able to pass through the smallest capillaries. Erythrocytes appear spherical in a genetic condition known as hereditary spherocytosis.

Normal RBCs are around 7 microns in diameter, whereas the diameter of capillaries is only around 5 microns. Red cells possess deformable walls and therefore become bullet-shaped as they pass through capillaries. This enables 'bolus flow' or 'plug flow' which eliminates some of the internal friction associated with lamina sliding over one another (Fahraeus–Lindqvist effect). The reduction in apparent viscosity means that capillaries have a lower resistance to flow than they would do if the blood were a uniform fluid containing the same amounts of protein without the red cell membrane to parcel it up. The efficiency of bolus flow depends critically on the deformability of the red cell, and this is impaired in many clinical conditions. The most dramatic of these is sickle cell anaemia.

Erythrocytes make a major contribution to the buffering capacity of the blood through the action of carbonic anhydrase and haemoglobin contained within the red cells. Indeed, red cells are responsible for most of the buffering power of whole blood.

Erythropoiesis (the production of red cells) is stimulated by the hormone erythropoietin, but the main source of erythropoietin is the kidney, not erythrocytes.

The capillary bed has a greater cross-sectional area than the venular bed. Blood therefore travels more slowly in capillaries compared to venules. This prolongs the time available for gaseous exchange. Red cells are not evenly distributed across the bloodstream in large blood vessels, but form an axial stream away from the vessel wall, leaving a cell-deficient layer of plasma at the margins. This marginal layer helps to ease the blood along.

119. **D: Is caused by a toxin which increases adenylate cyclase activity**

Cholera is caused by *Vibrio cholerae,* a Gram-negative, comma-shaped, flagellated bacterium. It is usually transmitted by contaminated water supplies, as deduced from the famous epidemiological work of John Snow in the 1850s, who was able to trace a cholera outbreak in London to a single water pump that had become contaminated with sewage. Removing the handle of the water pump led to a dramatic reduction in the number of new cases of cholera.

The diarrhoea of cholera is caused by the action of an exotoxin or enterotoxin (not endotoxin) called cholera toxin. The toxin increases the activity of adenylate cyclase resulting in the massive secretion of chloride, sodium and water (so-called 'rice-water diarrhoea'). The watery diarrhoea may be so extreme that death may occur from dehydration and electrolyte imbalance. The mucosa is not invaded by the bacteria (in contrast to *Salmonella, Shigella,* and *Campylobacter*) so that mucosal inflammation is only slight and there is no ulceration.

Overall absorption from the gut remains intact so that oral rehydration therapy can replace massive fluid and electrolyte losses, reducing the mortality from 50 per cent to less than 1 per cent. Antibiotics (such as tetracyclines) are used as an adjunct to fluid therapy. Antibiotics diminish the duration and volume of the fluid loss and hasten clearance of the organism from the stool.

120. **B: Buccinator**

    There are four muscles of mastication: temporalis, masseter, medial pterygoid, and lateral pterygoid. They are all 1st branchial arch derivatives and are therefore all innervated by the same nerve (mandibular division of trigeminal, or Vc).

    The buccinator muscle is regarded as a muscle of facial expression and is therefore a 2nd branchial arch derivative innervated by the facial, or 7th, cranial nerve. This is one of many situations in which a good knowledge of embryology and especially the branchial arches may help to predict the anatomy.

121. **C: It crosses the midline at the level of T5**

    The thoracic duct is 45 cm long and commences at T12 from the cisterna chyli, which lies to the right of the aorta. It drains all lymph below the diaphragm, left thorax, and left head and neck regions. Valves are present along the duct and encourage the propagation of chyle along the duct.

    It ascends behind the right crus and to the right of the aorta and oesophagus. It crosses the midline to the left, posterior to the oesophagus, at the level of T5. It passes over the dome of the left pleura, anterior to the left vertebral and subclavian arteries and enters the confluence of the left subclavian and internal jugular veins.

    The equivalent to the thoracic duct on the right is the right lymphatic trunk. This drains on the right into the confluence of the right subclavian and internal jugular veins.

    Injury to the thoracic duct may occur following trauma, or during insertion of a central venous catheter on the left-hand side. This may result in a chylothorax (a collection of lymph within the thoracic cavity). A haemothorax is a collection of blood.

122. **E: Emphysema results in increased lung compliance**

    Compliance is expressed as volume change per unit change in pressure. Elastance is the reciprocal of compliance. Compliance is extremely small in infants compared to adults. The pressure/volume curve of the lung is nonlinear with the lungs becoming stiffer at high volumes. The curves that the lungs follow in inflation and deflation are different. This behaviour is known as 'hysteresis'. The lung volume at any given pressure during deflation is larger than during inflation. This behaviour depends on structural proteins (collagen, elastin), surface tension, and the properties of surfactant.

    A sigh or yawn is a reflexively generated single, deep breath which occurs after a period of quiet breathing. The purpose of the lung inflation, which stretches and unfolds the alveolar surface area, is to spread out the surfactant molecules, returning the alveolar surface tension to its normal value.

Various disease states are associated with either a decrease or increase in the lung compliance. Fibrosis, atelectasis, and pulmonary oedema all result in a decrease in lung compliance (stiffer lungs). An increased lung compliance occurs in emphysema where an alteration in elastic tissue is probably responsible (secondary to the long-term effects of smoking). The lung effectively behaves like a 'soggy bag' so that a given pressure change results in a large change in volume (i.e., the lungs are more compliant). However, during expiration the airways are less readily supported and collapse at higher lung volumes, resulting in gas trapping and hyperinflation. Reduced gas transfer results from a loss of interstitial tissue, causing loss of available active alveolar area.

123. **D: Occlusion of the hepatic venous drainage**

Budd–Chiari syndrome is due to extensive occlusive fibrosis of the hepatic venous drainage. Patients present with ascites, hepatomegaly, and portal hypertension.

124. **B: Prospective studies allow direct determination of incidence rates**

In a prospective (or cohort) study, exposed and non-exposed individuals are identified and followed up over time to determine the incidence of a specific clinical disease, or event. For example, a population of smokers and non-smokers are followed up to provide comparison rates for lung cancer or heart disease. The incidence of a disease is the number of new cases per unit population per unit time.

Cross-sectional studies are like a snapshot in time and measure both exposure and outcome at one time point. They provide information on disease prevalence in a population. Prevalence of a disease is the proportion of a population that exhibits the disease at any one time.

Retrospective (or case–control) studies compare individuals with and without a disease to determine possible associations or risk factors for the disease in question. However, bias may influence the recall of exposure in these studies, especially if possible associations are known (recall bias). In addition, selection bias may impact on the study. A case–control study, on the other hand, is relatively easy and inexpensive to conduct because long-term follow up is not required and this type of study is therefore suitable for studying rare diseases.

125. **E: The lungs receive a dual blood supply**

The right and left lungs are not mirror images of each other. While the right lung is composed of three lobes, the left lung possesses only two. Each of the lobes, in turn, are separated by fissures or interlobar clefts. Thus, on the right, there must be two fissures separating three separate lobes (these are the oblique and the horizontal fissures, respectively). On the left there is only one fissure separating the two lobes and that is the oblique fissure. Thus the horizontal fissure exists only on the right.

There are typically ten anatomically definable bronchopulmonary segments within each lung, each containing a segmental (tertiary) bronchus, a segmental artery, a segmental vein, lymphatics, and autonomic nerves and separated from their adjacent segments by connective tissue. Each is pyramidal in shape with its apex towards the lung root and its base towards the surface of the lung, and each is anatomically and functionally separate from the rest. The importance of understanding bronchopulmonary segments is that diseased segments, since they are structural units, can be selectively removed surgically (segmentectomy). Nowadays, this can be performed by video-assisted thoracoscopic surgery (VATS).

The right bronchus is shorter, wider, and more vertical than the left bronchus so that foreign bodies that fall down the trachea are more likely to enter the right bronchus. Furthermore, material aspirated by a supine, comatose, or anaesthetised patient would tend to gravitate into the apical segment of the right lower lobe, which is consequently a common site for aspiration pneumonia and abscess formation.

The lungs receive a dual blood supply by way of the pulmonary artery and the bronchial arteries. Thus, obstruction of a small pulmonary arteriole by a pulmonary embolus has no effect in an otherwise healthy individual with an intact bronchial circulation. In such circumstances, pulmonary embolism usually results in infarction only when the circulation is already inadequate, as in patients with heart or lung disease. A large embolus that impacts in the main pulmonary artery, or that lodges at the bifurcation (as a saddle embolus), results in sudden death.

126. **C: Each haemoglobimolecule combines with eight oxygen atoms**

The formation of haemoglobin is:

- Four pyrrole rings $\rightarrow$ protoporphyrin IX
- Protoporphyrin IX + Fe^{2+} $\rightarrow$ haem
- Haem + polypeptide (globin) $\rightarrow$ haemoglobin chain (alpha or beta)
- Two alpha chains + two beta chains $\rightarrow$ haemoglobin A (normal adult Hb)

In normal adult haemoglobin, iron exists in the reduced, or ferrous (Fe^{2+}) state, rather than the ferric (Fe^{3+}) state. Oxygen combines with the ferrous iron that is present within the haem molecules and not with the globin chains. The globin molecules that surround the haem molecule serve two key functions; they form a microenvironment in which the Fe^{2+} is protected from oxidation and also contribute to the unique oxygen binding properties of haemoglobin (allosterism and cooperativity). When iron exists in the ferric state, instead of the normal ferrous state, the haemoglobin is known as methaemoglobin. This is abnormal and has a reduced oxygen-carrying capacity, resulting in cyanosis.

Haemoglobin consisting of two alpha and two gamma chains is foetal haemoglobin. Normal adult haemoglobin contains two alpha and two beta chains. Since each haemoglobin chain has a haem prosthetic group, there are four iron atoms in each haemoglobin molecule. Each of these can bind with one molecule of oxygen, making a total of four molecules of oxygen (or eight oxygen atoms) that can be transported by each haemoglobin molecule.

Why do we have red blood cells?

- Primarily for the transport of haemoglobin and oxygen. If haemoglobin molecules were free in the plasma (and not wrapped up inside red cells) they would get filtered through the capillary membrane into the tissue spaces, or through the glomerular membrane and would escape into the urine. For haemoglobin to remain in the bloodstream, it must exist inside RBCs.

- There are enzyme systems in the red cell that help to prevent haemoglobin breakdown. For example, methaemoglobin reductase converts ferric (Fe^{3+}) methaemoglobin back to ferrous (Fe^{2+}) haemoglobin.

- Carbonic anhydrase is restricted to the red cells and is crucial in CO_2 transport.

- The chemical environment in the cell, especially the presence of DPG, displaces the dissociation curve to the right so that oxygen unloads readily in active tissues.

- If haemoglobin were free in plasma, the viscosity of blood would rise to intolerable levels and colloid osmotic pressure would increase considerably. The viscosity effect is especially important in capillaries where the presence of red cells in blood gives it an anomalously low viscosity (Fahraeus–Lindqvist effect).

127. **C: Metaplasia in the bronchus involves a change from columnar to stratified squamous epithelium**

Metaplasia is the reversible change of one fully differentiated cell type into another fully differentiated cell type, in response to injury. It often represents as an adaptive response to environmental stress. Squamous metaplasia is by far the most common. Its significance lies in the fact that it can become dysplastic if the agent that caused the metaplasia persists and is capable of inducing dysplasia.

Important sites of metaplasia

- *Lower end of the oesophagus*: In response to acid reflux (Barrett's oesophagus). The normal stratified squamous epithelium is replaced by gastric-type columnar epithelium which is able to produce mucus and protect the epithelium from acid reflux.

- *Bronchi*: Where the normal respiratory (ciliated columnar) epithelium is replaced by stratified squamous epithelium under the influence of chronic irritation by cigarette smoke (squamous metaplasia).

- *Transformation zone of the cervix*: In response to environmental changes during the reproductive cycle and in response to human papilloma virus.

The normal columnar endocervical epithelium is replaced by stratified squamous epithelium.

- *Bladder*: Squamous metaplasia in response to chronic inflammation, infection, and irritation (schistosomiasis, calculi etc.).

128. C: Phaeochromocytoma

Phaeochromocytoma is a neoplasm of the adrenal medulla. Patients present with a triad of hypertension, adrenal mass, and elevated catecholamines.

129. D: Randomized controlled trial

Randomized controlled trials form the gold standard in epidemiological research. They resemble cohort studies in many respects, but include the randomization of participants to exposures. Randomization is an important part of the study design because it eliminates the effects of selection and confounding biases. Double-blinding (keeping trial participants and investigators oblivious to the assigned intervention) adds to the value of a randomized controlled trial by eliminating the effects of information bias.

Case reports are unreliable as they represent only single cases and do not have a comparison group to allow assessment of associations. However, they are often the first foray into a new disease or area of enquiry. Case-control studies are prone to bias. Cross-sectional studies measure both exposure and outcome simultaneously, so the temporal relationship between the two may be unclear.

130. B: It extends above the clavicle superiorly

The pleura clothes each lung and lines the thoracic cavity. It is composed of two layers. The visceral layer on the lung surface is in contact with parietal pleura that lines the thoracic wall (rib cage, vertebra, diaphragm), the surfaces being lubricated by a thin film of fluid. The space in between the two layers is known as the pleural space, or cavity.

The parietal pleura (along with the apex of the lung) projects 2.5 cm above the medial third of the clavicle superiorly. A penetrating wound above the medial end of the clavicle may therefore involve the apex of the lung, resulting in a pneumothorax or a collapsed lung. This is most commonly seen as an iatrogenic complication during the insertion of a subclavian (central) venous line. Owing to the obliquity of the thoracic inlet, the pleura does not extend above the neck of the first rib, which lies well above the clavicle.

It is also important to remember that the lower limit of the pleural reflection, as seen from the back, lies below the medial border of the 12th rib, behind the upper border of the kidney. It is vulnerable to damage here during removal of the kidney (nephrectomy) through an incision in the loin. Proper identification of the 12th rib is essential to avoid entering the pleural cavity.

The visceral pleura is poorly innervated, has an autonomic nerve supply, and is insensitive to ordinary stimuli. The parietal pleura, on the other hand, receives a rich innervation from the intercostal nerves and the phrenic nerve and is sensitive to pain. Thus, in tuberculosis or pneumonia pain may never be experienced. However, once lung disease crosses the visceral pleura to involve the parietal pleura, pain becomes a prominent feature. Lobar pneumonia with pleurisy is a good example. Since the lower part of the costal parietal pleura receives its innervation from the lower five intercostal nerves, which also innervate the skin of the lower anterior abdominal wall, pleurisy in this area commonly produces pain that is referred to the abdomen. This has sometimes resulted in a mistaken diagnosis of an acute abdominal lesion. In a similar manner, pleurisy of the central part of the diaphragmatic pleura, which receives sensory innervation from the phrenic nerve (C3, 4, 5), can lead to referred pain over the shoulder, since the skin of this region is supplied by the supraclavicular nerves (C3, 4).

The reflections (and therefore the surface anatomy) of the pleural linings and lungs may be remembered by the '2, 4, 6, 8, 10, 12 rule':

Pleura

- Starts 2.5 cm above the mid-point of the medial third of clavicle
- Meet in midline at rib **2**
- Left side diverges at rib **4** (to make room for the heart)
- Right side continues parasternally to rib **6**
- Both cross rib **8** in mid-clavicular line
- Both cross rib **10** in mid-axillary line
- Both reach posterior chest just below rib **12**

Lung

- Below rib **6**, the lungs extend to **2** rib spaces less than pleura (i.e., opposite rib **6** mid-clavicular line, rib **8** mid-axillary line, and rib **10** posteriorly).
- The parietal pleura extends a further **2** rib spaces inferiorly than the inferior lung edge to allow space for lung expansion.

Note how the right and left reflections are not identical to one another. On the left it is displaced by the central position of the heart.

131. **D: It acts via a secondary messenger**

Erythropoietin is a glycoprotein hormone, produced mainly by the juxtaglomerular apparatus of the kidney in adults. In the fetus, it is almost solely produced by the liver.

Once released, it acts on specific receptors which leads to activation of tyrosine kinase, which in turn promotes transcription towards the manufacture of more red cells from bone marrow.

The major factor causing erythropoietin release is local hypoxia in the kidney which may be derived from anaemia or systemic hypoxia. Erythropoietin secretion is a prominent feature of acclimatization to high altitude. A deficiency of erythropoietin partly explains the anaemia seen in individuals with chronic renal failure. Recombinant erythropoietin is now available, revolutionizing their treatment.

132. **D: Invasion beyond the basement membrane**

The defining and most reliable characteristic differentiating a benign from a malignant tumour is the ability of the latter to invade through the basement membrane into the surrounding tissues and metastasize to distant sites.

Both benign and malignant tumours increase in size with time. However, malignant tumours tend to grow more rapidly and aggressively than benign tumours. The result is that malignant tumours tend to outstrip their blood supply, leading to necrosis. Haemorrhage occurs as a result of the fragile new vasculature that forms in an attempt to increase blood supply to the tumour.

Chromosomal abnormalities do not define a tumour as malignant as this may be a feature of both benign and malignant tumours. The presence of a pseudo-capsule is typically a feature of benign lesions and results from the neoplasm expanding symmetrically and compressing the surrounding stroma. Such encapsulation tends to contain the benign neoplasm as a discrete, readily palpable, and easily movable mass that can be surgically enucleated since a well-defined cleavage plane exists around the tumour.

In general, benign tumours are well-differentiated, meaning the tumour cells resemble the normal mature cells of the tissue of origin of the neoplasm and display well-ordered maturation. Malignant tumours, in contrast, range from well-differentiated to undifferentiated, or poorly differentiated. Malignant tumours composed of undifferentiated cells are said to be anaplastic.

133. **C: It is responsible for the formation of the transverse and oblique sinuses**

The pericardium refers to the sac that encloses the heart. It comprises three layers: an outer fibrous pericardium and an inner serous pericardium (which comprises both an outer parietal layer and an inner visceral layer). There is a small amount of pericardial fluid between the visceral and parietal layers of the serous pericardium. This allows the heart to move freely within the pericardial sac.

The pericardium serves two main functions. First, it protects and lubricates the heart. Second, it contributes to diastolic coupling of the left and right ventricles. However, cardiac contractility functions normally (although maybe not optimally) in the absence of a pericardium. Indeed, after coronary artery bypass grafting surgery the pericardium is often left open (pericardiotomy) to prevent the build-up of fluid in the postoperative period causing a tamponade effect.

Between the parietal and visceral layers there are two pericardial sinuses. The transverse sinus lies in between the pulmonary artery and aorta in front and the pulmonary veins and superior vena cava behind. The oblique sinus is a space behind the heart between the left atrium in front and the fibrous pericardium behind, posterior to which lies the oesophagus. The transverse sinus is especially important in cardiac surgery. A digit and ligature can be passed through the transverse sinus and, by tightening the ligature, the surgeon can stop the blood flow through the aorta or pulmonary trunk while cardiac surgery is performed.

The fibrous pericardium and the parietal layer of the serous pericardium receive a rich innervation from the phrenic nerve. However, the visceral layer is insensitive. The pain of pericardial inflammation (pericarditis) is pronounced, originates in the parietal layer, and is transmitted by way of the phrenic nerve.

If extensive fluid collects within the pericardial cavity it interferes with the action of the heart since the fibrous pericardium is inelastic. The pericardial cavity, in this way, behaves like a rigid box with only a finite amount of space. Thus, if the pressure builds up within the compartment, something else has to give and this usually results in compression of the heart. Such a situation is most commonly encountered in the case of penetrating trauma where the build-up of blood within the pericardial space often results in a cardiac tamponade, manifesting as a precipitous fall in cardiac output (CO). Pericardiocentesis (removal, by needle, of pericardial fluid) may be a life-saving manoeuvre in such circumstances.

134. **B: Production is decreased by angiotensin-converting enzyme inhibitors**

Aldosterone is a steroid hormone secreted by the zona glomerulosa layer of the adrenal cortex. Secretion continues following the removal of the kidneys and their juxtaglomerular cells because other factors other than the renin-angiotensin system result in the secretion of aldosterone (e.g., hyperkalaemia).

Angiotensin-converting enzyme (ACE) inhibitors tend to reduce the level of angiotensin II, which normally stimulates the adrenal cortex to produce aldosterone. The reduction of angiotensin II and aldosterone, in part, explains the antihypertensive effect of ACE inhibitors.

Aldosterone increases the excretion of both potassium and hydrogen ions from the distal convoluted tubule and collecting ducts. This results in a potassium diuresis and an acidic urine of low pH.

135. **A: Hyperchromatism**

Both cytology and histology involve the study of cells at the microscopic level. Cytology studies individual cells and cell morphology. Histology studies cells within the context of tissues and provides information about tissue architecture. Only histology can provide definitive diagnosis of invasion.

The cytological features of malignancy include:

- Increased nuclear to cytoplasmic ratio
- Hyperchromatism (darkly staining nuclei due to increased amounts of DNA)
- Prominent nucleoli
- Variability in cellular and nuclear size and shape (cellular and nuclear pleomorphism)

- High mitotic index (increased mitotic rate)
- Abnormal mitotic figures
- Lack of differentiation (anaplasia)

The histological features of malignancy include all of the above, plus:

- Loss of normal tissue architecture
- Infiltrative borders, with a disordered growth pattern
- Invasion beyond the basement membrane
- Lymphovascular involvement
- Excessive necrosis and haemorrhage
- Loss of cell-to-cell cohesion, resulting in shedding

Pyknosis, karyorrhexis, and karyolysis are cytological features of cell death (necrosis and apoptosis), rather than malignancy.

136. **E: Amyloid**

Amyloid is an acellular material that is eosinophilic. After Congo red staining, there is apple-green birefringence under plane polarized light. Calcium salts tend to be deeply basophilic, not eosinophilic with routine stains. Cholesterol deposits tend to dissolve out of tissues with routine processing agents and only empty outlines are seen of where the crystals were once present. Myocyte fibrinoid necrosis would be moderately cellular and eosinophilic.

137. **E: The mean and standard deviation of a random sample will generally be different from the mean and standard deviation of the true population**

The standard error of the mean (SE) measures the variability of a sample statistic (i.e., mean or proportion) in relation to the true population characteristic (i.e., how accurate the sample mean is an estimate of the true population mean). The standard deviation (SD) is a measure of the variability of observations around the mean.

The SE is equal to the SD divided by the square-root of the sample size. The SE is therefore generally smaller than the SD. In addition, the SE is smaller when the sample size is larger.

- The mean is the arithmetic average
- The median is the middle value when the values are ranked
- The mode is the value that occurs most often

In a normal (Gaussian) distribution, the mean = median = mode. In skewed distributions, the following 3 rules apply:

- The median always lies between the mean and the mode
- The mode occurs at the maximum point in a frequency distribution curve
- The mean is affected by outliers

Thus:

- In a positively skewed distribution: mean>median>mode
- In a negatively skewed distribution: mode>median>mean

138. **D: Occlusion of the anterior interventricular artery (left anterior descending artery) results in an anterior myocardial infarction**

The heart is composed of cardiac muscle. This cardiac muscle receives the oxygen and nutrients that it requires to pump effectively through the coronary arteries. There are two principal coronary arteries: the right and the left. The right coronary originates from the anterior aortic sinus, whereas the left coronary artery originates from the left posterior aortic sinus. The left coronary artery divides into an anterior interventricular (or left anterior descending) artery and circumflex branches. The right coronary gives off the posterior interventricular (posterior descending) artery. The right coronary supplies the right atrium and part of the left atrium, the SA node in 60 per cent of cases, the right ventricle, the posterior part of the interventricular septum, and the AV node in 80 per cent of cases. The left coronary artery supplies the left atrium, left ventricle, anterior interventricular septum, SA node in 40 per cent of cases, and AV node in 20 per cent of cases.

Understanding the earlier, one is able to predict the consequences of a blockage within a particular coronary artery. Thus a lesion within the anterior interventricular artery (of the left coronary artery) leads to an anterior myocardial infarct and death of the left ventricular muscle, resulting in congestive cardiac failure. A lesion within the right coronary artery would be expected to produce arrhythmias since the dominant arterial supply to the SA and AV nodes is through the right coronary artery.

Angina pectoris originates in the muscle or the vessels and is transmitted by sympathetic nerves. The pain of angina is often referred to the left arm and shoulder, but also frequently to the neck, throat, and even side of the face. The reason for this is that the heart originates during embryonic life in the neck, as do the arms. Therefore, both these structures receive pain fibres from the same spinal segments. Angina is usually a result of the laying down of fatty deposits within the coronary arteries (atherosclerosis). However, angina may also occur in the absence of atherosclerosis, in cases such as aortic stenosis, cocaine misuse, vasculitis, and variant (Prinzmetal's) angina; the latter being due to vasospasm of the coronary arteries.

139. **C: Activation results in the stimulation of aldosterone release**

Angiotensinogen is synthesized by the liver. Renin catalyses the production of angiotensin I (a decapeptide) from angiotensinogen. Angiotensin I is further cleaved to an octapeptide, angiotensin II, by ACE found mainly in the capillaries of the lungs. Collectively, this is known as the renin–angiotensin system:

angiotensinogen $\rightarrow$ (renin) $\rightarrow$ angiotensin I $\rightarrow$ (ACE in lungs) $\rightarrow$ angiotensin II

The effects of activation of the renin–angiotensin system are the following:

- Stimulation of aldosterone release from the adrenal cortex; this increases sodium and water retention, helping to maintain the arterial pressure
- Enhanced NaCl and water reabsorption from the proximal convoluted tubule
- Angiotensin causing widespread vasoconstriction, increasing the systemic vascular resistance and so the arterial pressure (the resulting vasoconstriction also reduces the GFR at a time when water has to be conserved)
- Stimulation of ADH secretion from the posterior pituitary, leading to an increased solute-free water reabsorption
- Stimulation of thirst (dipsogenic effect)

140. B: Lymphatics

Metastasis is the seeding of tumour cells to sites distant and detached from the primary tumour. This is different from invasion which is spread in continuity.

As a general rule, carcinomas (malignant tumours of epithelial origin) most often metastasize via the lymph; sarcomas (malignant tumours of connective tissue origin) most often metastasize via the bloodstream.

Thus, breast carcinomas often spread to local lymph nodes (axillary and internal mammary), whereas osteosarcomas typically spread via the bloodstream, forming cannonball metastases in the lungs. However, this rule is slightly misleading because ultimately there are numerous interconnections between the vascular and lymphatic systems. In addition, every rule has exceptions (e.g., follicular carcinoma of the thyroid spreads by the haematogenous route).

Neoplasms, in general, may metastasize by several routes:

- Local invasion (direct spread)
- Via the bloodstream (haematogenous route)
- Via the lymphatics
- Trans-coelomic spread (e.g., across the peritoneal or pleural cavities)
- Via the CSF (for central nervous system tumours)
- Peri-neural spread (e.g., adenoid cystic carcinoma of the parotid)
- Implantation/accidental seeding during surgery – iatrogenic

141. C: Hepatic angiosarcoma

Environmental exposure to vinyl chloride is associated with the later development of hepatic angiosarcoma. Focal nodular hyperplasia and hepatic fibroma are not linked to any defined underlying carcinogen exposure. Hepatic adenomas occur sporadically in the setting of exogenous steroid hormone use. Hepatocellular carcinoma is associated with cirrhosis, chronic viral hepatitis, and aflatoxin exposure.

142. **D: p53 and Rb-1 are tumour suppressor genes**

Tumour suppressor genes encode proteins that negatively regulate cell proliferation and thus suppress tumour growth. p53 and Rb-1 are good examples located on chromosomes 17 and 13, respectively. Normal p53 is the so-called 'guardian of the genome' and triggers apoptosis and cell-cycle arrest in genetically damaged cells (i.e., it is pro-apoptotic). Mutations in p53 therefore result in the propagation of genetically damaged cells and tumourigenesis. Indeed, approximately 50 per cent of human tumours contain mutations in the p53 gene. p53-related cancers are more aggressive and have a poorer prognosis.

In contrast to oncogenes, tumours caused by tumour suppressor genes are generally caused by mutations that result in a loss of function of the gene product; neoplastic growth resulting from the loss of the protective role of tumour suppressor genes. Loss of tumour suppressor function usually requires the inactivation of both alleles of the gene, so that all of the protective effect of tumour suppressor genes is lost. That is, tumour suppressor genes are generally deemed to behave in a recessive manner.

Cellular proliferation is therefore tightly regulated by two sets of opposing functioning genes: the growth-promoting genes (proto-oncogenes) and the negative cell-cycle regulators (tumour suppressor genes). Abnormal activation of proto-oncogenes and/or loss of function of tumour suppressor genes leads to the transformation of a normal cell into a cancer cell.

143. **C: Buccinator**

Buccinator is a muscle of facial expression and is therefore innervated by the facial nerve. The lateral pterygoid, masseter, anterior belly of digastric, and temporalis are all muscles of mastication and therefore innervated by the mandibular division of the trigeminal nerve (Vc).

144. **D: It lies level with the hilum of the kidneys**

The transpyloric plane (of Addison) is an important landmark. It lies halfway between the suprasternal notch and the symphysis pubis at the level of L1. It coincides with the following:

- L1 vertebra
- Fundus of gallbladder
- Hilum of kidneys
- Hilum of spleen
- Pylorus of the stomach (hence the name transpyloric)
- Termination of the spinal cord in adults
- Neck of pancreas
- Origin of the portal vein

- Origin of the superior (not inferior) mesenteric artery
- Duodenojejunal flexure
- Attachment of transverse mesocolon
- Tip of 9th costal cartilage

The aorta bifurcates at the level of L4, not L1.

145. **B: It is potentiated by histamine**

There are 3 classic phases of gastric acid secretion:

Cephalic (preparatory) phase [significant]: This results in the production of gastric acid before food actually enters the stomach. It is triggered by the sight, smell, thought, and taste of food acting via the vagus nerve.

Gastric phase [most significant]: This is initiated by the presence of food in the stomach, particularly protein-rich food.

Intestinal phase [least significant]: The presence of amino acids and food in the duodenum stimulate acid production.

Gastric acid is *stimulated* by 3 factors:

- *Acetylcholine*: From parasympathetic neurones of the vagus nerve that innervate parietal cells directly
- *Gastrin*: Produced by pyloric G-cells
- *Histamine*: Produced by mast cells

Histamine stimulates the parietal cells directly and also potentiates parietal cell stimulation by gastrin and neuronal stimulation. H_2 blockers such as ranitidine are therefore an effective way of reducing acid secretion.

Gastric acid is *inhibited* by 3 factors:

- Somatostatin
- Secretin
- CCK

146. **D: The anterior surface of the right adrenal gland is overlapped by the inferior vena cava**

The adrenal glands lie anterosuperior to the upper part of each kidney. They weigh approximately 5 g each and measure 50 mm vertically, 30 mm across, and 10 mm thick. They are somewhat asymmetrical, with the right adrenal being pyramidal in shape and left adrenal being crescentic, and lie within their own compartment of (Gerota's) renal fascia. A fascial septum separates the adrenal gland from the kidney, which explains why in nephrectomy (removal of the kidney) the latter gland is not usually displaced (or even seen).

Each gland, although only weighing a few grams, has three arteries supplying it: a direct branch from the aorta, a branch from the renal artery, and a branch from the inferior phrenic artery. This reflects the high metabolic demands of the tissue. The single main suprarenal vein drains into the nearest available vessel: on the right it drains into the inferior vena cava and on the left directly into the renal vein. The right adrenal gland is tucked medially behind the inferior vena cava. In addition, the right suprarenal vein is particularly short and stubby. Both these features make the inferior vena cava vulnerable to damage in a right adrenalectomy.

The adrenal gland comprises an outer cortex and an inner medulla, which represent two developmentally and functionally independent endocrine glands within the same anatomical structure. The medulla is derived from the neural crest (ectoderm). It receives preganglionic sympathetic fibres from the greater splanchnic nerve and secretes adrenaline (70 per cent) and noradrenaline (30 per cent). The cortex is derived from mesoderm and consists of three layers, or zones. The layers from the surface inwards may be remembered by the mnemonic GFR (which also stands for glomerular filtration rate):

G = zona Glomerulosa (secretes aldosterone)

F = zona Fasciculata (secretes cortisol and sex steroids)

R = zona Reticularis (secretes cortisol and sex steroids)

147. **C: It stimulates gastric acid production**

Gastrin is secreted by gastrin-secreting cells (G-cells) found in two locations: the pyloric region of the stomach and the upper half of the small intestine. Gastrin is released by:

- Vagal stimulation
- Distension of the pyloric antrum
- Proteins (especially partially digested proteins) in the food

Gastrin is inhibited by:

- A low pH in the lumen of the pyloric antrum (negative feedback loop)
- Somatostatin

Gastrin has 3 main actions:

- It stimulates gastric acid secretion
- It stimulates gastric motility
- It stimulates exocrine pancreatic secretions

Overproduction of gastrin leads to excessive gastric acid secretion and the formation of multiple peptic ulcers. This is known as the Zollinger–Ellison syndrome and is often due to a gastrin-secreting tumour (gastrinoma).

148. **C: May produce paraneoplastic syndromes**

Currently, in the UK, lung cancer is the most common cause of death from cancer in both men and women. It is estimated that some 50 per cent of bronchial carcinomas have metastasized by the time of clinical presentation. Lung carcinoma is most commonly due to squamous cell carcinoma as a result of squamous cell metaplasia from smoking. Tobacco smoking is believed to account for 80–90 per cent cases of lung carcinoma; the remainder are associated with radon gas and asbestos exposure.

The pathological effects of any tumour may be local or distant; distant effects may be metastatic or non-metastatic (paraneoplastic). Applying this to lung carcinoma we have:

Local effects

- *Pulmonary involvement*: Cough (infection distal to airway blocked by tumour caused by disruption of the mucociliary escalator), haemoptysis (ulceration/ necrosis of tumour), breathlessness (local extension of tumour), chest pain (involvement of pleura and/or chest wall), wheeze (narrowing of airways)
- *Local invasion*: Hoarseness (recurrent laryngeal nerve infiltration), Horner's syndrome (infiltration of the ipsilateral sympathetic chain), wasting of the intrinsic hand muscles (brachial plexus infiltration), diaphragmatic paralysis (phrenic nerve invasion), pleural effusions (tumour spread into pleura), pericarditis (pericardial involvement), superior vena cava obstruction (direct compression by tumour)

Distant effects

- *Metastatic*: Pathological fractures (bone metastases), neurological symptoms (brain metastases), hepatomegaly or jaundice (liver metastases)
- *Non-metastatic (paraneoplastic) effects*: Ectopic hormone production (ADH, ACTH, PTHrP, serotonin, etc.), common generalized symptoms (weight loss, anorexia, lassitude) from the acute-phase response (IL-1, IL-6, TNFα)

Paraneoplastic syndromes are symptoms and signs associated with a malignant tumour that are not due to direct local effects of the tumour or the development of metastases.

149. **A: Peptidoglycan**

Prokaryotes have peptidoglycan in their cell walls, which makes them susceptible to penicillin. Sterol and endoplasmic reticulum are features of eukaryotic cells. Bacteria generally contain single, circular chromosomes (plasmids). Prokaryotes contain 70S, rather than 80S ribosomes, which are characteristic of eukaryotes.

150. **D: It is unimportant in humans**

The vermiform (worm-shaped) appendix is a blind-ending tube varying in length (commonly 6–9 cm) which opens into the posteromedial wall of the caecum, where the taeniae coli converge. The appendix is an intraperitoneal structure and therefore has its own short mesentery, the mesoappendix. Within the mesentery lies the appendicular artery, a branch of the ileocolic artery which arises from the superior mesenteric artery.

The surface marking of the base of the appendix is situated one-third of the way up the line joining the anterior superior iliac spine to the umbilicus (McBurney's point). This is an important landmark when making an appendicectomy (McBurney's or Gridiron) incision. The position of the free end of the appendix, however, is very variable. The most common, as found at operation, is the retrocaecal or retrocolic position (75 per cent of cases), with the subcaecal or pelvic position next in order of frequency (20 per cent of cases). Less commonly, in 5 per cent of cases it lies in the pre-ileal or retro-ileal positions, or lies in front of the caecum, or in the right paracolic gutter.

The appendix has no known physiological function in man and can therefore be removed without any consequences. It probably represents a degenerated portion of the caecum that, in ancestral forms, aided in cellulose digestion. In the other animals, the appendix is much larger and provides a pouch off the main intestinal tract, in which cellulose can be trapped and be subjected to prolonged digestion. The abundance of lymphoid tissue within the submucosa of the appendix has prompted the concept that the appendix is the human equivalent of the avian bursa of Fabricius as a site of maturation of thymus-independent lymphocytes. While no discernible change in immune function results from appendicectomy, the prominence of lymphatic tissue in the appendix of young adults seems important in the aetiology of appendicitis.

151. **D: The main stimulation for secretion occurs during the intestinal phase**

The pancreas is a mixed endocrine (ductless) and exocrine gland that forms embryologically from the fusion of separate dorsal and ventral pancreatic buds (endodermal outgrowths from the primitive foregut). The embryology helps to explain how aberrations of development lead to the formation of an annular pancreas, or pancreas divisum, either of which may lead to problems in later life.

The exocrine component of the pancreas consists of closely packed secretory acini which drain into a highly branched duct system. Approximately 1500 mL of pancreatic juice is secreted each day into the duodenum via the pancreatic duct. The alkaline pH of the pancreatic secretion (approximately 8.0) is due to a high content of bicarbonate ions and serves to neutralize the acidic chyme as it enters the duodenum from the stomach.

With regard to the secretion of gastric acid, it is possible to distinguish cephalic, gastric, and intestinal phases in the pattern of secretion. The weak cephalic phase contributes only 15 per cent of the total response, an enzyme-rich secretion caused by vagal efferents. The weak gastric phase also contributes only 15 per cent of the total response and is again enzyme-rich, caused by vaso-vagal reflexes originating in the stomach and gastrin secretion. The main stimulation (70 per cent of the total response) is the intestinal phase caused by food entering the duodenum from the stomach. Secretin, a hormone released by endocrine cells scattered in the duodenal mucosa, promotes the secretion of copious watery fluid rich in bicarbonate. The major stimulus for the release of secretin is acid. CCK, also derived from duodenal endocrine cells, stimulates the secretion of enzyme-rich pancreatic fluid. Secretin and CCK act synergistically.

152. D: Liver

After metastasing to the pericolonal lymph nodes, colonic tumour cells are then usually drained by the mesenteric lymphatics into blood vessels, the portal vein, and finally into the liver. The other choices are less likely sites of initial distant tumour spread.

153. B: It may result in thrombosis of the appendicular artery (endarteritis obliterans)

Acute appendicitis is the most common acute surgical condition of the abdomen. Approximately 7 per cent of the population will have appendicitis in their lifetime, with the peak incidence occurring between the ages of 10 and 30 years. Appendicitis is relatively uncommon at the two extremes of life since obstruction of the lumen is the usual cause of appendicitis and the lumen of the appendix is relatively wide in the infant and is frequently completely obliterated in the elderly.

Afferent nerve fibres concerned with the conduction of visceral pain from the appendix accompany the sympathetic nerves and enter the spinal cord at the level of T10. Consequently, the appendix refers visceral pain to the T10 dermatome which lies at the level of the umbilicus. Only later, when the parietal peritoneum overlying the appendix becomes inflamed, does the pain become more intense and localize to the right iliac fossa in the region of McBurney's point.

The following 3 factors contribute to why the appendix is prone to infection:

- It is a long, narrow blind-ended tube which encourages stasis of large bowel contents
- It has a large amount of lymphoid tissue in its wall (submucosa)
- The lumen has a tendency to become obstructed by hardened intestinal contents (enteroliths or faecoliths) which leads to further stagnation of its contents

The sequence of events underlying acute appendicitis is worth understanding. The initial event is probably related to obstruction of the mouth of the appendix. The most common cause of obstruction is a faecolith. This leads to formation of a closed system and the build-up of mucinous secretions (appendiceal mucocele). The distended appendix can become secondarily infected and inflamed (appendicitis). This may subsequently lead to the formation of an appendix mass, or abscess. Alternatively, the pressure within this closed system may begin to rise until the point is reached that it begins to compress the superficial veins in the wall of the appendix. Obstruction to venous outflow leads to oedema and a further increase in pressure. The pressure continues to rise until eventually the appendiceal artery is compressed and thromboses (endarteritis obliterans). Since the appendiceal artery is an end artery and does not anastomose with any other artery, it represents the entire vascular supply of the appendix. The appendix subsequently undergoes ischaemic necrosis and gangrene, which may eventually result in a perforated appendix.

Acute appendicitis almost always requires surgical intervention. This may be performed by open or laparoscopic techniques. It rarely resolves with conservative management and 'watchful waiting' risks progression to perforation and generalized peritonitis, which carries with it a high mortality. There is only one situation in which conservative management is a feasible alternative to surgery, and that is when an appendix mass (or abscess) is present and the patient is not compromised. Even then, however, it is advisable to remove the appendix later after an interval of 6–8 weeks.

154. **A: Trypsin is a powerful activator of other pancreatic proteolytic enzymes**

The pancreatic enzymes degrade proteins, carbohydrates, lipids, and nucleic acids. The pancreatic proteolytic enzymes, trypsin and chymotrypsin, are secreted as inactive proenzymes that require activation in the small intestine. Enterokinase (enteropeptidase), an enzyme secreted by the duodenal mucosa, activates trypsinogen to form trypsin; trypsin then activates chymotrypsinogen to form chymotrypsin and other proenzymes into active enzymes. Trypsin can also activate trypsinogen; therefore once some trypsin is formed, there is an autocatalytic chain reaction. By releasing the enzymes as inactive zymogens that become activated far from their site of origin, this mechanism prevents autodigestion of the pancreas.

However, the powerful nature of these proteolytic enzymes necessitates another mechanism to prevent digestion of the pancreas. The same cells that secrete the proteolytic enzymes also secrete another substance called trypsin inhibitor (not a trypsin activator which would be disastrous!). Trypsin inhibitor surrounds the enzyme granules and prevents activation of trypsin both inside the secretory cells and in the acini and ducts of the pancreas. It therefore acts as an additional safeguard should some of the trypsinogen be activated to trypsin. Following exocytosis this inhibitor is diluted out and becomes ineffective. Since trypsin activates the other pancreatic proteolytic enzymes too, trypsin inhibitor therefore also prevents the subsequent activation of the others.

When the pancreas becomes severely damaged or when the duct becomes blocked, large quantities of pancreatic secretion become pooled in the damaged areas of the pancreas. Under these circumstances, the effect of trypsin inhibitor is overwhelmed, in which case the pancreatic secretions rapidly become activated and literally digest the entire pancreas, giving rise to a condition known as acute pancreatitis. This can be lethal; even if not fatal, it may lead to a lifetime of pancreatic insufficiency.

155. E: Secondary carcinoma

Tumours or neoplasms may be benign or malignant. Malignant tumours may be primary or secondary. Secondary bone tumours (i.e., metastases) are the most common malignant tumour of bone, occurring in 70 per cent of patients with disseminated malignant disease. They are more common than all the primary malignant tumours put together. After the liver and lung, the bone is the third most common site for metastatic spread. The most common primary malignant tumour of bone is the osteosarcoma.

The 6 most common tumours that spread to bone are:

- Multiple myeloma
- Breast
- Bronchus (lung)
- Prostate
- Kidney
- Thyroid (follicular subtype)

Secondary bone tumours may be associated with an osteolytic (bone-dissolving) or osteoblastic (bone-forming) reaction within the bone. Interestingly both prostate and breast carcinoma have a propensity to form osteoblastic lesions within the bone. The direct effect of metastatic tumours on the bone is one explanation for the hypercalcaemia that is commonly seen in malignancy. Other factors seem to play a role, however, such as the release of parathyroid hormone-related protein (PTHrP) by tumour cells.

156. D: Autoclaving

Bacillus anthracis is a Gram-positive, spore-forming microbe. Autoclaving is the best option for killing vegetative cells and spores.

157. D: It provides a route of access to the lesser sac

The greater omentum (or gastrocolic omentum) is a double sheet of peritoneum, fused and folded on itself to form an integral structure comprising four layers. It contains adipose tissue of variable amount, depending on the nutritional status of the patient, and hangs down like an apron overlying loops of intestine. The anterior two layers descend from the greater curvature of the stomach (the lesser omentum, not the greater omentum, arises from the lesser curvature of the stomach) where they are continuous with the peritoneum on the anterior and posterior surfaces of the stomach. Posteriorly, they ascend to the transverse colon where they loosely blend with the peritoneum on the anterior and posterior surfaces of the transverse colon and the transverse mesocolon above it.

The right and left gastroepiploic arteries run between the layers of the greater omentum and supply it, close to the greater curvature of the stomach. The greater omentum may undergo torsion, and if this is extensive the blood supply to part of it may be cut off causing necrosis. The lesser sac may be accessed through the greater omentum (by incising between the greater curvature of the stomach and the transverse colon and lifting the stomach up).

The greater omentum is of paramount surgical importance. Surgeons sometimes use the omentum to buttress an intestinal anastomosis, or in the closure of a perforated gastric or duodenal ulcer ('omental patch repair'). One important function of the greater omentum is to attempt to limit the spread of intraperitoneal infections. Indeed, the greater omentum is often referred to by surgeons as the 'great policeman of the abdomen'. The lower, right, and left margins are free and it moves about the peritoneal cavity in response to peristaltic movements of the neighbouring gut. In an acutely inflamed appendix, for example, the inflammatory exudate causes the omentum to adhere to the appendix and wrap itself around the infected organ. By this means, the infection is often localized to a small area of the peritoneal cavity, thus saving the patient from a serious generalized peritonitis. The greater omentum is also commonly found plugging the neck of a hernial sac, thereby preventing the entry of coils of small intestine and strangulation of bowel. In the first two years of life, the greater omentum is poorly developed and thus is less protective in a young child.

158. C: Islets of Langerhans make up only 2 per cent of the volume of the gland

The endocrine tissue of the pancreas forms Islets of Langerhans. They make up about 2 per cent of the volume of the pancreas, whereas the exocrine portion makes up 80 per cent and ducts and blood vessels make up the rest. Pancreatic endocrine tissue, like all endocrine tissue, is ductless.

There are several different types of islet cell, each producing a different hormone:

- α-islet cells secrete glucagon
- β-islet cells secrete insulin
- δ-islet cells secrete somatostatin
- F-islet cells secrete pancreatic polypeptide

Each of these hormones passes directly into the bloodstream.

Glucagon has a reciprocal action to that of insulin. It is glycogenolytic, gluco-neogenic, lipolytic, and ketogenic.

159. **D: May be seen in histological section**

Apoptosis (from the Greek meaning 'to fall off', as the leaves from a tree) is programmed cell death. It acts to eliminate unwanted cells or damaged cells with abnormal DNA. It involves the death of individual cells, rather than large groups of adjacent cells (which is usually the case in necrosis). Apoptosis is usually unaccompanied by inflammation (as is the case in necrosis). A key feature of apoptosis is that cells can be eliminated with minimal disruption to adjacent cells.

Apoptosis may be physiological (as a normal part of growth and development), as well as pathological, where balancing the production of new cells enables a stable cell population. A good example of physiological apoptosis is the shaping of the hands in embryogenesis. Under normal conditions, apoptosis is precisely regulated by pro-apoptotic (p53, c-myc, Bax, Bad) and anti-apoptotic (Bcl-2, Bcl-XL) factors. Alteration in the fine balance of pro-apoptotic and anti-apoptotic factors may result in neoplasia (e.g., loss of p53 is found in many tumours).

Apoptosis is clearly visible in histological sections; apoptotic cells are seen as rounded membrane-bound bodies ('apoptotic bodies'). These bodies are eventually phagocytosed and digested by adjacent cells so that no clump of cellular debris is left permanently behind. The key differences between necrosis and apoptosis are summarized in Table 13.

160. **E: Destroys CD4 T-lymphocytes**

HIV is the virus responsible for causing AIDS. It multiplies in CD4 lymphocytes and this multiplication leads to severe lymphopenia due to the

Table 13 Apoptosis and necrosis compared

Apoptosis	Necrosis
Energy dependent (active process)	Energy independent
Internally programmed or 'suicide'	Response to external injury
Affects single cells	Affects groups of cells
No accompanying inflammation	Accompanied by inflammation
Physiological or pathological	Always pathological
Plasma membrane remains intact	Loss of plasma membrane integrity
Cell shrinkage, fragmentation, and formation of apoptotic bodies	Cell swelling and lysis

lysis of the CD4 cells. HIV is a member of the retrovirus group and contains single-stranded RNA and an enzyme that synthesizes DNA from RNA (reverse transcriptase). It also has an envelope.

161. **B: They enter the bladder obliquely, forming a flap valve**

The ureters are segmental muscular tubes, 25 cm long, composed of smooth (involuntary) muscle throughout their entire length. They are lined by transitional epithelium (urothelium) throughout their length. Indeed the whole urinary tract, including the renal pelvis and bladder, with the exception of the terminal urethra, is lined by transitional epithelium. The clinical significance of this is that the whole urinary tract epithelium is susceptible to widespread malignant change in response to carcinogens and, as a result, tumours of the urothelium are more often multifocal compared to other sites (the so-called 'field effect'). Only the terminal (glandular part of the urethra) is lined by stratified squamous epithelium.

It is important to recognize and distinguish the ureter from surrounding vessels and nerves in the living body during surgery in order to prevent inadvertent damage. The ureter is characteristically a whitish, non-pulsatile cord, which shows peristaltic activity when gently pinched with forceps (i.e., it vermiculates). There is no situation where it is more important to recognize and preserve the ureters than at hysterectomy where the ureters lie in close proximity to the uterine vessels and ligaments. Incorrect ligation of the ureters instead of the uterine vessels may be prevented by correctly identifying the ureters (by assessing for vermiculation) and by remembering the mnemonic 'water under the bridge' (e.g., the ureters are crossed above by the uterine arteries).

Blood supply to the ureters, like the oesophagus, is segmental. The upper third is supplied by the renal arteries, the middle third from branches given off from the descending abdominal aorta, and the lower third by the superior and inferior vesical arteries. Blood supply to the middle third is the most tenuous. Consequently, the middle third of the ureter is most vulnerable to postoperative ischaemia and stricture formation if blood supply to it is endangered by stripping the ureter clean of its surrounding tissue at surgery.

Along the course of the ureter are three constrictions worth remembering as they are often the site of hold-up for ureteric calculi (stones):

- The pelviureteric junction
- Where the ureter crosses the pelvic brim in the region of the bifurcation of the common iliac artery
- The vesicoureteric junction

The last is the point of narrowest calibre.

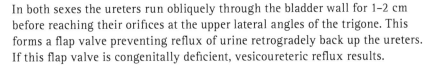

In both sexes the ureters run obliquely through the bladder wall for 1–2 cm before reaching their orifices at the upper lateral angles of the trigone. This forms a flap valve preventing reflux of urine retrogradely back up the ureters. If this flap valve is congenitally deficient, vesicoureteric reflux results.

162. **B: It is actively concentrated in the gallbladder**

The liver secretes approximately 500 mL of alkaline bile daily. It is composed of 97 per cent water, 0.7 per cent bile salts (sodium and potassium salts of bile acids), 0.2 per cent bile pigments (bilirubin and biliverdin), and 2 per cent of other substances (bicarbonate, fatty acids, cholesterol, lecithin). Bile salts are derived from cholesterol – do not confuse them with bile pigments which are the breakdown products of the haem component of haemoglobin. In addition it is the accumulation of bile pigments (bilirubin) that leads to jaundice.

Bile salts are responsible for the emulsification of fat in the chyme, by the formation of micelles. This aids in their absorption. Bile contains no digestive enzymes.

Between 90 and 95 per cent of the bile salts are absorbed from the small intestine and then excreted again from the liver; most are absorbed from the terminal ileum. This is known as the enterohepatic circulation. The entire pool recycles twice per meal and approximately 6–8 times a day. Disruption of the enterohepatic circulation, either by terminal ileal resection or through a diseased terminal ileum (e.g., Crohn's disease), results in decreased fat absorption and cholesterol gallstone formation. The latter is believed to result because bile salts normally make cholesterol more water-soluble through the formation of cholesterol micelles.

Between meals, the sphincter of Oddi which guards the opening of the bile duct into the duodenum is constricted and bile passes into the gallbladder. The gallbladder serves three main functions. It concentrates bile (5- to 20-fold) by the active reabsorption of salt and water through the gallbladder epithelium. It also stores bile and secretes mucus into the bile. The periodic discharge of bile from the gallbladder aids digestion but is not essential for it.

163. **B: Peripheral neurons**

Peripheral nerve cells, unlike nerve cells of the central nervous system, do regenerate following injury. It is a slow process that occurs at about 1 mm/day and may be followed with nerve conduction studies. Schwann cells are responsible for myelination of nerve fibres, which increases the axonal speed of conduction. Following injury (Wallerian degeneration), they are able to regenerate. Mucosal cells are epithelial cells, which behave like stem cells and can therefore continuously renew themselves. Liver cells (hepatocytes) under certain circumstances can be stimulated to divide. Renal tubular cells lack the ability to regenerate the following injury. This is why renal blood flow is so carefully autoregulated. It is also why acute tubular necrosis is taken so seriously, because damage to renal tubular cells is irreversible and will lead to end-stage renal failure, requiring renal replacement therapy in the form of dialysis or transplantation.

164. **E: Factor XII**

Deficiency of factor XII (Hageman factor) results in thrombosis rather than bleeding. The mechanism appears to be deficient activation of fibrinolysis and both thrombophlebitis and myocardial infarction have occurred in severe cases. It is inherited in an autosomal recessive manner. Deficiencies of the other factors listed are associated with bleeding.

165. **D: The gastroduodenal artery is a branch of the common hepatic artery**

The blood supply of the stomach is initially quite confusing, easily forgotten, and commonly asked about, but a few key rules make this a simple area of anatomy that will never be forgotten.

Rule 1

The coeliac trunk divides into 3 main branches, which can be easily remembered by the mnemonic Left-Hand Side (LHS):

- Left gastric artery (L)
- Common hepatic artery (H)
- Splenic artery (S)

Rule 2

For the purposes of remembering the blood supply to the stomach, the stomach can be divided into 3 main areas:

- Lesser curvature
- Greater curvature
- Fundus

Rule 3

The lesser curvature is supplied by the left and right gastric arteries. The left gastric, as already mentioned, comes directly off the coeliac trunk. The right gastric is a branch of the common hepatic artery.

Rule 4

The greater curvature is supplied by the right and left gastroepiploic arteries. The right gastroepiploic artery comes off the gastroduodenal artery. The left gastroepiploic artery comes off the splenic artery.

Rule 5

The fundus is supplied by the 6, or so, short gastric arteries which arise from the splenic artery.

Rule 6

The gastroduodenal artery is an important artery to remember for clinical purposes. It arises from the common hepatic artery and lies posterior to the first part of the duodenum. A posteriorly situated duodenal ulcer may erode through the duodenal wall into the blood vessel causing catastrophic, life-threatening haemorrhage. Urgent endoscopy or laparotomy may be required to stop the bleeding.

166. **D: It is an anabolic hormone**

Insulin acts via cell membrane spanning receptors which have intrinsic receptor tyrosine kinase activity. When insulin binds to the receptor, the tyrosine kinase is phosphorylated, resulting in a cascade of intracellular signalling mechanisms which results in glucose uptake into the cell. It is secreted by beta cells of the pancreas. Somatostatin is secreted by delta cells. Secretion is inhibited by somatostatin, which is always considered an inhibitory hormone. Insulin is considered an anabolic hormone; that is, it takes up glucose into the cell and converts it to larger 'building blocks' such as proteins and fats. Release of insulin is stimulated not only by the ingestion of glucose but also amino acids which it will convert into larger proteins.

167. **C: Liquefactive necrosis classically occurs in the brain**

Necrosis is abnormal tissue death during life. Necrosis is always pathological and is accompanied by inflammation. Groups of cells are involved and undergo swelling and lysis. Necrotic cells are phagocytosed by inflammatory cells. There are several different types of necrosis:

- *Coagulative* (structured) necrosis is the most common form. It results from interruption of blood supply. Tissue architecture is preserved. It is seen in organs supplied by end-arteries, such as the kidneys, heart, liver, and spleen.

- *Liquefactive* (colliquative) necrosis occurs in tissues rich in lipid where lysosomal enzymes denature the fat and cause liquefaction of the tissue. It characteristically occurs in the brain.

- *Caseous* (unstructured) necrosis has a gross appearance of soft, cheesy, friable material. Tissue architecture is destroyed. It is commonly seen in tuberculosis.

- *Fat* necrosis can occur following direct trauma (e.g., breast) or enzymatic lipolysis (e.g., pancreatitis).

- *Fibrinoid* necrosis is seen in the walls of arteries that are subjected to high pressures, as in malignant hypertension. The muscular wall undergoes necrosis and is associated with deposition of fibrin.

- *Gangrenous* necrosis is irreversible tissue death characterized by putrefaction. It may be wet, dry, or gaseous. The tissues appear green or black because of breakdown of haemoglobin.

168. **B: Left atrium**

Pressure in the left atrium can be approximated by wedging an arterial catheter in the small branch of the pulmonary artery. The pulmonary vascular tree abuts the left atrium anatomically. The pulmonary artery carries deoxygenated blood from the right ventricle into the pulmonary circulation where it is oxygenated and then returned into the left atrium via the pulmonary veins.

169. **E: Cloquet's node lies most medially within the femoral canal**

The boundaries of the femoral triangle are the inguinal ligament superiorly, the medial border of adductor longus medially and the medial border of sartorius laterally.

The contents of the femoral triangle from lateral to medial may be easily remembered by the mnemonic NAVY:

- N = Nerve (femoral) outside the femoral sheath
- A = Artery (femoral) within the femoral sheath
- V = Vein (femoral) within the femoral sheath
- Y = Y-fronts (most medially)

Within the femoral sheath lies the femoral artery, vein, and a space most medially known as the femoral canal. The purpose of the femoral canal is to allow the laterally placed femoral vein to expand into it, thereby encouraging venous return. However, a piece of bowel or omentum may extend down into the femoral space, causing a femoral hernia. Within the space of the femoral canal normally lies extraperitoneal fat and a lymph node which is often given its eponymous name: Cloquet's lymph node. Cloquet's lymph node drains the lower limb, perineum, and anterior abdominal wall inferior to the umbilicus. It may be enlarged (as inguinal lymphadenopathy) in cases of carcinoma and infection at these sites.

The femoral artery lies at the mid-inguinal point (halfway between the anterior superior iliac spine and symphysis pubis), as opposed to mid-point of the inguinal ligament (halfway between the anterior superior iliac spine and the pubic tubercle) which is the surface marking of the deep inguinal ring. The surface marking of the femoral artery is imperative to understand as, not only does it provide a site for the clinician to assess the femoral pulse, but it also provides the clinician with a surface landmark for gaining access to the femoral artery for procedures such as coronary angioplasty and lower limb angiography and embolectomy.

170. **B: Prolactin is under dominant inhibitory regulation**

Oxytocin and ADH are synthesized in the paraventricular and supraoptic nuclei of the hypothalamus. They are transported from the hypothalamus down into the posterior pituitary gland (or neurohypophysis) via magnocellular neurones and are stored in the posterior pituitary as vesicles prior to release into the bloodstream.

GH, ACTH, TSH, prolactin, and LH/FSH are released from the anterior pituitary gland. Prolactin is under inhibitory control by dopamine but can also be stimulated by TRH/TSH. Catecholamines, serotonin, and thyroxine are amine hormones, whereas cortisol, aldosterone, androgens, oestrogens, progesterone, and vitamin D are steroid hormones. All other hormones are peptide hormones.

Insulin, growth hormone, and prolactin act via tyrosine kinase receptors. Adrenaline, ACTH, TSH, LH/FSH, glucagon, and somatostatin act via G-protein receptors coupled to cAMP. The G-protein-coupled receptor activates adenylate cyclase, which in turn generates cAMP in an amplification process. GnRH and TRH act via G-protein receptors coupled to intracellular calcium as a second messenger. This is undertaken through activation of phospholipase C. It is the steroid hormones which bind to intracellular receptors.

171. **B: Digestion of dead tissue by saprophytic bacteria**

In gangrene, tissue that is dead is digested by bacteria which are incapable of invading and multiplying in living tissue (saprophytes), a process known as putrefaction. Gas production may be present in some forms of gangrene (e.g., gas gangrene from clostridial anaerobic infection), but not others.

Necrosis of tissue is an essential prerequisite for gangrene. Necrosis, however, may be caused by ischaemia (secondary gangrene, or dry gangrene), or by bacterial toxins (primary gangrene, or moist gangrene).

172. **D: Cholecystokinin**

Cholecystokinin (CCK) is responsible for stimulation of gallbladder contraction. The release of CCK is stimulated by dietary fat. It is produced in the I-cells of the duodenum and jejunum. Moreover, CCK also stimulates the release of pancreatic enzyme secretion and decreases the rate of gastric emptying.

173. **B: It has high mobility at the expense of stability**

The shoulder joint, like the hip joint, is a synovial joint of the ball and socket variety. The joint cavity, as is the case with all synovial joints, is lined by articular hyaline cartilage and not fibrocartilage. As with all joints, stability is brought about by the way the various bones articulate with one another (through their incongruous surfaces) and through the various ligaments, tendons, and muscles that surround the joint. Clearly, it is impossible to have a joint that is both highly mobile and perfectly stable, as a highly mobile joint requires a wide range of movement, in all possible degrees of freedom, which is in itself intrinsically unstable. In contrast to the hip joint where stability is of paramount importance, in the shoulder joint, mobility comes at the expense of stability.

The rotator cuff muscles are the most important factor in maintaining the stability of the shoulder joint and preventing dislocation. The ligaments and bones are less important in the case of the shoulder joint. There are only four muscles of the rotator cuff, and these may be remembered by the mnemonic SITS:

- Supraspinatus
- Infraspinatus

- Teres minor
- Subscapularis

Note that teres major is not a rotator cuff muscle. Note also that the first three muscles are placed posteriorly, behind the shoulder joint, while only one of the rotator cuff muscles (subscapularis) is positioned anteriorly. This may in part explain why the shoulder more commonly dislocates anteriorly, rather than posteriorly. An alternative explanation may relate to the deficiency of the joint capsule inferiorly, which makes the shoulder susceptible to antero-inferior dislocation when in the abducted, externally rotated position. The previous two explanations are not mutually exclusive.

It should never be forgotten that the axillary nerve lies in close proximity to the shoulder joint and the surgical neck of the humerus. Consequently, it is vulnerable to injury at the time of a shoulder dislocation, or while attempting to reduce the shoulder back into its normal position following a dislocation. It is therefore imperative (from both clinical and medicolegal points of view) that the integrity of the axillary nerve be documented, both after seeing the patient who has a dislocated shoulder and following successful reduction.

174. **E: It has a peak hormonal concentration in the morning**

Cortisol is a steroid hormone that is released in stress to cause an increase in blood glucose. It is a catabolic hormone. It is stimulated by ACTH released from the anterior pituitary. ACTH is stimulated by CRH released from the median eminence of the hypothalamus. It has a diurnal variation and peaks on waking up in the morning. Its lowest level is around midnight and this is why a 'midnight cortisol' is used to detect excess cortisol production in Cushing's syndrome.

175. **A: Immobility**

A thrombus is solid material formed from the constituents of blood in flowing blood. Three primary influences predispose to thrombus formation, the so-called Virchow's triad:

- *Damaged vessel wall*: Denuded endothelium
- *Changes in blood flow*: Turbulence, stasis
- *Alterations in blood constituents*: Platelets, clotting factors, blood, hyperlipidaemia, hyperviscosity, etc.

The normal, intact endothelium is anti-thrombotic. This prevents the clotting of blood within the normal circulation. When the endothelium is injured, thrombosis occurs. Under physiological circumstances this prevents haemorrhage, as part of the normal haemostatic response to injury. Only when the formation of thrombus becomes excessive does it become pathological, resulting in vascular obstruction or migration of the thrombus to a distant site (embolization).

Heparin and warfarin both reduce the risk of thrombosis by their action on the clotting cascade. Thrombocytopenia means a low platelet count which also reduces the risk of thrombosis. Increased blood viscosity increases the risk of thrombosis ('thicker blood clots more easily'). Immobility increases the risk of thrombosis by stasis.

176. **B: It may refer pain to knee**

The hip joint, like the shoulder joint, is a synovial joint of the ball and socket variety. In general it can be said that in all joints stability and range of movement are inversely proportional to one another. The shoulder joint is the most commonly dislocated joint in the body because it has adapted for a high degree of mobility at the expense of stability. The hip joint is an exception to the rule and provides a remarkable example of a joint that has a high degree of both mobility and stability. Its stability is largely a result of the adaptation of the acetabulum and femoral head to one another, with a snug fit of the femoral head into the acetabulum, deepened by the labrum and further reinforced by three ligaments on the outside of the capsule (the iliofemoral, ischiofemoral, and pubofemoral ligaments). The iliofemoral ligament (of Bigelow) is the strongest of the three ligaments. The short muscles of the gluteal region are important muscular stabilizers. Since the hip is such a stable joint, it requires considerable force to become dislocated. When it does occur, it usually dislocates in the setting of a road traffic accident, where typically the hip joint dislocates posteriorly. The hip's great range of mobility results from the femur having a long neck that is much narrower than its head.

The hip joint lies deep to the pulsation of the femoral artery at the mid-inguinal point (halfway between the anterior superior iliac spine and the symphysis pubis, in contrast to the middle of the inguinal ligament which is halfway between the anterior superior iliac spine and the pubic tubercle, which marks the site of the deep inguinal ring). The mid-inguinal point is the surface marking of the hip joint and pain at this point may indicate pathology originating in the hip joint. Posterior to the hip lies the important sciatic nerve. Consequently, the sciatic nerve is at risk in a posterior surgical approach to the hip, or in a posterior dislocation.

The hip joint is innervated by the sciatic, femoral, and obturator nerves (Hilton's law). The knee joint is also innervated by the same nerves. This may explain why hip pathology commonly refers pain to the knee. In a child who presents with a painful knee, examination should always consist of examination of the ipsilateral hip joint, in addition to examination of the knee, so as not to miss a diseased hip.

The blood supply to the femoral head originates from 3 important sources.

- The most important is via retinacular vessels that run up from the trochanteric anastomosis and then along the neck of the femur to supply the major part of the head. The trochanteric anastomosis is formed by an anastomosis of the medial and lateral circumflex femoral arteries and the superior and inferior gluteal arteries

- The second supply is from the obturator artery in the ligamentum teres (round ligament). This is usually more important in the young child
- A third supply is via the nutrient, or diaphyseal, artery of the femur, originating from the profunda femoris artery

A fractured neck of femur may disrupt these vessels and consequently disrupt the blood flow to the femoral head, resulting in avascular necrosis. This condition frequently occurs in osteoporotic elderly women following a fall. The femoral head must be taken out and replaced with a prosthesis quickly so that mobility may be regained.

177. **D: PTH acts directly on osteoblasts in bone**

Four hormones are primarily concerned with the regulation of calcium metabolism:

- PTH
- Activated vitamin D (1,25-dihydroxycholecalciferol)
- Calcitonin (secreted from the parafollicular cells – also known as the clear or C-cells – of the thyroid gland, and relatively unimportant in humans)
- PTHrP, important in the hypercalcaemia of malignancy

The main regulatory tissues are bone, kidney, and intestine.

Activated vitamin D

The 25-hydroxylation step of vitamin D activation occurs in the liver, whereas the 1-hydroxylation step occurs in the kidneys. Activation of vitamin D requires both activation steps and PTH.

- *Intestine*: 1,25-dihydroxycholecalciferol promotes the intestinal absorption of calcium and phosphate. Absence leads to rickets in children and osteomalacia in adults
- *Kidneys*: Increased tubular reabsorption of calcium and phosphate
- *Bone*: Mobilization of calcium and phosphate

Effects of PTH

PTH is secreted from the chief cells (also known as principal cells) of the parathyroid glands. The major regulator of PTH secretion is extracellular calcium. Circulating ionized calcium acts directly on the parathyroid glands in a negative-feedback fashion to regulate the secretion of PTH. The pituitary gland does not play a role in the secretion of PTH.

- *Bone*: Resorption with calcium and phosphate release into the bloodstream. PTH acts directly on osteoblasts and osteocytes that contain membrane receptors

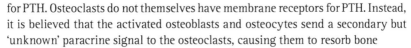

for PTH. Osteoclasts do not themselves have membrane receptors for PTH. Instead, it is believed that the activated osteoblasts and osteocytes send a secondary but 'unknown' paracrine signal to the osteoclasts, causing them to resorb bone

- *Kidney*: PTH acts on the kidneys to increase calcium reabsorption and increase phosphate excretion (phosphaturic effect). There is one caveat to this; although PTH enhances renal calcium reabsorption, in hyperparathyroidism urinary calcium excretion is paradoxically increased because the reabsorbing mechanism is saturated. This increases the tendency to renal stone formation in hyperparathyroidism
- *Intestine*: PTH increases the formation of activated vitamin D and this increases calcium absorption from the gut

178. **E: It generally has a worse outcome than thrombus**

- A thrombus is an organized mass of blood constituents that forms in flowing blood (e.g., in the living body)
- A clot is a solid mass of blood constituents formed in stationary blood when blood is allowed to coagulate outside the body or post-mortem
- An embolus is an abnormal mass of undissolved material (of solid, liquid, or gaseous origin) that is carried in the bloodstream from one place to another

Thrombus and clot can be readily distinguished from one another at post-mortem (Table 14). Veins, rather than arteries, are the most common source of emboli.

Table 14 Distinguishing thrombus and post-mortem clot

Thrombus	Post-mortem clot
Grey	Dark purple-red
Organized structure forming lines of Zahn (the pale lines are platelet aggregates enmeshed in fibrin, whilst the intervening dark lines are composed of RBCs)	Separation of RBCs and plasma producing a 'chicken fat' appearance since red cells often gravitate to the bottom of post-mortem clot
Dull surface and firm consistency	Shiny surface and gelatinous consistency ('redcurrant jelly')
Adherent to vessel wall	Peels away easily from the vessel wall
Dry, granular, and friable	Moist and rubbery
Conforms to shape of vessel	Does not conform to shape of vessel
May show features of recanalization	

Emboli most commonly arise from thrombosis formed within the deep veins of the lower limb and pelvis; thrombus formed here is known as a deep vein thrombosis. Anatomy ensures that emboli of venous origin lodge in pulmonary arteries. The size of the pulmonary artery blocked depends on the size of the thrombo-embolus. Usually, they are small and lodge in small pulmonary arteries, but sometimes an extensive thrombus from the deep veins ends up as a saddle embolus blocking the main pulmonary artery. This massive pulmonary embolus is the most common preventable cause of death in hospitalized, bed-bound patients.

An embolus is not always due to thrombus, although about 95 per cent of all emboli are thrombotic. Other emboli include:

- *Solid material*: Fat, tumour cells, atheromatous material, foreign matter
- *Liquid material*: Amniotic fluid
- *Gaseous material*: Air, nitrogen bubbles

The ischaemia resulting from an embolus tends to be worse than that due to thrombosis because the blockage is so sudden. Thrombi tend to slowly occlude the vessel lumen. Thrombi are therefore less likely to cause infarction since they provide time for the development of alternative perfusion pathways by way of collaterals.

179. B: Left suprarenal

The left suprarenal vein empties into the left renal vein which crosses the vertebral column to reach the inferior vena cava. The left renal vein also receives the left gonadal vein.

180. E: The pulsation of the radial artery may be felt at its base

The contents and boundaries of the anatomical snuffbox are shown in Table 15.

The anatomical snuffbox is an important region clinically for three reasons. First, tenderness within the anatomical snuffbox may indicate a fractured scaphoid bone. This is important to recognize since X-rays are often unremark-able in the early stages and, if left untreated, there is a risk of avascular necrosis of the scaphoid (in fact, the proximal scaphoid segment necroses since it receives its blood supply from distal to proximal). Second, tendonitis of the abductor pollicis longus and extensor pollicis brevis tendons may occur; this is known as DeQuervain's tenovaginitis stenosans. Third, the cephalic vein is almost invari-ably found in the region of the anatomical snuffbox. The anatomical snuffbox therefore forms a useful landmark for the purpose of gaining intravenous access.

181. C: Thyroxine promotes the growth and development of the brain

The thyroid gland primarily produces T4 which is converted to T3 (the more active form) in the periphery. Thyroxine is released when TSH, produced from the anterior pituitary, binds to cell surface receptors on the thyroid gland. TRH is a hypothalamic hormone which causes TSH secretion. TSH release is under

Table 15   Anatomical snuffbox

Base	From proximal to distal – radial styloid, scaphoid, trapezium, base of 1st metacarpal
Roof	Skin Fascia
Medially (ulnar side)	Extensor pollicis longus tendon
Laterally (radial side)	Extensor pollicis brevis tendon Abductor pollicis longus tendon
Contents	Cephalic vein (beginning in its roof) Terminal branches of radial nerve (supplying the overlying skin) Radial artery (on its floor)

inhibitory control by dopamine. Thyroxine increases basal metabolic rate. Protein, carbohydrate, and fat metabolism is increased. Thyroxine, although not a steroid, does not act on cell surface receptors, but acts on intracellular receptors bound to promoters of genes. It directly affects gene transcription in this way. Thyroxine plays an extremely important role in the myelination of axons during brain development. Neonatal deficiency leads to reduced axonal conduction velocities at the critical time in development when the brain is growing and maturing, resulting in developmental delay and mental retardation. This is known as cretinism or congenital hypothyroidism. Thyroid replacement therapy must be initiated soon after birth if mental retardation is to be prevented. Affected infants should be identified on neonatal biochemical screening (Guthrie test).

182. **C: It is an abnormal reduction of the blood supply to, or drainage from, an organ or tissue**

- *Ischaemia* is an abnormal reduction of the blood supply to, or drainage from, an organ or tissue
- *Infarction* is the death of tissues specifically caused by ischaemia or loss of blood supply
- *Necrosis* refers to generalized tissue death due to toxins, trauma, or vascular occlusion

Ischaemia is most commonly due to vascular narrowing or occlusion from atherosclerosis. However, blood supply to tissues may be inadequate for a variety of reasons, besides vascular occlusion. Thus, ischaemia may also result from states of shock (i.e., circulatory collapse with low arterial blood pressure). The most common causes of shock are insufficient blood volume (hypovolaemia), sepsis, and heart failure. In all cases there is a low blood pressure. All tissues may therefore become ischaemic and any organ may fail as a result.

The outcome of ischaemia is determined by a variety of factors:

- The nature of the vascular supply (the most important factor). The presence of collaterals is protective against the effects of ischaemia. Conversely, blockage of an end-artery will almost always cause infarction
- The tissue involved. The brain and heart are more susceptible to the effects of hypoxia
- The speed of onset. Slowly developing occlusions are less likely to cause infarction since they provide time for the development of alternative perfusion pathways
- The degree of obstruction and the calibre of the vessel occluded
- The oxygen content of the blood supplying the ischaemic tissue
- The presence of concomitant heart failure
- The state of the microcirculation, as in diabetes mellitus

183. E: The submucosa of the duodenum

The Brunner glands are located in the submucosa of the duodenum. These glands are connected to the interstitial lumen by ducts that open into certain crypts. They secrete an alkaline product that protects the duodenal mucosa from the acidic chyme and helps achieve an optimal pH for the enzymes.

184. C: The suprapatellar bursa (pouch) communicates with the knee joint

The knee joint is a synovial joint (the largest in the body), of the modified hinge variety. The bony contours contribute little to the stability of the joint. Nevertheless, the ligaments and muscles make it a very stable joint which rarely dislocates.

The cruciate ligaments are two very strong ligaments that cross each other within the joint cavity, but are excluded from the synovial cavity by a covering of synovial membrane (they are therefore described as being intracapsular, but extrasynovial). They are crucial in the sense that they are essential for stability of the knee. They are named anterior and posterior according to their tibial attachments. Thus the anterior cruciate ligament is attached to the anterior intercondylar area of the tibia and runs upwards, backwards and laterally to attach itself to the medial surface of the lateral femoral condyle. The anterior cruciate prevents anterior displacement of the tibia on the femur. Backward displacement of the tibia on the femur is prevented by the stronger posterior cruciate ligament. The integrity of the latter is therefore important when walking down stairs or downhill. Tears of the anterior cruciate ligament are common in sports injuries, whereas tears of the posterior cruciate ligament are rare since it is much stronger than the anterior cruciate.

Bursae are lubricating devices found wherever skin, muscle, or tendon rubs against bone. There are approximately a dozen bursae related to the knee joint. The details are not important, only the salient points. For instance, it would be important to remember that the suprapatellar bursa communicates with the knee joint. An effusion of the knee may therefore extend some 3–4 finger-breadths above the patella into the suprapatellar pouch. The prepatellar and infrapatellar bursae do not communicate with the knee joint, but may become inflamed causing a painful bursitis. Inflammation of the prepatellar bursa is known as housemaid's knee, whereas that of the infrapatellar bursa is called clergyman's knee.

The menisci, or semilunar cartilages, are crescent-shaped laminae of fibrocartilage, the medial being larger and less curved than the lateral. They have an important role in:

• Distributing the load by increasing the congruity of the articulation
• Contributing to stability of the knee by their physical presence and by acting as providers of proprioceptive feedback
• Acting as shock absorbers through a 'cushioning' effect
• Probably assisting in lubrication

However, the menisci do not play a role in the locking/unlocking mechanism of the knee joint. This is primarily the responsibility of the popliteus muscle.

The menisci are liable to injury from twisting strains applied to a flexed weight-bearing knee. The medial meniscus is much less mobile than the lateral meniscus (because of its strong attachment to the medial collateral ligament of the knee joint) and it cannot as easily accommodate abnormal stresses placed on it. This, in part, explains why meniscal lesions are more much common on the medial side than on the lateral.

The menisci are so effective that if they are removed, the force taken by the articular hyaline cartilage during peak loading increases by about five-fold. Meniscectomy (removal of the menisci), or damage to the menisci, therefore exposes the articular hyaline cartilage to much greater forces than normal and evidence of degenerative osteoarthritis is seen in 75 per cent of patients 10 years after meniscectomy.

185. C: Hyperkalaemia occurs

Diabetic ketoacidosis results from insulin deficiency. Insulin is normally responsible for the uptake of glucose by cells in the body. Most of the pathological features can be attributed to one of the following effects of insulin lack:

• Hyperglycaemia in the blood
• Intracellular glucose deficiency

A good way of thinking about diabetic ketoacidosis is therefore 'starvation in the midst of plenty'.

Insulin deficiency results in lipolysis, glycogenolysis, gluconeogenesis, and ketogenesis, in an analogous way to starvation. The production of ketone bodies results in an acetone breath and a metabolic acidosis with a fall in blood pH. The resulting acidosis stimulates the respiratory centre. This leads to a characteristic breathing pattern seen in diabetic ketoacidosis known as Kussmaul's breathing. Glucose spills over into the urine (glycosuria) when glucose levels exceed the capacity of the kidneys to reabsorb glucose. This produces an osmotic diuresis (with consequent polyuria and polydipsia). The overall effect is a massive loss of fluid in the urine causing dehydration and circulatory collapse. Dehydration is worsened by the vomiting and hyperventilation that may also occur. Circulatory failure in itself worsens the metabolic acidosis (through lactic acidosis, acute renal failure, etc.) and leads to uraemia. A vicious circle is set up leading to coma and death.

Insulin is normally responsible for driving potassium into cells. Insulin deficiency therefore results in hyperkalaemia. This is worsened by any dehydration, metabolic acidosis, or renal impairment from circulatory failure, that may also be present. Despite the hyperkalaemia, total body potassium content is actually low (secondary to vomiting, renal losses, etc.).

The aims of treatment in diabetic ketoacidosis are three-fold: insulin replacement, rehydration with intravenous fluids, and potassium replacement. The latter requires special attention; although potassium is initially high, when insulin is given potassium is rapidly driven into cells resulting in hypokalaemia. Potassium therefore needs to be cautiously and judiciously replaced during the treatment of ketoacidosis.

186. C: It induces acute inflammatory changes, maximal at 1–3 days post-infarct

Myocardial infarction is infarction of the myocardium as a result of severe ischaemia leading to necrosis of the myocardium. It is usually due to coronary artery occlusion secondary to atherosclerosis, with or without superimposed thrombosis or plaque haemorrhage. Only rarely is a myocardial infarct due to an embolic event. In at least 10 per cent of patients, myocardial infarction is painless or 'silent'; this is particularly true in diabetics and elderly patients because of the accompanying autonomic neuropathy.

If a patient survives an acute infarction, the infarct heals through the formation of scar tissue. The infarcted tissue is not replaced by new cardiac muscle because cardiac myocytes are permanent (non-dividing) cells and cardiac muscle is therefore unable to regenerate. Scar tissue does not possess the usual contractile properties of normal cardiac muscle; the result is contractile dysfunction or congestive cardiac failure.

The macroscopic and microscopic changes of myocardial infarcts follow a predictable sequence of events. The chief features are coagulative necrosis, inflammatory cell infiltration, followed by organization and repair where granulation tissue replaces dead muscle and is gradually converted into scar tissue. The entire process from coagulative necrosis to the formation of well-formed scar tissue takes 6–8 weeks (Table 16).

Table 16 Macroscopic and microscopic changes

Time	Macroscopic changes	Microscopic changes
0–12 hours	None	None
12–24 hours	Infarcted area appears pale with blotchy discolouration	Infarcted muscle brightly eosinophilic with intercellular oedema; beginning of neutrophilic infiltrate
24–72 hours	Infarcted area appears soft and pale; mottling with a yellow-tan infarct centre	Coagulation necrosis and acute inflammatory response most prominent; loss of nuclei and striations; marked infiltration by neutrophils
3–10 days	Hyperaemic border develops around yellow dead muscle	Organization of infarcted area and replacement with granulation tissue; dying neutrophils with macrophages predominating; disintegration and phagocytosis of dead myofibres
Weeks to months	Tough grey-white scar	Progressive collagen deposition; infarct replaced by dense acellular scar

187. **D: Calcaneo-fibular ligament**

The most common ankle sprain is lateral which occurs as a result of excessive inversion of the foot and dorsiflexion of the ankle. The deltoid ligament, also known as the medial ligament of the ankle, is very strong and located at the medial malleolus. Excessive eversion would be the most likely mechanism of injury.

188. **E: Roots lie in the neck between the scalenus anterior and medius muscles**

There are two principal enlargements of the spinal cord, the cervical and lumbar enlargements, that give rise to the brachial and lumbrosacral plexuses, respectively, that innervate the upper and lower limbs. Both enlargements are due to the greatly increased mass of motor cells in the anterior horns of grey matter in these situations.

The brachial plexus has root values C5–8 and T1. In 10 per cent of cases the brachial plexus may be either pre-fixed (C4–8) or post-fixed (C6–T2) as an anatomical variant. The anatomical relations of the different parts of the brachial plexus are important:

- *Roots*: Exit their respective intervertebral foraminae between the scalenus anterior and medius muscles (interscalene space)
- *Trunks*: At the base of the posterior triangle of the neck, lying on the 1st rib posterior to the third part of the subclavian artery

- *Divisions*: Behind the middle third of the clavicle
- *Cords*: In the axilla, in intimate relation to the second part of the axillary artery
- *Terminal branches*: In relation to the third part of the axillary artery

The relationships of the roots, trunks, and divisions of the brachial plexus to the scalene muscles, 1st rib, and clavicle are important. Compression within a fixed space (the thoracic outlet) may lead to symptoms resulting from compression of the brachial plexus and/or nearby vascular structures (subclavian artery and vein). This is known as the thoracic outlet syndrome.

The serratus anterior muscle is innervated by the long thoracic nerve of Bell (C5, 6, 7). This may be remembered by the old aphorism 'C5, 6, 7 – Bell's of heaven'. Denervation of the serratus muscle may result in winging of the scapula.

There are two recognized types of brachial plexus palsy; both usually occur as a result of trauma or obstetric injury. The first type follows injury to the upper roots of the brachial plexus (typically C5–7) and is known as the Erb–Duchenne palsy. The arm typically lies in a waiter's tip position. The second type follows injury to the lower roots of the brachial plexus (typically C8, T1) and is known as Klumpke's palsy. The hand in this case typically takes on the position of a 'claw'.

189. **E: Congenital adrenal hyperplasia (adrenogenital syndrome) results in virilization and salt wasting**

Disorders of the adrenal gland may relate to the adrenal cortex, medulla, or both. There is only one disorder worth mentioning that selectively affects the adrenal medulla. That is a phaeochromocytoma – a tumour of the adrenal medulla that results in the overproduction of catecholamines (such as adrenaline and noradrenaline). This leads to hypertension, headaches, palpitations, and sweating (all known effects of adrenaline).

Conditions of the adrenal cortex may result from an overproduction or an underproduction of hormones. An overproduction of cortisol is known as Cushing's syndrome. There are several causes of Cushing's syndrome, the most common being iatrogenic (the use of exogenous steroids). However, the term Cushing's disease is strictly used to describe Cushing's syndrome as a result of an ACTH-producing pituitary tumour, or adenoma.

An overproduction of aldosterone from the zona glomerulosa of the adrenal cortex, as a result of a functioning adenoma, is known as Conn's syndrome. The overproduction of aldosterone leads to increased excretion of potassium and hydrogen ions from the distal convoluted tubule and collecting ducts of the kidney, resulting in a hypokalaemic metabolic alkalosis.

Adrenal insufficiency (also known as Addison's disease) results in decreased production of glucocorticoids and mineralocorticoids from the adrenal cortex. It is most commonly a result of destruction of the adrenal cortex by autoimmune adrenalitis. Decreased mineralocorticoid activity results in sodium loss and decreased potassium excretion, with consequent hyperkalaemia, hyponatraemia, volume depletion, and hypotension. Hypoglycaemia may occasionally occur as a result of glucocorticoid deficiency and impaired gluconeogenesis. Stresses such as infections, trauma, or surgery may precipitate a life-threatening adrenal crisis, which may prove fatal unless corticosteroid therapy is begun immediately.

Congenital adrenal hyperplasia (or adrenogenital syndrome) represents a group of autosomal recessive, inherited metabolic disorders characterized by a deficiency in a particular enzyme involved in the biosynthesis of cortical steroids, particularly cortisol and aldosterone. 21-hydroxylase deficiency accounts for 90 per cent of cases. Steroidogenesis is then channelled into other pathways leading to increased production of androgens, leading to virilization in females and genital enlargement and/or precocious puberty in males. Simultaneously, the deficiency of cortisol results in increased secretion of ACTH, resulting in adrenal hyperplasia. Impaired aldosterone secretion leads to salt wasting. Patients are treated with exogenous steroids which, in addition to providing adequate levels of glucocorticoids, suppress ACTH levels and thus decrease the synthesis of the steroid hormones responsible for many of the clinical abnormalities.

190. B: Most commonly occurs at branching points within the circulation

Atherosclerosis is a focal disease of the tunica intima of large and medium-sized arteries and consists of the gradual accumulation of focal raised patches (plaques) on the arterial lining in response to arterial wall injury. Its complications are the main cause of death in urbanized societies.

The anatomical sites of atherosclerosis are somewhat predictable. Plaques generally occur at branching points and bends in arteries exposed to high pressure, pulmonary arteries being relatively spared, veins completely so. The turbulence and eddy currents set up at branching points exposes the intimal surface to haemodynamic injury and encourages the uptake of circulating lipoproteins and macrophages into the vessel wall. Thus atherosclerotic plaques are common at sites of bifurcation such as:

- The entrance to the coronary ostia (causing a myocardial infarction)
- Close to where the descending abdominal aorta bifurcates into the common iliac arteries (resulting in an abdominal aortic aneurysm)
- In the internal carotid artery close to where the common carotid bifurcates into internal and external branches (resulting in a cerebrovascular accident)
- Close to where the renal arteries break off the aorta (resulting in renal artery stenosis)
- In the ileo-femoral arteries of the lower limb (causing lower limb ischaemia)

The lesions are essentially foci of chronic inflammation in which the macrophages seem to be doing harm. The basic lesion consists of a raised focal plaque within the intima with a core of lipid (mainly cholesterol) and a covering fibrous cap.

The 4 most important risk factors for atherosclerosis to remember are those that are potentially controllable, namely high cholesterol, diabetes mellitus, smoking and hypertension. All are associated with intimal injury and accelerate atherosclerosis. Atherosclerosis is a reversible disease process so that risk-factor modification ameliorates the size of atherosclerotic plaques. Risk-factor modification forms an essential part of the management of patients with known atherosclerotic disease.

191. **E: Tibial nerve**

Tarsal tunnel syndrome results from entrapment of the tibial nerve as it passes deep to the flexor retinaculum between the medial malleolus and calcaneus.

192. **C: The musculocutaneous nerve arises from the lateral cord**

This is a common question! The three cords of the brachial plexus lie in close relation to the second part of the axillary artery. Thus the posterior, lateral, and medial cords lie posteriorly, laterally, and medially to the second part of the axillary artery, respectively, in the axilla. There is no anterior cord:

- *Lateral cord*: Musculocutaneous nerve
- *Medial cord*: Ulnar nerve
- *Posterior cord*: Radial nerve, axillary nerve
- *Medial and lateral cords*: Median nerve

193. **D: It is essential for spermatogenesis**

Testosterone is a steroid hormone, secreted by the interstitial cells (of Leydig) within the mature testis. It is essential for the growth and division of the germinal cells in forming sperm and in the development of the secondary sexual characteristics. Sertoli cells, on the other hand, are postulated to act as 'nurse' cells, providing structural and metabolic support for the developing spermatogenic cells.

Whereas follicle stimulating hormone (FSH) is trophic to Sertoli cells, luteinizing hormone (LH) is trophic to the Leydig cells. LH, secreted by the anterior pituitary, stimulates the Leydig cells to secrete testosterone through the formation of cyclic AMP via the G-protein coupled serpentine LH receptor. The secretion of LH in turn depends on the pulsatile release of gonadotrophin-releasing hormone (GnRH) from the hypothalamus. Androgen production from the adrenal cortex (and to a lesser extent from the ovaries) of females is normal and is responsible for the growth of pubic and axillary hair.

194. **C: One of the first signs of toxicity is perioral paraesthesia**

Two separate classes of local anaesthetics exist: amides and esters. Amides account for the majority of local anaesthetics in clinical use, although cocaine is an ester. Local anaesthetics work by blocking sodium channels. This prevents depolarization and thereby propagation of pain impulses along the nerve.

Local anaesthetics tend to block the smaller fibres before the larger ones; that is the smaller pain fibres are blocked first (Aδ and C fibres) with sparing of the larger neurones such as the motor fibres.

The addition of adrenaline to local anaesthetic has three effects. First, it prevents bleeding by a direct effect of adrenaline on the local vasculature causing vaso-constriction. Second, by way of vasoconstriction it prevents systemic absorption of the local anaesthetic thereby preventing toxicity/side effects and increasing the local duration of action. Third, by preventing systemic absorption it allows larger doses to be used than would otherwise be allowed in the absence of adren-aline. However, because of this 'vasoconstrictive effect', adrenaline must never be used on pedicles that contain an end artery (e.g., digits, nose tips, earlobe, penis) where ischaemic necrosis may result.

It is important that the maximum dose of local anaesthetic not be exceeded, otherwise the consequences may be lethal. This is because local anaesthetics are cardiotoxic by way of blocking sodium channels and interfering with cardiac conduction. One of the earliest and reliable signs of systemic toxicity is perioral tingling. This may be followed by cardiovascular collapse and death.

195. **E: Caudate lobe of the liver**

The greater sac communicates with the lesser sac through the epiploic foramen of Winslow. The superior boundary is the caudate lobe of the liver. The common bile duct lies in the free edge of the lesser omentum, that forms the anterior boundary. The first part of the duodenum is the inferior boundary. The posterior boundary is the inferior vena cava.

196. **D: It contains ten tendons within it**

The carpal tunnel is a fibro-osseous tunnel situated on the flexor aspect of the proximal part of the hand and lying between the flexor retinaculum and the carpal bones. It contains the median nerve and ten flexor tendons that include:

- Four tendons of flexor digitorum superficialis
- Four tendons of flexor digitorum profundus
- Flexor carpi radialis tendon
- Flexor pollicis longus tendon

The flexor retinaculum is attached to the tubercle of the scaphoid and pisiform proximally and the hook of the hamate and trapezium distally. Its function is to prevent bow-stringing of the flexor tendons at the wrist.

Since the carpal tunnel exists as a confined space, entrapment of the median nerve may occur within it. This is commonly due to a build-up of fluid within the carpal tunnel, or because of hypertrophy of the bones/ligaments/tendons that surround, or are contained within, the carpal tunnel. Compression of the median nerve within the carpal tunnel is known as carpal tunnel syndrome. Note this is different from cubital tunnel syndrome, which refers to compression of the ulnar nerve behind the medial epicondyle at the elbow. The ulnar artery and nerve do not pass through the carpal tunnel, but instead pass superficial to the carpal tunnel in their own fibro-osseous tunnel commonly given the name Guyon's canal. The ulnar nerve and artery are therefore unaffected in carpal tunnel syndrome.

The clinical features of carpal tunnel syndrome relate to loss of function of the median nerve. There are both motor and sensory components. The median nerve supplies 4 muscles in the hand, given by the mnemonic LOAF:

- Lateral two lumbricals
- Opponens pollicis
- Abductor pollicis brevis
- Flexor pollicis brevis

All four muscles are weak in someone with carpal tunnel syndrome. In addition, there is loss of sensation over the lateral three-and-a-half digits, which is median nerve territory. However, since the palmar cutaneous branch of the median nerve passes superficial to the carpal tunnel, there is no loss of sensation over the thenar eminence in someone with carpal tunnel syndrome.

197. **A: Subcapital neck fracture**

Intracapsular femoral neck fractures are at risk of avascular necrosis if left untreated due to interruption of the blood supply that runs from a distal to proximal direction.

198. **A: It is devoid of valves**

Most veins in the body contain veins to maintain the direction of flow. The valves also provide restriction in spread of cancer metastasis. The internal vertebral venous plexus is devoid of veins allowing free movement of cancer cells.

199. **D: Infraspinatus**

The rotator cuff muscles/tendons are: supraspinatus, infraspinatus, subscapularis, and teres minor.

200. **A: Osteoarthritis**

Heberden and Bouchard's nodes form secondary to marginal osteophytes at the distal interphalangeal and proximal interphalangeal joints, respectively. Erosions are more typically seen in inflammatory arthritis, including rheumatoid arthritis, psoriatic arthritis, and gout.

Index

Note: Page numbers in *italic* and **bold** refer to figures and tables, respectively.

Milton Keynes UK
Ingram Content Group UK Ltd.
UKHW020315030124
435381UK00013B/55